Medical
Terminology

a systems approach

THIRD EDITION

BARBARA A. GYLYS, BS, MEd, CMA-A
Professor of Health and Human Services
Medical Assisting Technology
University of Toledo Community and Technical College
Toledo, Ohio

MARY ELLEN WEDDING, BS, MT(ASCP), MEd, CMA
Professor of Health and Human Services
Director of Medical Assisting Technology
University of Toledo Community and Technical College
Toledo, Ohio

F. A. DAVIS COMPANY • Philadelphia

F. A. Davis Company
1915 Arch Street
Philadelphia, PA 19103

MAI 35/ 3936

Cover Art: Frank Kupka
Disks of Newton, 1912
Philadelphia Museum of Art: The Louise and Walter Arensberg Collection
Accession number: '50-134-122

Printed in the United States of America

Last digit indicates print number: 10 9 8 7 6 5 4 3 2 1

Publisher: Jean-François Vilain
Developmental Editor: Ralph Zickgraf
Production Editor: Marianne Fithian
Cover Designer: Donald B. Freggens, Jr.

As new scientific information becomes available through basic and clinical research, recommended treatments and drug therapies undergo changes. The author(s) and publisher have done everything possible to make this book accurate, up to date, and in accord with accepted standards at the time of publication. The authors, editors, and publisher are not responsible for errors or omissions or for consequences from application of the book, and make no warranty, expressed or implied, in regard to the contents of the book. Any practice described in this book should be applied by the reader in accordance with professional standards of care used in regard to the unique circumstances that may apply in each situation. The reader is advised always to check product information (package inserts) for changes and new information regarding dose and contraindications before administering any drug. Caution is especially urged when using new or infrequently ordered drugs.

Library of Congress Cataloging-in-Publication Data

Gylys, Barbara A.
    Medical terminology: a systems approach / Barbara A. Gylys, Mary
Ellen Wedding. — 3rd ed.
        p.   cm.
    Includes bibliographical references and index.
    ISBN 0-8036-4500-7
    1. Medicine—Terminology.   I. Wedding, Mary Ellen.   II. Title.
    [DNLM: 1. Nomenclature—problems.   W 15 G996m 1994]
R123.G94   1995
610'.14—dc20
DNLM/DLC
for Library of Congress   94-28995
                                                                                CIP

This book is dedicated with love

to my husband, Julius A. Gylys
and
to my children, Regina Maria and Julius A., II

B.G.

to my sister, Sr. M. Adele Karwacki
and
to my children, Carol Ann, Don II, Vicki, and Daniel
and
to my husband, Don

M.E.W.

Acknowledgments

We wish to thank Jean-François Vilain, Publisher, Allied Health, and the editorial and production staffs of the F. A. Davis Company for their combined efforts in guiding and contributing to this project. In addition, we want to recognize the efforts of the following individuals, who contributed to this textbook.

- Joseph R. Bittengle, MEd, BS, RT(R), who reviewed the diagnostic imaging procedures
- Lydia D. Schafer, PhD, Assistant Professor at Medical College of Ohio, Pathology Department, who edited the pathology and general vocabulary
- Buford T. Lively, EdD, RPh, Professor of Pharmacy and Health Care Administration at the University of Toledo, who reviewed the pharmacology and provided constructive suggestions
- Regina Masters, MEd, CMA, RN, instructor and colleague at The University of Toledo Community and Technical College, for reviewing the entire manuscript and providing constructive suggestions
- Julius A. Gylys, PhD, who edited various parts of the manuscript and provided encouragement and support for the project
- Judith A. Shook, CMT, AD, Pathology Department, Toledo Hospital and Cheryl Homan, MBA, RRA, Director of Health Information Services, Riverside Hospital, for their help with the case studies
- Patricia Goshorn, MA, RN, CMA-C, Cosumnes River College, Sacramento, California, for developing the case studies
- Kathryn Larson, PhD, West Valley College, California, for developing multiple choice test questions in the *Instructor's Guide*
- Ralph Zickgraf, Senior Developmental Editor, for his expert editing of the manuscript, helping it along at every stage of the way, and for developing the crossword puzzles

Finally, we would like to express our appreciation of the following educators, whose careful reviews of the manuscript guided us as we revised:

- Patrick J. Debold, BS, MS, Vice President of Education, Concorde Career Colleges, Kansas City, Missouri
- Joan F. Glasheen, RN, MS, Community College of Rhode Island
- Mary Ann Woods, RN, BSN, MEd, PhD, CMA, Director of Medical Assisting, Fresno City College, California.

Preface

Although we have made several additions to the third edition of *Medical Terminology: A Systems Approach,* the basic features remain the same as in previous editions. We have incorporated several insightful suggestions from educators in order to develop a complete learning and teaching package. We have updated and strengthened various topics in each chapter and provided a comprehensive *Instructor's Guide.*

Like previous editions, the third edition teaches basic principles of medical word building following the criteria of a competency-based curriculum. The book is designed as a classroom teaching text with the underlying pedagogy of a textbook-workbook format. However, a variety of self-teaching features allow a student to work through the chapters at his or her own pace without any outside guidance.

The principal objectives of the textbook are twofold. First, it provides basic principles of medical word building. These principles, once learned, can readily be applied to building an extensive medical vocabulary. In writing and revising the book, we considered both the objectives of students who want to proceed at their own pace and the needs of instructors who employ traditional lecture and recitation methods. Secondly, it presents material at a level that is easily understood by the average student. Thus, no previous knowledge of anatomy, physiology, or pathology is necessary. Once the course is completed, the student will have a basic knowledge of these disciplines.

The third edition is designed as follows:

- **Chapter 1** explains the method by which basic elements form medical words.
- **Chapter 2** categorizes major suffixes in the following groups: surgical, diagnostic, symptomatic, and related suffixes. Pronunciations and definitions of suffixes are included as they are presented.
- **Chapter 3** contains suffixes denoting adjective, noun, singular, and plural forms of medical words.
- **Chapter 4** includes major prefixes in the following groups: position, number and measurement, negation, direction, and other prefixes.
- **Chapter 5** introduces anatomical, physiological, and pathological terms as a foundation for understanding the body systems chapters.
- **Chapters 6 to 16** are organized according to body systems and may be taught in any sequence. These chapters include anatomy and physiology; combining forms, suffixes, and prefixes; pathology; diagnostic, symptomatic, and related terms; special procedures, such as, diagnostic imaging, endoscopic, clinical, surgical and laboratory; pharmacology terms; abbreviations; a case study; and worksheets.

The worksheets provide a means of self-testing and evaluation of material included in each chapter.

v

- **Appendix A: Answer Key** contains worksheet answers to validate medical terminology competency and provides immediate feedback for a student's progress.
- **Appendix B: Abbreviations** includes a comprehensive list of medical abbreviations and their meanings.
- **Appendix C: Index of Medical Word Elements** contains alphabetical lists of medical word elements with corresponding pronunciations and meanings. This appendix employs two methods for word-element indexing—first by medical word element, then by English term.
- **Appendix D: Index of Genetic Disorders** lists the genetic disorders covered in the textbook.
- **Appendix E: Index of Diagnostic Imaging Procedures** lists the radiographic and other diagnostic imaging procedures covered in the textbook.
- **Appendix F: Index of Pharmacology** lists the medications covered in the textbook.
- **Appendix G: Index of Oncological Terms** lists the terms related to oncology covered in the textbook.
- **Flash Cards** for suffixes, prefixes, and combining forms are found in the back of the book. The flash cards, which are labeled according to the chapter in which the element was first presented, can be organized in various ways for study purposes.
- **Audiocassette Tapes** are included with the text or (at the instructor's option*) available through the instructor; use them to strengthen and reinforce spelling and pronunciation of medical words.
- **Anatomical Color Plates** in the front of the textbook consist of 24 comprehensive colored plates that provide detailed structures of various organs of the body.

OTHER TEACHING AIDS

We are pround to offer, to instructors who adopt the third edition of *Medical Terminology: A Systems Approach,* F.A. Davis's new CyberTest™ test-generating program. A DOS-based program that can also be run from Windows, CyberTest™ allows instructors to create chapter, midterm, and final tests in a flash. Users can specify question format and choose (or randomly select) from over 800 questions. A demo diskette is available to any interested educator.

Also included in the *Instructor's Guide to Medical Terminology: A Systems Approach* are: a complete hard copy of the CyberTest™ testbank, consisting of over 800 questions in a variety of formats; case studies with an analysis of each case study; crossword puzzles to reinforce material covered in each chapter; and a list of journals, films, and community resources to help instructors develop various teaching activities.

Taber's Cyclopedic Medical Dictionary is the recommended companion reference because it includes etymologies for nearly all the main entries presented in this textbook.

B.A.G.
M.E.W.

---

*The instructor may choose to adopt 1) the book/cassette package, with the two audiocassettes shrink-wrapped with each copy of the book; or 2) the book by itself (at less cost to the student). Instructors who adopt the book alone may make copies, for their students, of the two audiocassette masters included in the complimentary instructor's package.

Contents

CHAPTER 5

BODY STRUCTURE

CHAPTER 6

INTEGUMENTARY SYSTEM

CHAPTER 11

CHAPTER 16

APPENDIX A

APPENDIX B

APPENDIX C

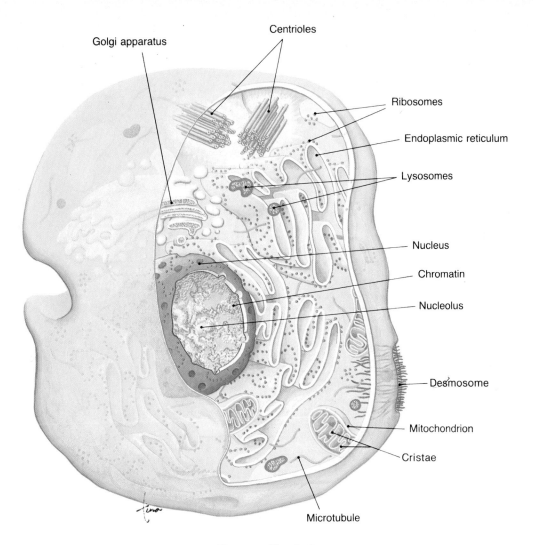

Golgi apparatus

Centrioles

Ribosomes

Endoplasmic reticulum

Lysosomes

Nucleus

Chromatin

Nucleolus

Desmosome

Mitochondrion

Cristae

Microtubule

Plate 1.   The Cell.

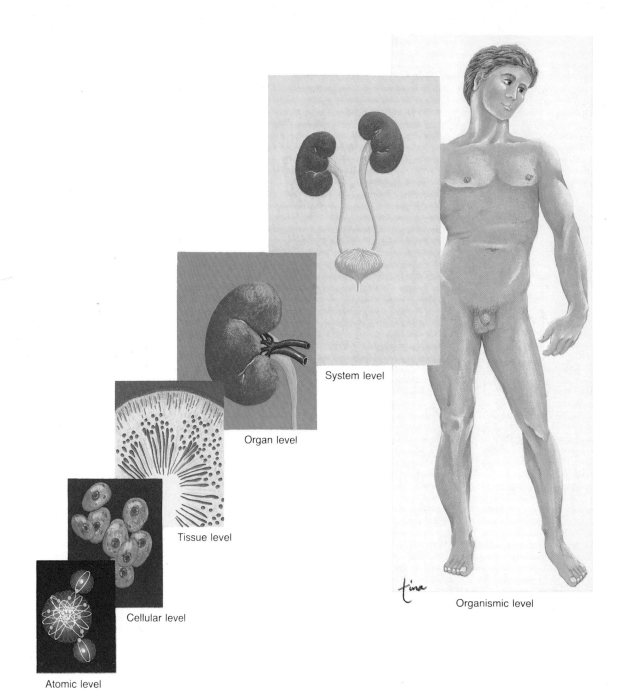

Atomic level

Cellular level

Tissue level

Organ level

System level

Organismic level

Plate 2.   Levels of Organization of the Body.

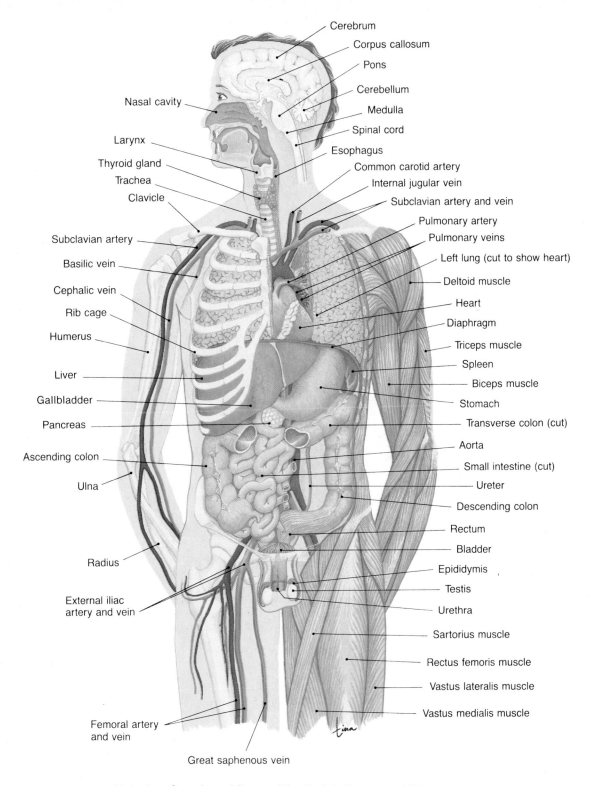

Plate 3. Overview of Some of the Body's Organs and Structures.

Cerebrum
Corpus callosum
Pons
Cerebellum
Medulla
Spinal cord
Esophagus
Common carotid artery
Internal jugular vein
Subclavian artery and vein
Pulmonary artery
Pulmonary veins
Left lung (cut to show heart)
Deltoid muscle
Heart
Diaphragm
Triceps muscle
Spleen
Biceps muscle
Stomach
Transverse colon (cut)
Aorta
Small intestine (cut)
Ureter
Descending colon
Rectum
Bladder
Epididymis
Testis
Urethra
Sartorius muscle
Rectus femoris muscle
Vastus lateralis muscle
Vastus medialis muscle

Nasal cavity
Larynx
Thyroid gland
Trachea
Clavicle
Subclavian artery
Basilic vein
Cephalic vein
Rib cage
Humerus
Liver
Gallbladder
Pancreas
Ascending colon
Ulna
Radius
External iliac
artery and vein
Femoral artery
and vein
Great saphenous vein

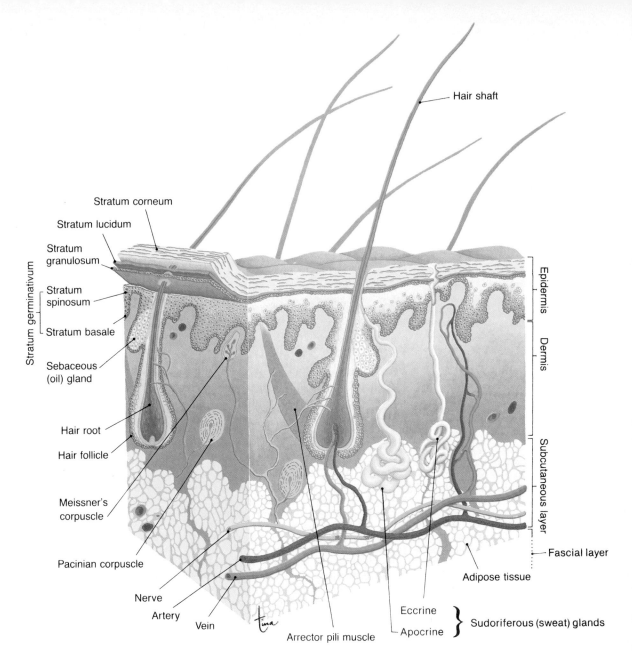

Hair shaft

Stratum corneum
Stratum lucidum
Stratum granulosum
Stratum germinativum
Stratum spinosum
Stratum basale
Sebaceous (oil) gland
Hair root
Hair follicle
Meissner's corpuscle
Pacinian corpuscle
Nerve
Artery
Vein

Epidermis
Dermis
Subcutaneous layer
Fascial layer
Adipose tissue

Arrector pili muscle
Eccrine
Apocrine
} Sudoriferous (sweat) glands

Plate 4.   Cross-Section of the Skin.

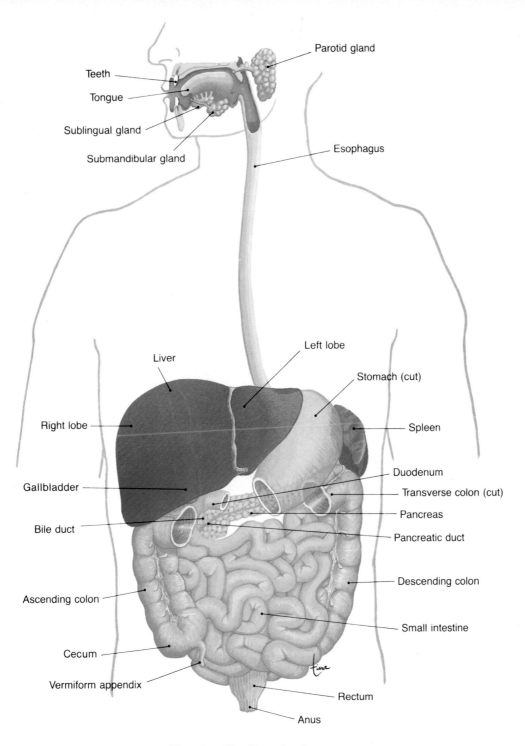

Plate 5.   The Digestive System.

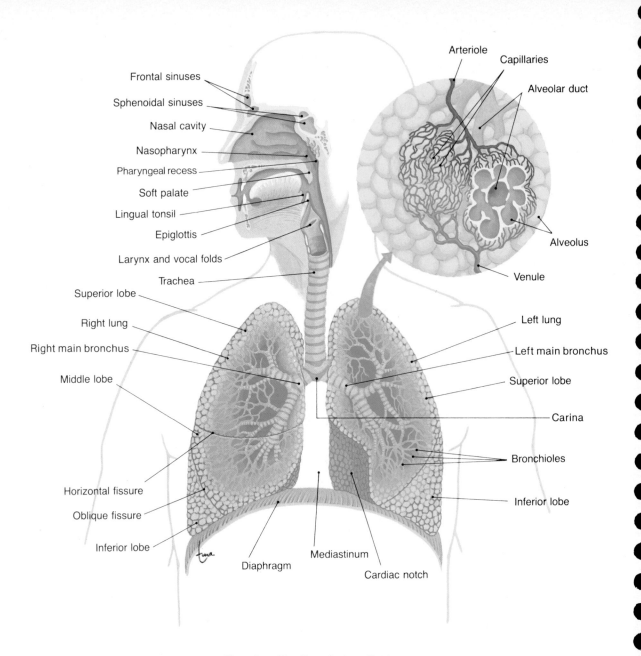

Plate 6. The Respiratory System.

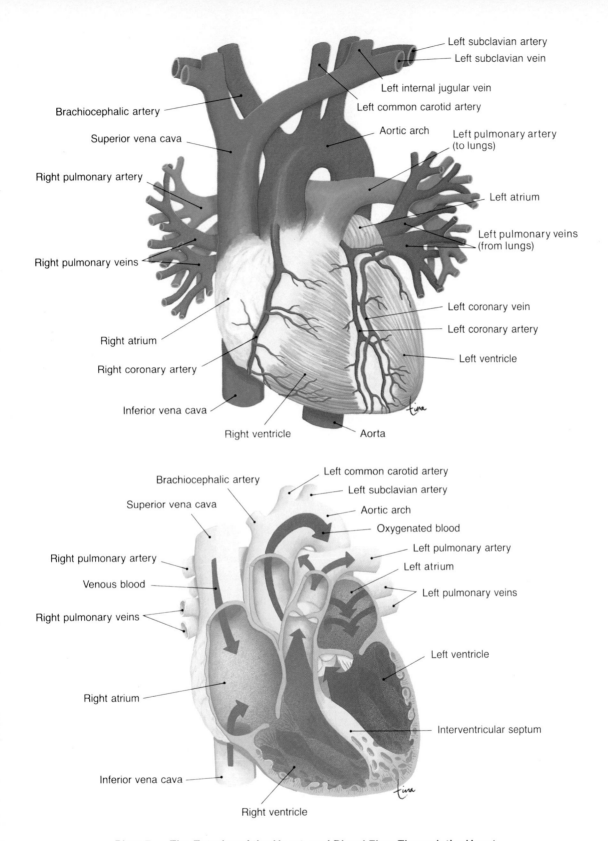

Plate 7. The Exterior of the Heart, and Blood Flow Through the Heart.

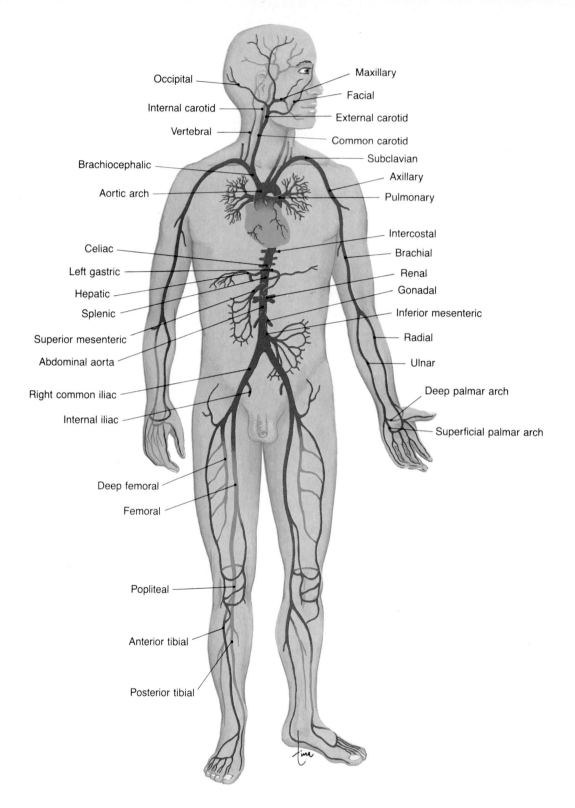

Occipital

Maxillary

Facial

Internal carotid

External carotid

Vertebral

Common carotid

Brachiocephalic

Subclavian

Aortic arch

Axillary

Pulmonary

Celiac

Intercostal

Left gastric

Brachial

Hepatic

Renal

Splenic

Gonadal

Superior mesenteric

Inferior mesenteric

Abdominal aorta

Radial

Right common iliac

Ulnar

Internal iliac

Deep palmar arch

Superficial palmar arch

Deep femoral

Femoral

Popliteal

Anterior tibial

Posterior tibial

Plate 8.   The Arteries.

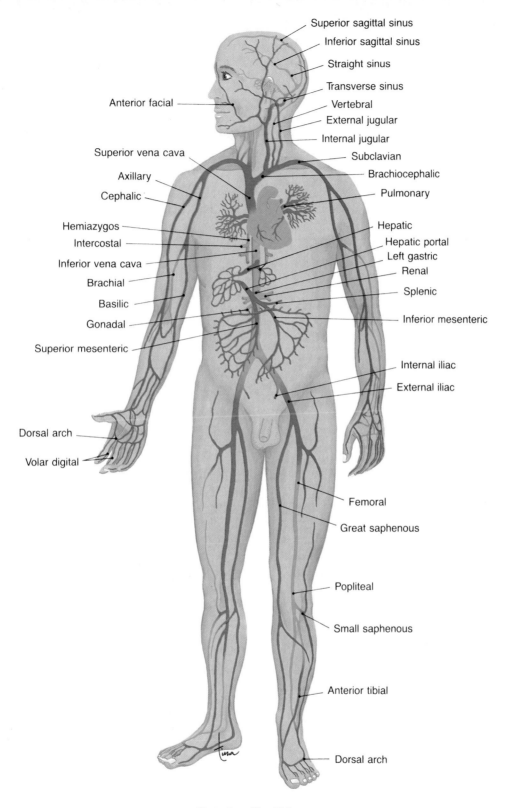

Plate 9. The Veins.

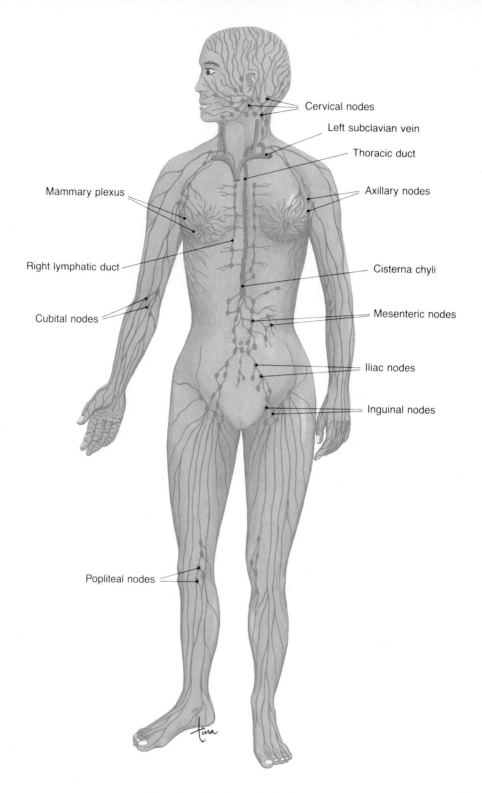

Cervical nodes

Left subclavian vein

Thoracic duct

Mammary plexus

Axillary nodes

Right lymphatic duct

Cisterna chyli

Cubital nodes

Mesenteric nodes

Iliac nodes

Inguinal nodes

Popliteal nodes

Plate 10.   The Lymphatic System.

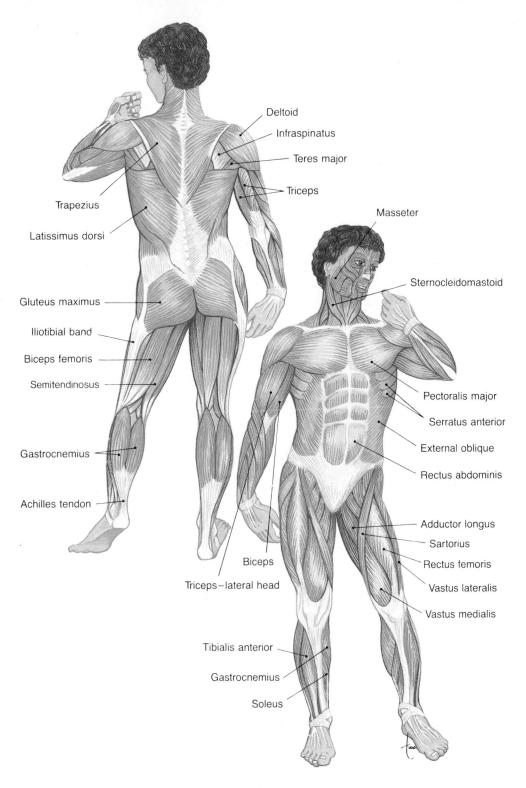

Deltoid

Infraspinatus

Teres major

Triceps

Trapezius

Latissimus dorsi

Masseter

Sternocleidomastoid

Gluteus maximus

Iliotibial band

Biceps femoris

Semitendinosus

Pectoralis major

Serratus anterior

External oblique

Rectus abdominis

Gastrocnemius

Achilles tendon

Adductor longus

Sartorius

Rectus femoris

Vastus lateralis

Vastus medialis

Biceps

Triceps–lateral head

Tibialis anterior

Gastrocnemius

Soleus

Plate 11.   Posterior and Anterior Views of the Muscles.

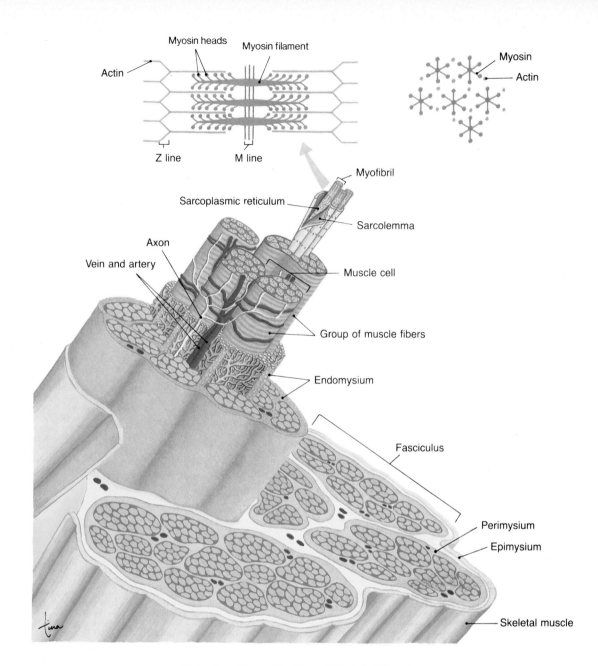

Plate 12.   Cross-Section of Skeletal Muscle.

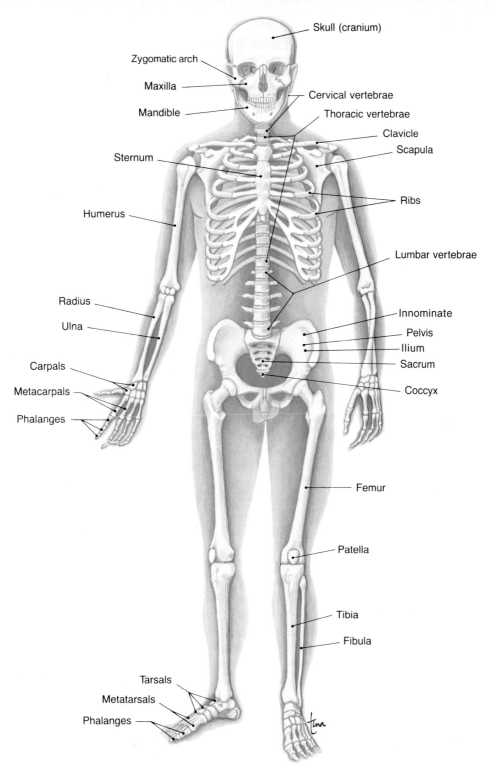

Plate 13.   Anterior View of the Skeleton.

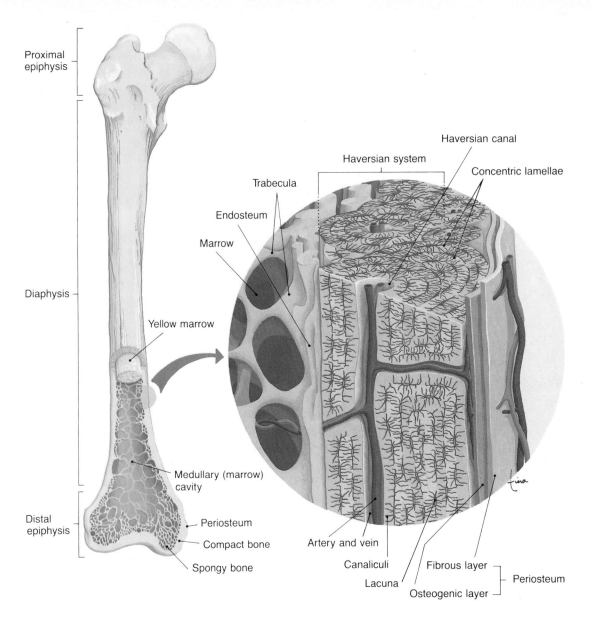

Plate 14.   Longitudinal Section of a Long Bone.

Proximal epiphysis

Diaphysis

Distal epiphysis

Yellow marrow

Medullary (marrow) cavity

Periosteum

Compact bone

Spongy bone

Trabecula

Endosteum

Marrow

Haversian system

Haversian canal

Concentric lamellae

Artery and vein

Canaliculi

Lacuna

Fibrous layer

Osteogenic layer

Periosteum

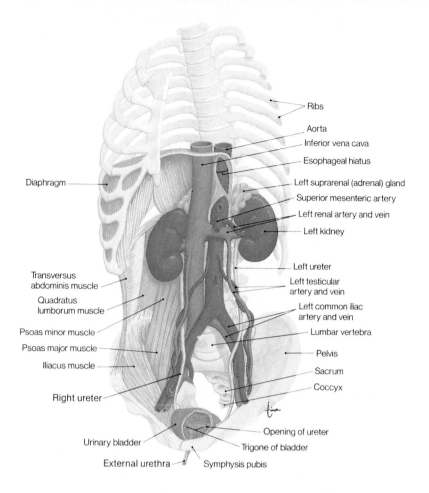

Ribs
Aorta
Inferior vena cava
Esophageal hiatus
Left suprarenal (adrenal) gland
Superior mesenteric artery
Left renal artery and vein
Left kidney

Diaphragm

Left ureter
Left testicular artery and vein
Left common iliac artery and vein
Lumbar vertebra
Pelvis
Sacrum
Coccyx

Transversus abdominis muscle
Quadratus lumborum muscle
Psoas minor muscle
Psoas major muscle
Iliacus muscle
Right ureter

Opening of ureter
Urinary bladder
Trigone of bladder
External urethra
Symphysis pubis

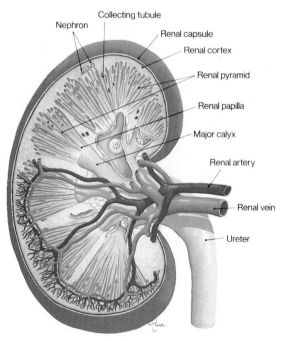

Collecting tubule
Nephron
Renal capsule
Renal cortex
Renal pyramid
Renal papilla
Major calyx
Renal artery
Renal vein
Ureter

Plate 15.   The Urinary System, and the Kidney.

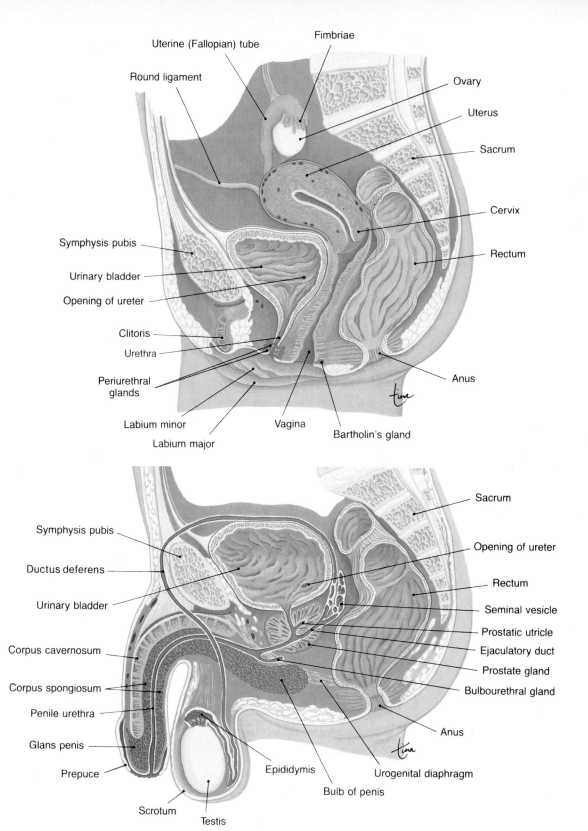

Plate 16.   The Female and Male Reproductive Systems.

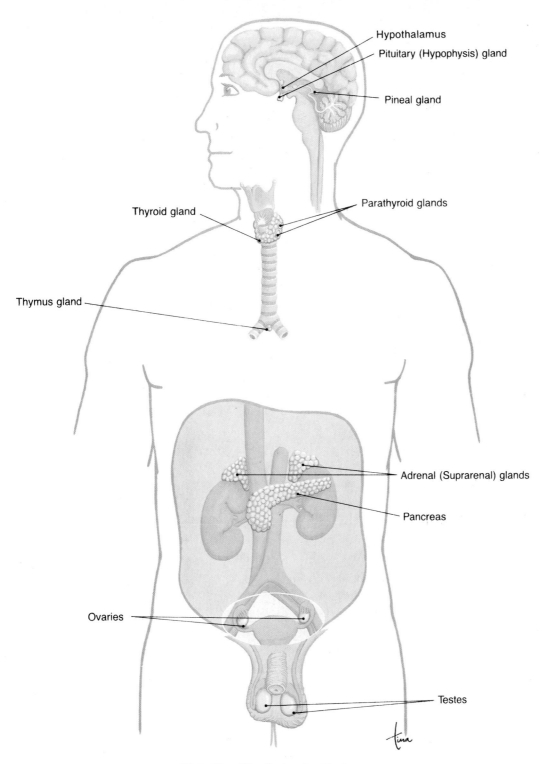

Plate 17.   The Endocrine System.

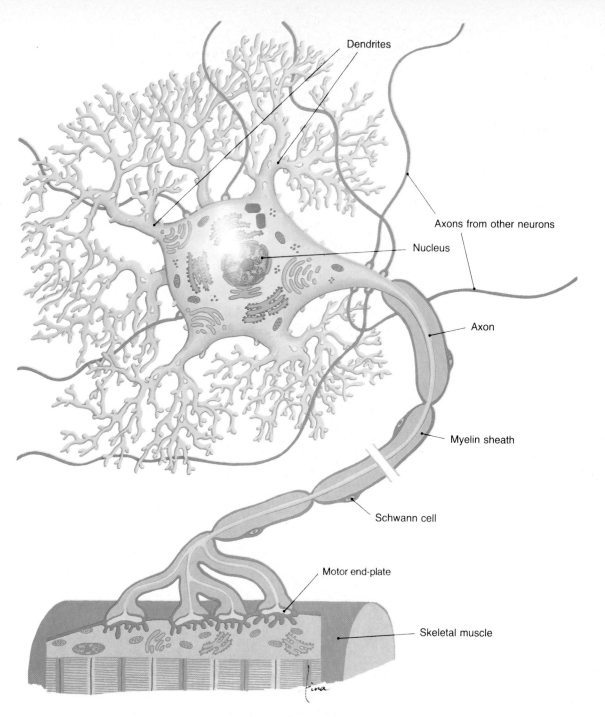

Dendrites

Axons from other neurons

Nucleus

Axon

Myelin sheath

Schwann cell

Motor end-plate

Skeletal muscle

Plate 18.   A Motor Neuron.

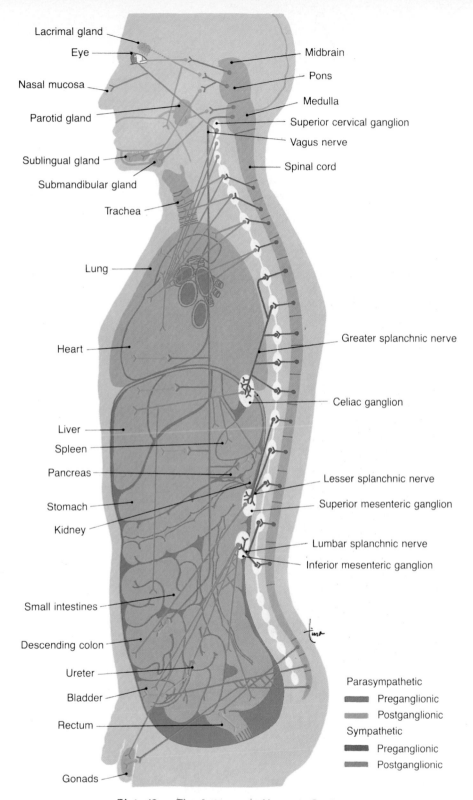

Lacrimal gland

Eye

Nasal mucosa

Parotid gland

Sublingual gland

Submandibular gland

Trachea

Lung

Heart

Liver

Spleen

Pancreas

Stomach

Kidney

Small intestines

Descending colon

Ureter

Bladder

Rectum

Gonads

Midbrain

Pons

Medulla

Superior cervical ganglion

Vagus nerve

Spinal cord

Greater splanchnic nerve

Celiac ganglion

Lesser splanchnic nerve

Superior mesenteric ganglion

Lumbar splanchnic nerve

Inferior mesenteric ganglion

Parasympathetic
- Preganglionic
- Postganglionic

Sympathetic
- Preganglionic
- Postganglionic

Plate 19.   The Autonomic Nervous System.

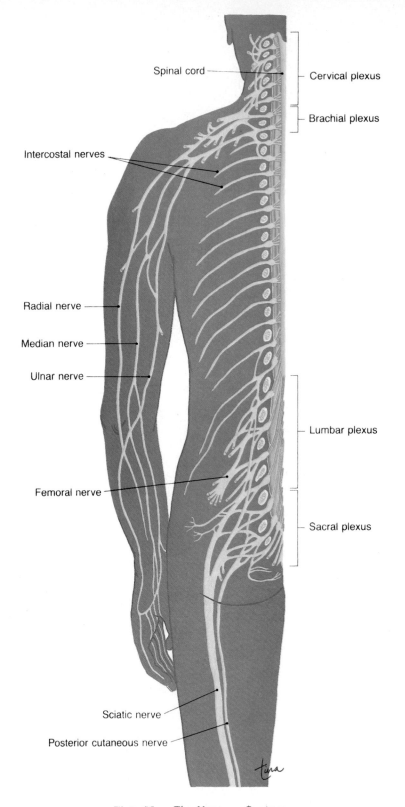

Plate 20.   The Nervous System.

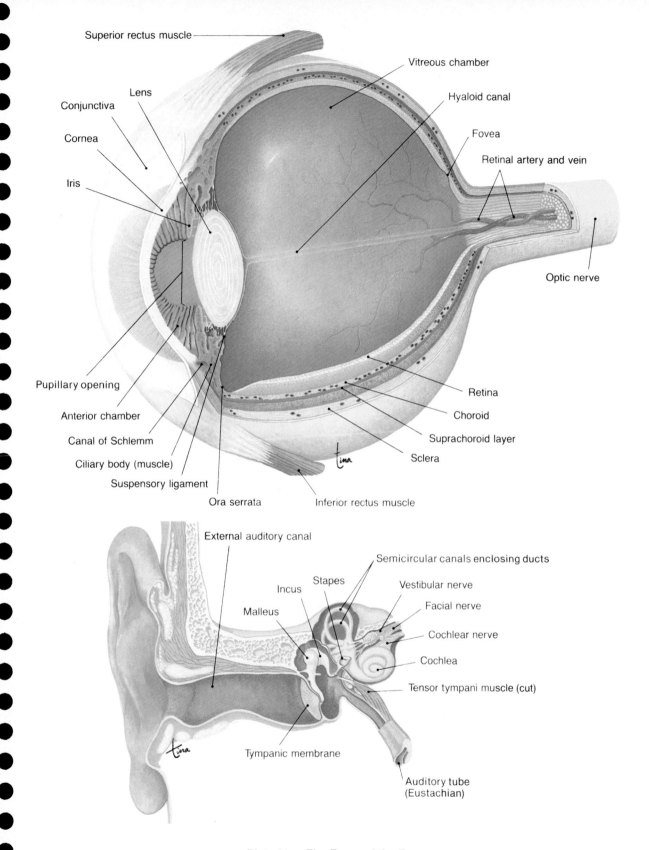

Superior rectus muscle

Vitreous chamber

Hyaloid canal

Lens

Conjunctiva

Cornea

Fovea

Retinal artery and vein

Iris

Optic nerve

Pupillary opening

Anterior chamber

Canal of Schlemm

Ciliary body (muscle)

Suspensory ligament

Ora serrata

Inferior rectus muscle

Retina

Choroid

Suprachoroid layer

Sclera

External auditory canal

Semicircular canals enclosing ducts

Incus

Stapes

Vestibular nerve

Malleus

Facial nerve

Cochlear nerve

Cochlea

Tensor tympani muscle (cut)

Tympanic membrane

Auditory tube
(Eustachian)

Plate 21.   The Eye, and the Ear.

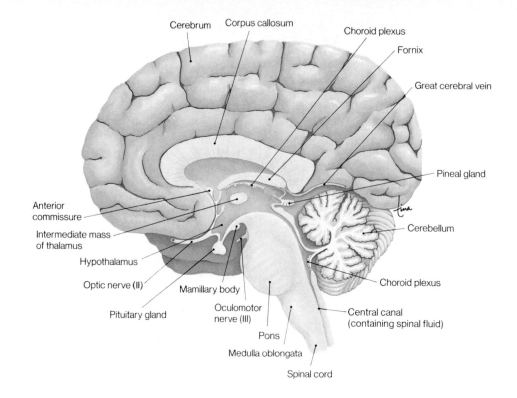

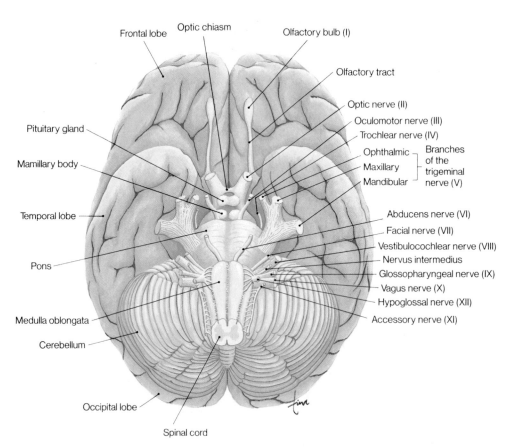

Plate 22.   Cross-Sections of the Brain, and the Cranial Nerves.

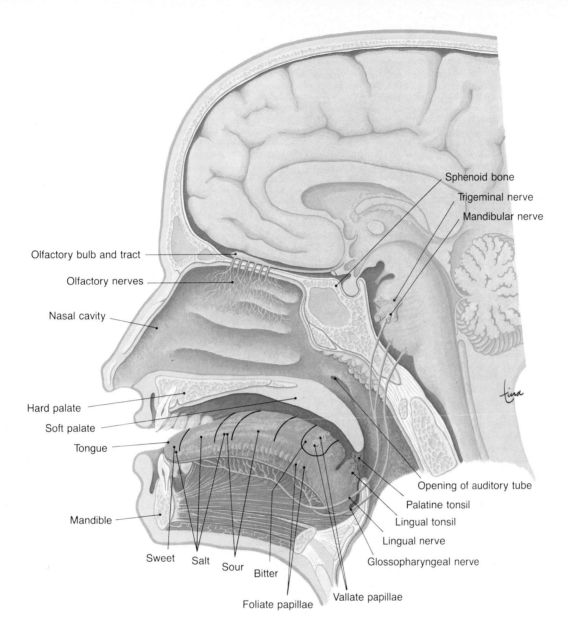

Plate 23.   The Centers of Smell and Taste.

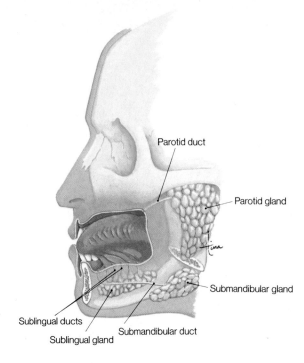

Parotid duct

Parotid gland

Submandibular gland

Sublingual ducts

Sublingual gland

Submandibular duct

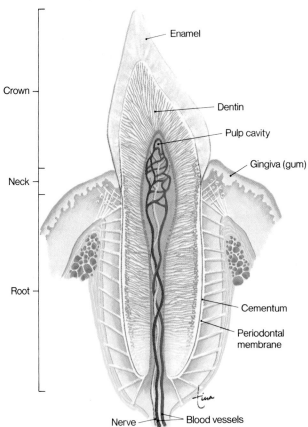

Enamel

Crown

Dentin

Pulp cavity

Gingiva (gum)

Neck

Root

Cementum

Periodontal
membrane

Nerve

Blood vessels

Plate 24.   The Salivary Glands, and the Tooth.

Chapter 1

Basic Elements of a Medical Word

Chapter Outline

Student Objectives

Upon completion of this chapter, you will be able to do the following:

Define and provide several examples of word roots, combining forms, suffixes, and prefixes.

Divide medical words into their component parts.

Describe how medical words are formed.

Explain the two basic rules for building medical words.

Explain the three basic guidelines for defining medical words.

Demonstrate your knowledge of the chapter by completing the worksheets.

Medical word building follows simple rules. Once these rules are learned, numerous medical terms can be formed and defined. As in all languages, some words are exceptions to such rules. Fortunately, in medical terminology few words are subject to irregularities.

To analyze medical words, you need to identify the four elements that are used to form words: word root, combining form, suffix, and prefix.

Word Roots

The main part or stem of a word is called a **word root (WR).** A word root is usually derived from the Greek or Latin language and frequently indicates a body part. All medical words have one or more roots.

EXAMPLES OF WORD ROOTS

Greek Word	Word Root
kardia (heart)	cardi
erythros (red)	erythr
gastros (stomach)	gastr
nephros (kidney)	nephr
osteon (bone)	oste

Combining Forms

The **combining form (CF)** is a word root plus a vowel, usually an "o." Like the word root, the combining form usually indicates a body part. In this text, a combining form will be listed as word root/vowel (e.g., cardi/o), as illustrated in the following chart.

EXAMPLES OF COMBINING FORMS

Word Root	+	Combining Vowel	=	Combining Form	Meaning
cardi/	+	o	=	cardi/o	heart
erythr/	+	o	=	erythr/o	red
gastr/	+	o	=	gastr/o	stomach
nephr/	+	o	=	nephr/o	kidney
oste/	+	o	=	oste/o	bone

Try to learn the combining form rather than the word root because the combining form makes many words easier to pronounce. For example, in the previous list, the word roots erythr, gastr, and nephr are difficult to pronounce, whereas their combining forms erythr/o, gastr/o, and nephr/o are easy to pronounce.

Suffixes

A **suffix** is a word ending. In the words work/*er,* and work/*ing,* the suffixes are *-er* and *-ing.* Changing the suffix gives the word a new meaning. This is also true in medical terminology. Whenever you change the suffix, the medical word takes on a new meaning. In medical terminology, a suffix usually indicates a procedure, condition, disease, or part of speech. Many suffixes are derived from Greek or Latin words.

EXAMPLES OF SUFFIXES

Combining Form	+	Suffix	=	Medical Word	Meaning
arthr/o (joint)		-centesis (puncture)		arthrocentesis	puncture of a joint
thorac/o (chest)		-tomy (incision)		thoracotomy	incision of the chest
gastr/o (stomach)		-megaly (enlargement)		gastromegaly	enlargement of the stomach

Prefixes

A **prefix** is a word element located at the beginning of a word. Prefixes occur frequently in general language as well as in medical and scientific terminology. When a medical word contains a prefix, the meaning of the word is influenced. The prefix usually indicates a number, time, position, direction, or sense of negation.

EXAMPLES OF PREFIXES

Prefix	+	Word Root	+	Suffix	=	Medical Word	Meaning
hyper- (excessive)		therm (heat)		-ia (condition)		hyperthermia	condition of excesssive heat
macro- (large)		gloss (tongue)		-ia (condition)		macroglossia	condition of a large tongue
micro- (small)		card (heart)		-ia (condition)		microcardia	condition of a small heart

Basic Rules for Building and Defining Medical Words

BUILDING MEDICAL WORDS

There are two basic rules for building medical words.

Rule 1. A word root is used before a suffix that begins with a vowel.

WORD ROOT		SUFFIX		MEANING
scler/	+	osis	=	abnormal condition of hardening
(hardening)		(abnormal condition)		

Rule 2. A combining vowel is used to link a word root to a suffix that begins with a consonant, and to link a word root to another word root to form a compound word.

- Here is an example of a combining vowel linking a word root to a suffix that begins with a consonant.

WORD ROOT AND COMBINING VOWEL		SUFFIX		MEANING
therm/o	+	meter	=	instrument for measuring heat
(heat)		(instrument for measuring)		

- Here are two examples of a combining vowel linking one word root to another word root to form a compound word.

WORD ROOT	COMBINING VOWEL	WORD ROOT		SUFFIX		MEANING
oste/	o/	chondr/	+	itis	=	inflammation of bone and cartilage
(bone)		(cartilage)		(inflammation)		

WORD ROOT	COMBINING VOWEL	WORD ROOT	+	SUFFIX		MEANING
oste/	o/	arthr/	+	itis	=	inflammation of bone and joint
(bone)		(joint)		(inflammation)		

In most instances, the combining vowel is retained between two roots even if the second root begins with a vowel, as illustrated in the preceding example, oste/o/arthr/itis.

DEFINING MEDICAL WORDS

There are three basic steps to defining medical words.
- First, define the **suffix,** or last part of the word.
- Second, define the **prefix,** or **first part of the word.**
- Last, define the **middle** of the word.

Here is an example.

gastr/	o/	enter/	itis
stomach		intestine	inflammation
(2)		(3)	(1)

Read as follows:

1. Inflammation (of) [suffix]

2. stomach (and) [first part of the word]
3. intestine [middle]

The definition of gastr/o/enter/itis is "inflammation (of) stomach and intestine."

Pronunciation Guidelines

Although medical words usually follow the rules that govern the pronunciation of English words, they may be difficult to pronounce when you first encounter them. Here are some general rules you will find helpful:

- For **ae** and **oe,** only the second vowel is pronounced. Examples: burs**ae**, pleur**ae**, r**oe**ntgen
- **c** and **g** are given the soft sound of s and j, respectively, before e, i, and y in words of both Greek and Latin origins.
  Examples: **c**erebrum, **c**ircumcision, **c**ycle, **g**el, **g**ingivitis, **g**iant, **g**yrate
- **c** and **g** have a hard sound before other letters.
  Examples: **c**ardiac, **c**ast, **g**astric, **g**onad
- **e** and **es,** when forming the final letter or letters of a word, are often pronounced as separate syllables.
  Examples: syncop**e**, systol**e**, nar**es**
- **ch** is sometimes pronounced like k.
  Examples: **ch**olesterol, **ch**olera, **ch**olemia
- **i** at the end of a word (to form a plural) is pronounced "eye."
  Examples: bronch**i**, fung**i**, nucle**i**
- **pn** at the beginning of a word is pronounced with only the n sound.
  Examples: **pn**eumonia, **pn**eumotoxin
- **pn** in the middle of a word is pronounced with a hard p and a hard n.
  Examples: ortho**pn**ea, hyper**pn**ea
- **ps** is pronounced like s.
  Examples: **ps**ychology, **ps**ychosis
- All other vowels and consonants have ordinary English sounds.

Most medical words in this textbook are spelled phonetically in order to teach their correct pronunciation. Diacritical marks, the macron and breve, are used for long and short vowel pronunciations, respectively.

The macron (¯) indicates the long sound of vowels, as in the following:

ā in rate
ē in rebirth
ī in isle
ō in over
ū in unite

The breve (˘) indicates the short sound of vowels, as in the following:

ă in apple
ĕ in ever
ĭ in it
ŏ in not
ŭ in cut

Capitalization is used to indicate emphasis on certain syllables, as in LĔT - ter.

Worksheet 1

1. List the four elements used to form words: _____

   _____

2. A root is the main part or foundation of a word. In the words teacher, teaches, and teaching, the root is _____ .

Answer the following statements either true or false.

3. _____ A combining vowel is usually an "e."

4. _____ A combining vowel is not used before a suffix that begins with a vowel.

5. _____ A combining vowel is used to link one root to another root.

6. _____ A combining vowel is not used before a suffix that begins with a consonant.

7. _____ To define a medical word, first define the prefix.

Check your answers in Appendix A. Review any material that you did not answer correctly.

Worksheet 2

Underline the word root in each of following combining forms.

1. rhin/o (nose)
2. splen/o (spleen)
3. hyster/o (uterus)
4. enter/o (intestine)
5. neur/o (nerve)
6. ot/o (ear)
7. dermat/o (skin)
8. hydr/o (water)
9. hepat/o (liver)
10. toxic/o (poison)

Worksheet 3

Underline the word root in the following words. Recall that in most instances the root designates a body part.

Word	Meaning
1. nephritis	inflammation of the kidneys
2. arthrodesis	surgical fixation of a joint
3. phlebotomy	incision of a vein
4. dentist	specialist in teeth
5. gastrectomy	excision of the stomach

Word	Meaning
6. lumpectomy	excision of a lump
7. hepatoma	tumor of the liver
8. cardiologist	specialist in the heart
9. gastria	condition of the stomach
10. thermometer	instrument for measuring heat

Worksheet 4

Underline the elements that are combining forms.

1. hepat
2. pancreat
3. cardi/o
4. oste/o
5. gastr/o

6. nephr/o
7. cyt
8. arthr
9. erythr/o
10. dent/o

Worksheet 5

In the space provided, change the roots to combining forms.

Root	Combining Form
1. mast (breast)	*mast/o*
2. hepat (liver)	
3. arthr (joint)	
4. cyst (bladder)	
5. phleb (vein)	
6. thorac (chest)	
7. abdomin (abdomen)	

Root   **Combining Form**

8. trache
    (trachea)   _____

9. leuk
    (white)   _____

10. gastr
    (stomach)   _____

Chapter 2

Suffixes: Surgical, Diagnostic, Symptomatic, and Related

Chapter Outline

STUDENT OBJECTIVES
SUFFIXES
SURGICAL SUFFIXES
Suffixes Denoting Incisions
Suffixes Denoting Reconstructive Surgeries

Suffixes Denoting Refracturing, Loosening, or Crushing
DIAGNOSTIC, SYMPTOMATIC, AND RELATED SUFFIXES
WORKSHEETS

Student Objectives
Upon completion of this chapter, you will be able to do the following:

Define and provide examples of operative, diagnostic, and symptomatic suffixes.

Determine the use of a combining form and word root when linking these elements to a suffix.

Demonstrate your knowledge of the chapter by completing the worksheets.

Suffixes

In medical words a *suffix* is added to the end of a root or combining form to change its meaning. For example, the combining form **gastr/o** means stomach. The suffix **-megaly** means enlargement, and **-itis** means inflammation. Gastr/o/megaly is an enlargement of the stomach, gastr/itis is an inflammation of the stomach. Whenever you change the suffix, the word takes on a new meaning. Suffixes are also used to denote singular and plural forms of a word as well as a part of speech.

Following are additional examples applying Rule 1 (Chapter 1, page 4) of medical word building.

A WORD ROOT IS USED BEFORE A SUFFIX THAT BEGINS WITH A VOWEL

Word Root	+	Suffix	=	Medical Word
gastr (stomach)	+	itis (inflammation)	=	gastritis inflammation of the stomach
cephal (head)	+	algia (pain)	=	cephalalgia pain in the head, headache
mast (breast)	+	ectomy (excision)	=	mastectomy excision of a breast

Following are additional examples applying rule 2 (Chapter 1, page 4) of medical word building.

A COMBINING VOWEL IS USED BEFORE A SUFFIX THAT BEGINS WITH A CONSONANT

Combining Form (WR + o)	+	Suffix	=	Medical Word
phleb + o (vein)	+	tomy (incision)	=	phlebotomy incision of a vein
colon + o (colon)	+	scopy (visual examination)	=	colonoscopy visual examination of colon
arthr + o (joint)	+	centesis (puncture)	=	arthrocentesis puncture of a joint
thorac + o (chest)	+	tomy (incision)	=	thoracotomy incision of the chest

A COMBINING VOWEL IS USED TO LINK A WORD ROOT TO ANOTHER WORD ROOT TO FORM A COMPOUND WORD

Combining Form (WR + o)	+	WR	+	Suffix	=	Medical Word
gastr + o (stomach)	+	enter (intestine)	+	itis (inflammation)	=	gastroenteritis inflammation of stomach and intestine
oste + o (bone)	+	arthr (joint)	+	itis (inflammation)	=	osteoarthritis inflammation of bone and joint
encephal + o (brain)	+	mening (meninges)	+	itis (inflammation)	=	encephalomeningitis inflammation of brain and meninges

An effective strategy in mastering medical terminology is learning the major suffixes first. To become proficient in medical terminology, review the examples in each section and say each word by referring to its phonetic pronunciation. Define medical words by following the three basic steps outlined in Chapter 1: *First, define the suffix,* or end of the word; *second, define the prefix,* or *first part of the word. Last, define the middle* of the word. For example, gastr/o/enter/itis is defined as inflammation of the stomach and intestine; append/ectomy is defined as excision of the appendix.

Surgical Suffixes

SUFFIXES DENOTING INCISIONS

Suffix	Meaning	Example	Pronunciation
-centesis	puncture	arthr/o/<u>centesis</u> joint	ăr-thrō-sĕn-TĒ-sĭs
-ectomy	excision, removal	append/<u>ectomy</u> appendix	ăp-ĕn-DĔK-tŏ-mē
-stomy	forming an opening (mouth)	col/o/<u>stomy</u> colon	kŏ-LŎS-tō-mē
-tome	instrument to cut	oste/o/<u>tome</u> bone	ŎS-tē-ō-tōm
-tomy	incision, cut into	phleb/o/<u>tomy</u> vein	flĕ-BŎT-ō-mē

SUFFIXES DENOTING RECONSTRUCTIVE SURGERIES

Suffix	Meaning	Example	Pronunication
-desis	binding, fixation (of a bone or joint)	arthr/o/desis joint	ăr-thrō-DĒ-sĭs
-pexy	fixation (of an organ)	mast/o/pexy breast	MĂS-tō-pĕks-ē
-rrhaphy	suture	my/o/rrhaphy muscle	mī-ŌR-ă-fē
-plasty	surgical repair	rhin/o/plasty nose	RĪ-nō-plăs-tē

SUFFIXES DENOTING REFRACTURING, LOOSENING, OR CRUSHING

Suffix	Meaning	Example	Pronunciation
-clasis	break, fracture	oste/o/clasis bone	ŏs-tē-ŎK-lăh-sĭs
-lysis	separation, destruction, loosening	enter/o/lysis intestine	ĕn-tĕr-ŎL-ĭ-sĭs
-tripsy	crushing	lith/o/tripsy stone, calculus	LĬTH-ō-trĭp-sē

Diagnostic, Symptomatic, and Related Suffixes

Suffix	Meaning	Example	Pronunciation
-algia	pain	cephal/algia head	sĕf-ăh-LĂL-jē-ăh
-cele	hernia, swelling	hepat/o/cele liver	HĔP-ă-tō-sēl
-dynia	pain	gastr/o/dynia stomach	găs-trō-DĬN-ē-ăh
-ectasis	dilation, expansion	bronchi/ectasis bronchus	brŏng-kē-ĔK-tăh-sĭs
-emesis	vomiting	hyper/emesis excessive	hī-pĕr-ĔM-ĕ-sĭs

Diagnostic, Symptomatic, and Related Suffixes (Continued)

Suffix	Meaning	Example	Pronunciation
-emia	blood	leuk/emia white	loo-KĒ-mē-ăh
-gen	forming, producing, origin	carcin/o/gen cancer	kăr-SĬN-ō-jĕn
-genesis	forming, producing, origin	oste/o/genesis bone	ŏs-tē-ō-JĔN-ĕ-sĭs
-gram	record, a writing	cardi/o/gram heart	KĂR-dē-ō-grăm
-graph	instrument for recording	cardi/o/graph heart	KĂR-dē-ō-grăf
-graphy	process of recording	cardi/o/graphy heart	kăr-dē-ŎG-ră-fē
-iasis	abnormal condition (produced by something specified)*	chole/lith/iasis gall stone	kō-lē-lĭ-THĪ-ăh-sĭs
-itis	inflammation	gastr/itis stomach	găs-TRĪ-tĭs
-lith	stone, calculus	chol/e/lith gall	KŌ-lē-lĭth
-logist	specialist in the study of	dermat/o/logist skin	dĕr-mă-TŎL-ō-jĭst
-logy	study of	psych/o/logy mind	sī-KŎL-ō-jē
-malacia	softening	oste/o/malacia bone	ŏs-tē-ō-măh-LĀ-shē-ăh
-megaly	enlargement	hepat/o/megaly liver	hĕp-ăh-tō-MEG-ăh-lē
-meter	instrument for measuring	therm/o/meter heat	thĕr-MŎM-ĕ-tĕr
-metry	act of measuring	pelv/i/metry pelvis	pĕl-VĬM-ĕt-rē
-oid	resembling	lip/oid fat	LĬP-oid
-oma	tumor	aden/oma gland	ăd-ĕ-NŌ-măh

*There are a few exceptions to this rule.

Diagnostic, Symptomatic, and Related Suffixes (Continued)

Suffix	Meaning	Example	Pronunciation
-osis	abnormal condition, increase (used primarily with blood cells)	dermat/osis skin erythr/o/cyt/osis red cell	dĕr-măh-TŌ-sĭs ĕ-rĭth-rō-sī-TŌ-sĭs
-para	to bear (offspring)	multi/para many, much	mŭl-TĬP-ă-ră
-paresis	partial paralysis	hemi/paresis half	hĕm-ē-PĂR-ĕ-sĭs
-pathy	disease	neur/o/pathy nerve	nū-RŎP-ă-thē
-penia	decrease, deficiency	leuk/o/penia white (cell)	loo-kō-PĒ-nē-ăh
-phagia	eating, swallowing	dys/phagia difficult, painful	dĭs-FĀ-jē-ăh
-phasia	speech	a/phasia without	ăh-FĀ-zē-ăh
-philia	attraction for	hem/o/philia blood	hē-mō-FĬL-ē-ăh
-phobia	fear	claustr/o/phobia confined place	klaws-trō-FŌ-bē-ăh
-plasia	formation, growth	hyper/plasia excessive	hī-pĕr-PLĀ-zē-ăh
-plegia	paralysis	hemi/plegia half	hĕm-ĕ-PLĒ-jē-ăh
-poiesis	formation, production	hem/o/poiesis blood	hē-mō-poy-Ē-sĭs
-ptosis	prolapse, downward displacement	hyster/o/ptosis uterus	hĭs-tĕr-ŏp-TŌ-sĭs
-rrhage -rrhagia }	bursting forth	hem/o/rrhage blood men/o/rrhagia menses	HĔM-or-ĭj mĕn-ō-RĀ-jē-ăh

Diagnostic, Symptomatic, and Related Suffixes (Continued)

Suffix	Meaning	Example	Pronunciation
-rrhea	discharge, flow	dia/rrhea through	dī-ă-RĒ-ăh
-rrhexis	rupture	angi/o/rrhexis vessel	ăn-jĭ-ō-RĔK-sĭs
-scope	instrument to view or examine	gastr/o/scope stomach	GĂS-trō-skōp
-scopy	visual examination	proct/o/scopy anus, rectum	prŏk-TŎS-kō-pē
-spasm	involuntary contraction, twitching	blephar/o/spasm eyelid	BLĔF-ăh-rō-spăzm
-stasis	standing still	hem/o/stasis blood	hē-mō-STĀ-sĭs
-stenosis	narrowing, stricture	arteri/o/stenosis artery	ăr-tē-rē-ō-stĕ-NŌ-sĭs
-trophy	development, nourishment	a/trophy without	ĂT-rō-fē
-toxic	poison	thyr/o/toxic thyroid	thī-rō-TŎKS-ĭk

Worksheet 1

SURGICAL SUFFIXES DENOTING INCISIONS*

Use the meaning column to complete the words on the left.

Incomplete Word	Meaning
1. episi/o/ _t o m y_	incision of the perineum
2. col _ _ _ _ _ _ _	excision (of all or part) of the colon
3. arthr/o/ _ _ _ _ _ _ _ _ _	puncture of a joint (to remove fluid)
4. splen _ _ _ _ _ _ _	excision of the spleen
5. col/o/ _ _ _ _ _	forming a permanent opening into the colon
6. derma _ _ _ _ _	instrument to cut skin
7. tympan/o/ _ _ _ _ _	incision of the tympanic membrane
8. trache/o/ _ _ _ _ _ _	forming an opening into the trachea
9. mast _ _ _ _ _ _ _	excision of a breast
10. lith/o/ _ _ _ _ _	incision to remove a stone or calculus
11. hemorroid _ _ _ _ _ _ _	excision of hemorrhoids

Cover the meaning column in the previous section. Use the word list to build words meaning:

12. forming an opening into the colon _colostomy_ _____

13. excision of the colon _____

14. instrument to cut skin _____

15. puncture of a joint _____

16. incision to remove a stone _____

17. excision of a breast _____

---

*In Worksheets 1 and 2 the word roots are underlined.

18. incision of the tympanic membrane _____

19. forming an opening into the trachea _____

20. excision of the spleen _____

Worksheet 2

SURGICAL SUFFIXES DENOTING RECONSTRUCTIVE SURGERIES*

Use the meaning column to complete the words on the left.

Incomplete Word	Meaning
1. arthr/o/ _ _ _ _ _	fixation or binding of a joint
2. rhin/ _ / _ _ _ _ _ _ _	surgical repair of the nose
3. ten/o/ _ _ _ _ _ _ _	surgical repair of tendons
4. my/o/ _ _ _ _ _ _ _ _	suture of muscle
5. mast/ _ / _ _ _ _ _	fixation of a (pendulous) breast
6. cyst/ _ / _ _ _ _ _ _ _ _	suture of the bladder

SURGICAL SUFFIXES DENOTING REFRACTURING, LOOSENING, OR CRUSHING

7. oste/o/ _ _ _ _ _ _ _	to break or fracture a bone
8. lith/ _ / _ _ _ _ _ _ _	crushing a stone
9. enter/ _ / _ _ _ _ _ _	separating intestinal (adhesions)
10. neur/ _ / _ _ _ _ _ _ _	crushing a nerve

Cover the meaning column in the previous section. Use the word list to build medical words meaning:

11. surgical repair of the nose _____

12. fixation of a joint _____

13. suture of (a torn) muscle _____

14. fixation of a (pendulous) breast _____

15. suture of the bladder _____

16. repair of tendons _____

---

*In Worksheets 1 and 2 the word roots are underlined.

17. refracturing a bone _____

18. crushing stones _____

19. freeing intestinal (adhesions) _____

20. crushing a nerve _____

Worksheet 3

DIAGNOSTIC, SYMPTOMATIC, AND RELATED SUFFIXES

Fill in the blanks to complete each medical word.

Incomplete Word	**Meaning**
1. bronchi_____	dilation of a bronchus
2. gastr/o/_____	pain in the stomach
3. nephr_____	abnormal condition of the kidneys
4. chole_____	gallstone
5. carcin/o/____	forming or producing cancer
6. psych/o/_____	study of the mind
7. oste/__/_____	softening of bone
8. hepat/__/_____	enlargement of the liver
9. cholelith_____	abnormal condition of gallstones
10. therm/__/_____	instrument for measuring heat
11. hepat/__/_____	herniation of the liver
12. lip____	resembling fat
13. neur/o/_____	disease of the nerves
14. dermat_____	abnormal condition of the skin
15. hemi_____	paralysis of one half of the body
16. proct/o/_____	visual examination of the colon
17. dys_____	difficult swallowing
18. a_____	without speech or absence of speech
19. cephal_____	pain in the head; headache
20. blephar/__/_____	twitching of the eyelid
21. angi/__/_____	rupture of a blood vessel

Incomplete Word	Meaning
22. hem/__/ _ _ _ _ _ _ _ _ _	formation of blood
23. hyster/o/ _ _ _ _ _ _ _	prolapse of the uterus
24. hemi _ _ _ _ _ _ _ _	partial paralysis of one half (of the body)
25. hyper _ _ _ _ _ _ _	excessive formation (of an organ or tissue)

Worksheet 4

SURGICAL SUFFIXES REVIEW

-centesis	-plasty
-clasis	-rrhaphy
-desis	-stomy
-ectomy	-tome
-lysis	-tomy
-pexy	-tripsy

Use the suffixes in the table to form surgical terms meaning:

1. crushing a stone   lith/o/_____

2. puncture of a joint (to remove fluid)   arthr/o/_____

3. excision of the spleen   splen/_____

4. forming an opening into the colon   col/o/_____

5. instrument to cut skin   derma/_____

6. forming an opening into the trachea   trache/o/_____

7. incision to remove a stone or calculus   lith/__ /_____

8. excision of a breast   mast/_____

9. excision of hemorrhoids   hemorrhoid/_____

10. incision of the trachea   trache/__ /_____

11. fixation of a (pendulous) breast   mast/__ /_____

12. excision (of part or all) of the colon   col/_____

13. suture of the stomach (wall)   gastr/__ /_____

14. fixation of the uterus   hyster/__ /_____

15. surgical repair of the nose   rhin/__ /_____

16. fixation or binding of a joint   arthr/__ /_____

17. to break or fracture a bone   oste/__ /_____

18. loosening of nerve (tissue)   neur/__/_____

19. suture of muscle   my/o/_____

20. incision of the tympanic membrane   tympan/__/_____

Worksheet 5

DIAGNOSTIC, SYMPTOMATIC, AND RELATED SUFFIXES REVIEW

-algia	-malacia	-phasia
-cele	-megaly	-plegia
-dynia	-metry	-poiesis
-ectasis	-oid	-rrhage
-emia	-oma	-rrhea
-genesis	-osis	-rrhexis
-graph	-pathy	-spasm
-iasis	-penia	-stenosis
-itis	-phagia	

Use the suffixes in the table to form diagnostic and symptomatic terms meaning:

1. dilation of a bronchus   bronchi/_____

2. pain (along the course) of a nerve   neur/_____

3. inflammation of the stomach   gastr/_____

4. headache; pain in the head   cephal/o/_____

5. tumor of the liver   hepat/_____

6. producing or forming cancer   carcin/o/_____

7. abnormal condition of the skin   dermat/_____

8. resembling fat   lip/_____

9. enlarged kidney   nephr/o/_____

10. narrowing or stricture of the pylorus   pylor/__ /_____

11. discharge or flow from the ear   ot/__ /_____

12. production or formation of blood   hem/o/_____

13. rupture of the uterus   hyster/__ /_____

14. spasm or twitching of the eyelid   blephar/__ /_____

15. herniation of the bladder   cyst/__ /_____

16. bursting forth (of) blood   hem/o/_____

17. abnormal condition of a stone or calculus   lith/_____

18. paralysis affecting one side (of the body)   hemi/_____

19. diseases of muscle (tissue)   my/__/_____

20. difficult or painful eating   dys/_____

21. softening of the bones   oste/__/_____

22. without, or absence of, speech   a/_____

23. white blood   leuk/_____

24. deficiency in number of red blood cells   erythr/__/_____

25. measuring the pelvis   pelv/i/_____

Chapter 3

Suffixes: Adjective, Noun, Diminutive, Singular, Plural

Chapter Outline

STUDENT OBJECTIVES

ADJECTIVE SUFFIXES

NOUN SUFFIXES

DIMINUTIVE SUFFIXES

PLURAL SUFFIXES

WORKSHEETS

Student Objectives

Upon completion of this chapter, you will be able to do the following:

List and define diminutive suffixes.

List and define adjective suffixes, and apply this knowledge by completing Worksheet 1.

List and define nouns suffixes, and apply this knowledge by completing Worksheet 2.

Define the rules for changing singular words to plural words, and apply this knowledge by completing Worksheets 3 and 4.

The suffixes discussed in this chapter are added to word roots to indicate either a part of speech or a singular or plural form of a medical word.

Adjective Suffixes

The adjective suffixes that mean "pertaining to" or "relating to," or both, are as follows.

Adjective Suffix	Example	Adjective Suffix	Example
-ac*	cardi/ac heart	-ic	hypo/ derm/ic under skin
-al	neur/al nerve	-ical[†]	med/ical medicine
-ar	muscul/ar muscle	-ory	audit/ory hearing
-ary	saliv/ary saliva	-ous	cutane/ous skin
-eal	mening/eal meninges	-tic	acous/tic sound

*-ac ending is rarely used.
[†]-ical is a combination of -ic and -al.

Noun Suffixes

The suffixes added to word roots to indicate a noun as follows.

Noun Suffix	Meaning	Example
-ia	condition	pneumon/ia lung
-iatry	treatment, medicine	pod/iatry foot
-ism	condition	alcohol/ism alcohol
-ist	specialist	ur/o/ log/ist urine study [of]
-y	condition	path/y disease

Diminutive Suffixes

A diminutive suffix forms a word designating a smaller version of the object indicated by the word root.

Dimunitive Suffix	Meaning	Example
-ole		arteri/ole artery
-icle		part/icle piece
-ula	small, minute	mac/ula spot
-ule		ven/ule vein

Plural Suffixes

The rules for forming plural words from singular words are listed in the following chart.

Form		Rule	Example	
SINGULAR	PLURAL		SINGULAR	PLURAL
a	ae	Retain the a and add e.	pleura	pleurae
ax	aces	Drop the x and add ces.	thorax	thoraces
en	ina	Drop en and add ina.	lumen	lumina
is	es	Drop the is and add es.	diagnosis	diagnoses
ix ex	ices	Drop the ix or ex and add ices.	appendix apex	appendices apices
on	a	Drop on and add a.	ganglion	ganglia
um	a	Drop um and add a.	bacterium	bacteria
us	i	Drop us and add i.	bronchus	bronchi
y	ies	Drop y and add ies.	deformity	deformities
ma	mata	Retain the ma and add ta.	carcinoma	carcinomata

Worksheet 1

Use the following adjective suffixes to complete a medical term. When in doubt about the validity of a medical term, refer to a medical dictionary.

-ac   -ic
-al   -ous
-ary   -tic
-eal   -tix

Element	Medical Term	Meaning
1. thorac/	*thoracic*	pertaining to the chest
2. gastr/	_____	pertaining to the stomach
3. bacteri/	_____	pertaining to bacteria
4. aqua/	_____	pertaining to water
5. axill/	_____	pertaining to the armpit
6. cardi/	_____	pertaining to the heart
7. spin/	_____	pertaining to the spine
8. membran/	_____	pertaining to a membrane

Worksheet 2

Use the following noun suffixes to form a medical term. When in doubt about the validity of a medical term, refer to a medical dictionary.

-er	-ism
-ia	-ist
-is	-y

Element	Medical Term	Meaning
1. intern/	*internist*	specialist in internal medicine
2. leuk/em/	_____	condition of "white" blood
3. sigmoid/o/scop/	_____	visual examination of the sigmoid colon
4. alcohol/	_____	condition of (excessive) alcohol
5. allerg/	_____	specialist in allergies
6. senil/	_____	condition associated with aging
7. man/	_____	condition of madness
8. orth/o/ped/	_____	specialist in orthopedics

Worksheet 3

Write the plural form for each word and briefly state the pertinent rule. Use the dictionary as a reference.

Singular	Plural	Rule
1. diagnosis	*diagnoses*	*Drop the is and add es.*
2. fornix		
3. bursa		
4. vertebra		
5. keratosis		
6. bronchus		
7. spermatozoon		
8. septum		
9. coccus		
10. apex		
11. ganglion		
12. prognosis		
13. thrombus		
14. appendix		
15. bacterium		
16. radius		
17. testis		
18. nevus		

Chapter 4

Prefixes

Chapter Outline

Student Objectives

Upon completion of this chapter, you will be able to do the following:

Define the concept of prefix and provide several examples.

Identify prefixes of position, number and measurement, negation, and direction.

Demonstrate your knowledge of this chapter by completing the worksheets.

33

This chapter emphasizes the major prefixes used in building a medical vocabulary. It completes the information necessary to develop a basic foundation for learning medical words. Once you have learned their basic components, medical terms will be much easier to define.

Prefixes

A prefix is a word element located at the beginning of a word. The prefix can affect the meaning of the word. Not all medical words contain a prefix. Review the following examples to see how the prefix influences the meaning of a word.

PREFIX		WORD ROOT		SUFFIX		
pre (before)	+	nat (birth)	+	al (pertaining to)	=	pertaining to before birth
peri (around)	+	nat (birth)	+	al (pertaining to)	=	pertaining to the period around birth
post (after)	+	nat (birth)	+	al (pertaining to)	=	pertaining to after birth

PREFIXES OF POSITION

Prefix	Meaning	Example	Pronunciation
ante-	before, in front	ante/cubit/ al elbow pertaining to	ăn-tē-KŪ-bĭ-tăl
pre-		pre/operative operation	prē-ŎP-ĕr-ă-tĭv
pro-		pro/ot/ ic ear pertaining to	prō-ŎT-ĭk
epi-	above, upon	epi/derm/ is skin noun ending	ĕp-ĭ-DĔR-mĭs
hypo-	under, below	hypo/derm/ic skin relating to	hī-pō-DĔR-mĭk
infra-		infra/pub/ ic pubis relating to	ĭn-fră-PŪ-bĭk
sub-		sub/nas/ al nose pertaining to	sŭb-NĀ-zăl
inter-	between	inter/cost/ al ribs pertaining to	ĭn-tĕr-KŎS-tăl
meso-	middle	meso/derm skin	MĔS-ō-dĕrm
medi-		medi/al pertaining to	MĒ-dē-ăl

PREFIXES OF POSITION (Continued)

Prefix	Meaning	Example	Pronunciation
post-	after, behind	post/nat/ al 　　birth pertaining to	pōst-NĀ-tăl
retro-	backward, behind	retro/peritone/ al 　　peritoneum pertaining to	rĕt-rō-pĕr-ĭ-tō-NĒ-ăl

PREFIXES OF NUMBER AND MEASUREMENT

Prefix	Meaning	Example	Pronunciation
bi-	two	bi/later/ al 　　side relating to	bī-LĂT-er-ăl
dipl- diplo-	double, twofold	dipl/opia 　　vision diplo/cocci 　　spherical-shaped 　　bacteria	dĭp-LŌ-pē-ă dĭp-lō-KŎK-sī
hemi- semi-	one half	hemi/plegia 　　paralysis semi/circul/ ar 　　circle pertaining to	hĕm-ĕ-PLĒ-jē-ăh sĕm-ē-SŬR-kū-lăr
hyper-	excessive, above normal	hyper/glyc/ emia 　　glucose, blood 　　sugar	hī-pĕr-glī-SĒ-mē-ăh
macro-	large	macro/cephal/y 　　head noun ending	măk-rō-SĔF-ăh-lē
micro-	small	micro/scope 　　instrument to view	MĪ-krō-skōp
mono- uni-	one	mono/cyte 　　cell uni/para 　　to bear (offspring)	MŎN-ō-sīt ū-NĬP-ă-ră
multi- poly-	many, much	multi/para 　　to bear (offspring) poly/phobia 　　fear(s)	mŭl-TĬP-ăh-răh pŏl-ē-FŌ-bē-ăh
primi-	first	primi/gravida 　　pregnancy	prī-mĭ-GRĂV-ĭ-dă
quadri-	four	quadri/plegia 　　paralysis	kwŏd-rĭ-PLĒ-jē-ăh
tri-	three	tri/ceps 　　heads	TRĪ-sĕps

PREFIXES OF NEGATION

Prefix	Meaning	Example	Pronunciation
a-* an-†	without, not	a/mast/ ia — breast condition	ă-MĂS-tē-ăh
		an/esthes/ ia — sensation condition	ăn-ĕs-THĒ-zē-ăh
im-	not	im/potency — potent	ĬM-pō-tĕn-sĭ
in-	in, not	in/sane — sound	ĭn-SĀN

*Usually used before a consonant.
†Usually used before a vowel.

PREFIXES OF DIRECTION

Prefix	Meaning	Example	Pronunciation
ab-	away from	ab/norm/ al — regular, pertaining to usual	ăb-NŎR-măl
ad-	toward	ad/stern/ al — sternum, relating to breastbone	ăd-STĔR-năl
circum- peri-	around	circum/or/ al — mouth pertaining to	sĕr-kŭm-Ō-răl
		peri/oste/ itis — bone inflammation	pĕr-ē-ŏs-tē-Ī-tĭs
ec- ex-	out, out from	ec/top/ ia — place condition	ĕk-TŌ-pē-ăh
		ex/cise — to cut	ĕk-SĪZ
dia- trans-	through, across	dia/rrhea — flow	dī-ăh-RĒ-ăh
		trans/fusion — a pouring	trăns-FŪ-zhŭn
ecto- exo- extra-	outside	ecto/derm — skin	ĔK-tō-dĕrm
		exo/trop/ ia — turning condition	ĕks-ō-TRŌ-pē-ăh
		extra/ocul/ ar — eye pertaining to	ĕks-tră-ŎK-ū-lăr
endo- intra-	in, within	endo/cardi/ um — heart noun ending	ĕn-dō-KĂR-dē-ŭm
		intra/muscul/ ar — muscle relating to	ĭn-trăh-MŬS-kū-lăr

PREFIXES OF DIRECTION (Continued)

Prefix	Meaning	Example	Pronunciation
para-*	near, beside, beyond	para/nas/ al nose pertaining to	păr-ă-NĀ-săl
super-	above, excessive	super/sensitive sensation	soo-pĕr-SĔNS-ĭ-tĭv
supra-		supra/ren/ al kidney pertaining to	soo-pră-RĒ-năl

*Para- may also be used as a suffix, at which time it means "to bear (offspring)."

OTHER PREFIXES

Prefix	Meaning	Example	Pronunciation
anti-	against	anti/bacteri/ al bacteria pertaining to	ăn-tĭ-băk-TĒ-rē-ăl
contra-		contra/ception conceiving	kŏn-tră-SĔP-shŭn
brady-	slow	brady/card/ ia heart noun ending, condition	brăd-ē-KĂR-dē-ăh
dys-	bad, painful, difficult	dys/pepsia digestion	dĭs-PĔP-sē-ăh
eu-	good, normal	eu/pnea breathing	ūp-NĒ-ăh
hetero-	different	hetero/sex/ual sex pertaining to	hĕt-ĕr-ō-SĔK-shū-ăl
homo-	same	homo/sex/ual sex pertaining to	hō-mō-SĔK-shū-ăl
mal-	bad	mal/nutrition food substances	măl-nū-TRĬSH-ŭn
pan-	all	pan/hyster/ ectomy uterus excision	păn-hĭs-tĕr-ĔK-tō-mē
pseudo-	false	pseudo/plegia paralysis	soo-dō-PLĒ-jē-ăh
syn-*	union, together, joined	syn/arthr/osis joint abnormal condition	sĭn-ăr-THRŌ-sĭs
tachy-	rapid	tachy/pnea breathing	tăk-ĭp-NĒ-ăh

*Appears as sym- before b, p, ph, or m.

Worksheet 1

Place a slash after each prefix, and then define the prefix.*

Word	Definition of Prefix
1. inter/dental	*between*
2. hypodermic	
3. epigastrium	
4. retroactive	
5. subnasal	
6. medial	
7. infrapatellar	
8. postnatal	
9. quadriplegia	
10. hyperlipidemia	
11. primipara	
12. microcephaly	
13. triceps	
14. polydipsia	
15. impotent	
16. anaerobic	
17. macrocephaly	
18. intramuscular	
19. suprarenal	
20. diarrhea	

*Before you complete the worksheets, use the flash cards at the end of this book to review the prefixes.

Word	Definition of Prefix
21. circumrenal	_____
22. adhesion	_____
23. perirenal	_____
24. bradycardia	_____
25. tachypnea	_____
26. dyspnea	_____
27. eupnea	_____
28. heterograft	_____
29. malfunction	_____
30. periosteum	_____

Worksheet 2

Match the medical words that follow with the definitions in the numbered list.

diarrhea   impotent   monocyte   primigravida
ectoderm   intercostal   periosteum   quadriplegia
epidermis   macrocephaly   polyphobia   retroperitoneal
hemiplegia   medial   postoperative   subnasal
hypodermic   microscope   preoperative   suprarenal

Prefixes of Position and Direction

1. _____ behind the peritoneum

2. _____ pertaining to under the skin

3. _____ before surgery

4. _____ pertaining to under the nose

5. _____ after surgery

6. _____ between the ribs

7. _____ pertaining to the middle

8. _____ around the bone

9. _____ flow through (watery bowel movement)

10. _____ outside the skin

11. _____ above the kidney

Prefixes of Number and Measurement

12. _____ paralysis of one half of the body

13. _____ one cell

14. _____ paralysis of four limbs

15. _____ abnormally large head

16. _____ instrument to view minute objects

17. _____ many fears

18. _____ first pregnancy

Worksheet 3

Prefixes of Negation and Other Prefixes

Match the following medical words with the definitions in the numbered list.

amastia   eupnea
anesthesia   heterosexual
antibacterial   homosexual
bradycardia   malnutrition
contraception   pseudomembranous
dyspepsia   synarthrosis
dysphagia   tachycardia

1. _____ difficult digestion

2. _____ pertaining to the opposite sex

3. _____ pertaining to a false membrane

4. _____ against bacteria

5. _____ slow heartbeat

6. _____ poor or bad nutrition

7. _____ without a breast

8. _____ without sensation

9. _____ good or normal breathing

10. _____ abnormal condition of a united joint

11. _____ rapid heartbeat

12. _____ against conception

13. _____ pertaining to the same sex

Chapter 5

Body Structure

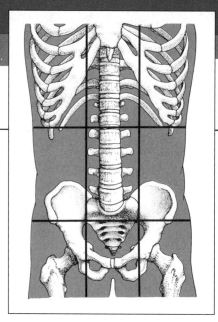

Chapter Outline

Student Objectives

Upon completion of this chapter, you will be able to do the following:

List and briefly define the levels of organization in the human body.

Demonstrate an understanding of the disease process by defining medical terms associated with pathology.

Define and identify four body planes.

List two dorsal cavities and two ventral cavities, and identify at least one organ within each cavity.

43

Student Objectives (Continued)

List and locate nine abdominopelvic regions and the four quadrants of the same area.

Demonstrate an understanding of body imaging by defining terms associated with radiology, computed tomography, magnetic resonance imaging, and ultrasonography.

Define directional terms and be able to use them correctly.

Identify combining forms, suffixes, and prefixes related to body structure.

Demonstrate your knowledge of the chapter by completing the worksheets.

This chapter is an overview of body structure and presents terms related to the body as a whole, rather than to any specific body system. Review the material carefully because it provides a foundation for the remaining chapters of the book.

Levels of Organization

The body is composed of different levels of structure and function. Each of these levels incorporates the structures and functions of the previous level, contributing to the entire organism. The levels of organization are as follows:

Cells → Tissues → Organs → Systems → Organism

CELLS

The **cell** is the structural and functional unit of life. All activities that we associate with living (eating, eliminating waste, breathing, reproducing) are performed by individual cells. The way different cells undertake these activities may vary considerably, but the end result is the same. The study of the body at the cellular level is called **cytology.** An understanding of cytology is important because the disease process originates at the cellular level.

TISSUES

Groups of cells that perform a specialized activity are called **tissues.** The study of tissues is called **histology.** The four major tissues of the body are:
- **epithelial tissue,** composed of cells arranged in a continuous sheet consisting of one or several layers; forms the epidermis of the skin, covers surfaces of organs, lines cavities and canals, forms tubes, ducts, and secreting portions of glands
- **connective tissue,** supports and connects other tissues and organs
- **muscle tissue,** all contractile tissue of the body
- **nervous tissue,** all tissue capable of transmitting electrical impulses

ORGANS

Organs are body structures composed of at least two different tissue types that perform specialized functions. For example, the stomach is composed of muscle tissue and epithelial tissue. The muscle tissue moves food through the stomach, and epithelial tissue secretes enzymes and gastric products for digestion.

SYSTEMS

The next level of organization is a **system.** A body system is composed of at least one organ and accessory structures that have similar or interrelated functions. For example, the organs and accessory structures of the gastrointestinal system include the esophagus, stomach, and small intestine. The purpose of this system is to digest food, extract nutrients from it, and eliminate waste products. Some of the other body systems are the reproductive, respiratory, and cardiovascular systems.

ORGANISM

The highest level of organization is the **organism.** This is a complete living entity capable of independent existence. All complex organisms, including humans, are composed of several body systems that work together to sustain life.

The Disease Process

Although most people understand the concept of **disease,** a clinical definition is quite complex. From the clinical point of view, disease is a **pathological** or **morbid condition** of the body that presents a group of **signs, symptoms,** and **clinical findings.** Signs are objective indicators that are observable by others. A palpable mass or tissue redness are examples of signs. In contrast, a symptom is subjective and is experienced only by the patient. Dizziness, pain, and malaise are examples of symptoms. Clinical findings are results of laboratory examinations and other tests performed on the patient.

All body cells require oxygen and nutrients for survival. They also need a stable internal environment that provides a narrow range of temperature, water, acidity, and salt concentration. This stable internal environment is called **homeostasis.** When homeostasis is significantly interrupted and cells, tissues, organs, or systems are unable to meet the challenges of everyday life, the condition is called **pathology.** As each phase of pathology progresses, signs, symptoms, and clinical findings change. The study of the progression of a disease is called **pathogenesis.** Pathogenesis varies from disease to disease.

Etiology is the study of all factors involved in the development of a disease. The following list identifies several types of diseases.

- Metabolic (diabetes)
- Infectious (measles, mumps)
- Congenital (harelip)
- Hereditary (hemophilia)

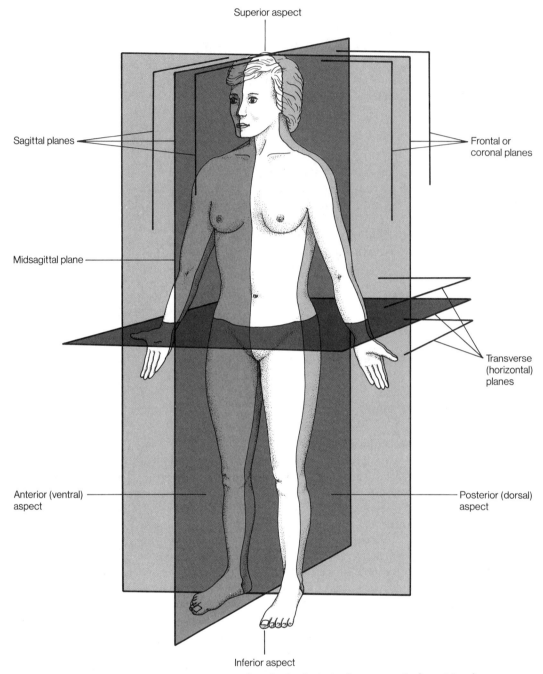

Figure 5–1   Body planes. (Note that the body is in the anatomical position.)

- Environmental (burns, trauma)
- Neoplastic (cancer)

Establishing the cause and nature of a disease is referred to as **diagnosis.** Determining a diagnosis helps the physician select a method of treatment. A **prognosis** is the prediction of the course of a disease and its probable outcome. Any disease whose cause is unknown is said to be **idiopathic.**

Anatomical Position

The **anatomical position** is placement of the body in a stance that is accepted by anatomists throughout the world. In this position, the body is erect and the eyes are looking forward. The upper limbs hang to the sides, with the palms facing to the front; the lower limbs are parallel, with the toes pointing forward. Regardless of whether the body actually lies facing upward or downward, or how the limbs are actually placed, the positions and relationships of a structure are always described as if the body were in the anatomical position.

Planes of the Body

An anatomical **plane** of the body is an imaginary flat surface that passes through the body at different places in order to divide it for anatomical purposes. Several commonly used anatomical planes are illustrated in Figure 5–1. Table 5–1 lists body planes and describes their anatomical divisions.

Body Cavities

The body is divided into four major cavities. A coronal plane divides these four cavities into two **dorsal cavities** and two **ventral cavities** (Fig. 5–2). Table 5–2 lists the body cavities and some of the major organs found within them. The thoracic cavity is separated from the abdominopelvic cavity by a muscular wall, the diaphragm.

The Abdominopelvic Region

The abdominopelvic region may be divided into nine major sections by constructing an imaginary "tic-tac-toe" over this region. This provides divisions to locate the placement of internal or **visceral** organs. Operative reports frequently refer to these divisions as a point of reference to designate exact locations of tumors, ulcers, and body structures. The

Table 5–1   **Planes of the Body**

Body Plane	Anatomical Division
Midsagittal or median	Right and left halves
Sagittal	Unequal right and left sides
Coronal or frontal	Front side (anterior or ventral aspect) and back side (posterior or dorsal aspect)
Transverse or horizontal	Upper portion (superior aspect) and lower portion (inferior aspect)

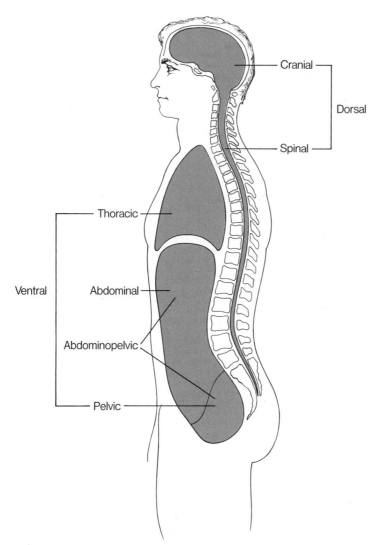

Figure 5–2 Body cavities.

Table 5–2 **Body Cavities**

Cavity	Major Organ(s) Found in the Cavity
Dorsal	
Cranial	Brain
Spinal	Spinal cord
Ventral	
Thoracic	Heart, lungs, and associated structures
Abdominopelvic	Digestive, excretory, and reproductive systems and associated structures

nine regions (Fig. 5–3), from left to right and top to bottom, are as follows:

Right hypochondriac	Upper right region beneath the ribs
Epigastric	Region of the stomach
Left hypochondriac	Upper left region beneath the ribs
Right lumbar	Right middle lateral region
Umbilical	Region of the navel
Left lumbar	Left middle lateral region
Right inguinal (iliac)	Right lower lateral region
Hypogastric	Lower middle region beneath the navel
Left inguinal (iliac)	Left lower lateral region

For purposes of clinical evaluation, the abdominopelvic region may be divided into four quadrants (sections) by an imaginary cross (Fig. 5–4):

Right upper quadrant (RUQ)	Left upper quadrant (LUQ)
Right lower quadrant (RLQ)	Left lower quadrant (LLQ)

Diagnostic Imaging

Recent advances in body imaging procedures have greatly reduced the need for exploratory surgery. Current techniques for examining underlying structures include radiogra-

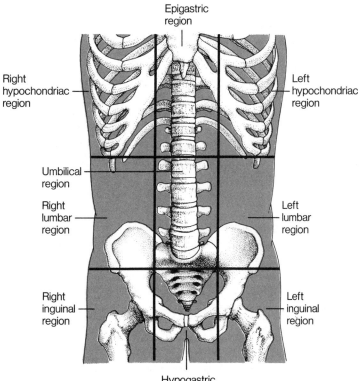

Figure 5–3 Anatomical divisions of the abdominopelvic region.

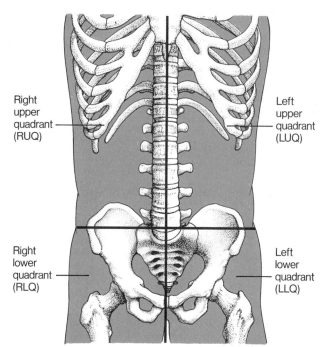

Right upper quadrant (RUQ)

Left upper quadrant (LUQ)

Right lower quadrant (RLQ)

Left lower quadrant (LLQ)

Figure 5–4 Abdominal quadrants.

phy, computed tomography (CT) scan, magnetic resonance imaging (MRI), and ultrasonography (echography, sonography).

The oldest and most widely used of these methods is **radiography (roentgenography),** more commonly called **x-ray examination.** In this technique, an energy beam in the x band of the radiation spectrum passes through the area of the body to be examined. Although some x-rays are absorbed by the structures through which the beam passes, the remainder of the x-rays falls on the radiographic film placed behind the area to be examined. Denser tissue absorbs more of the beam than does tissue of a lesser density. Because of the difference in densities of various tissues, an image, called a radiograph or x-ray film, is produced. It is a negative image similar to a photographic negative produced by a camera.

In its early applications, radiography was used almost exclusively to visualize bones because bones are very dense and abnormalities are easily seen. With the advent of **radiopaque materials** (substances that absorb x-rays), the use of radiography expanded to include visualization of many soft tissues of the body.

Computed tomography (CT) scan is a variation of the radiographic technique just described. CT scan, however, is more sensitive than conventional x-ray examination and is particularly valuable in detecting soft body tissue diseases. In this procedure the x-ray beam circles around a central axis of the body or an organ. The data obtained are computerized and then reconstructed to generate an image. This image appears as a "slice" of an organ or body part. The term tomography literally means "a recording or record of a slice."

Magnetic resonance imaging (MRI) is another type of scanning technique. However, a magnetic field rather than an x-ray beam is used to produce the image. A magnetic field induces tissue to produce **radiofrequency (RF)** waves. These waves are sensed by a receiving device called an **RF detector coil,** which sends them to a computer. The computer then generates an image of the tissue and provides three views from different angles: axial, sagittal, and coronal. Different tissues can be distinguished because each emits a different radio signal. MRI often produces sharper images of soft tissue than those obtained using CT scans. MRI also has the advantage over CT scans in that it does not employ the potentially harmful radiation associated with x-rays.

Ultrasonography is a technique that reflects high-frequency sound (ultrasonic) waves off internal tissues. The ultrasonic waves are received by a detector called a **transducer,** where they are converted to electrical impulses and then displayed on a video monitor. The resultant images are not as clear as those produced with x-rays or RF waves, but ultrasonography is easy to use, inexpensive, and associated with little or no risk to the patient. Ultrasonography is used extensively in maternofetal diagnostics.

The Spine

The spine is divided into sections corresponding to the vertebrae, which are located in the spinal column. (For a more complete discussion, refer to Chapter 11, Musculoskeletal System.) These divisions are as follows:

Cervical (neck)
Thoracic (chest)
Lumbar (loin)
Sacral (lower back)
Coccyx (tailbone)

Directional Terms

Directional terms are used to indicate the position of a structure in relation to another structure. For example, the kidneys are superior to (above) the urinary bladder. The directional term "superior to" denotes "above" the structure, which, in this example, is the urinary bladder. In the following list, opposing terms are presented consecutively to aid in memorization.

Superficial	Toward the surface of the body
Deep	Away from the surface of the body (internal)
Abduction	Movement away from the median plane of the body or one of its parts
Adduction	Movement toward the median plane of the body
Medial	Pertaining to the midline of the body or structure
Lateral	Pertaining to a side
Superior	Toward the head or upper portion of a structure (cephalad, cranial)
Inferior	Away from the head, or toward the tail or lower part of a structure (caudal or caudad)
Proximal	Near the attachment of an extremity to the trunk or a structure
Distal	Farther from the attachment of an extremity to the trunk or a structure

Anterior	Near the front of the body (ventral)
Posterior	Near the back of the body (dorsal)
Parietal	Pertaining to the outer wall of the body cavity
Visceral	Pertaining to the covering of an organ
Prone	Lying horizontal with the face downward, or denoting the hand with palms turned downward
Supine	Lying on the back with the face upward, or denoting the position of the hand or foot with the palm or foot facing upward
Inversion	Turning inward or inside out
Eversion	Turning outward

COMBINING FORMS

Combining Form	Meaning	Example	Pronunciation
anter/o	anterior, front	anter/o/posterior behind	ăn-tĕr-ō-pŏs-TĒ-rē-or
cyt/o	cell	cyt/o/logist specialist in the study of	sī-TŎL-ō-jĭst
hist/o	tissue	hist/o/logy study of	hĭs-TŎL-ō-jē
home/o	same	home/o/stasis standing still	hō-mē-ō-STĀ-sĭs
idi/o	unknown, peculiar	idi/o/path/ ic disease pertaining to	ĭd-ē-ō-PĂTH-ĭk
later/o	to one side, side	later/o/abdomin/al abdomen pertaining to	lăt-ĕr-ō-ăb-DŎM-ĭ-năl
medi/o	middle, median	medi/o/later/al side pertaining to	mē-dē-ō-LĂT-ĕr-ăl
nucle/o	nucleus	nucle/o/toxin poison	NŪ-klē-ō-tŏk-sĭn
path/o	disease	path/o/gen to produce	PĂTH-ō-jĕn
poster/o	back (of body), behind, posterior	poster/o/later/al side pertaining to	pŏs-tĕr-ō-LĂT-ĕr-ăl
proxim/o	near, nearest	proxim/al pertaining to	PRŎK-sĭm-ăl
radi/o	radiation, x-ray	radi/o/graphy process of recording	rā-dē-ŎG-ră-fē

COMBINING FORMS (Continued)

Combining Form	Meaning	Example	Pronunciation
ventr/o	belly, belly-side	ventr/al pertaining to	VĔN-trăl
viscer/o	internal organs	viscer/o/megaly enlargement	vĭs-ĕr-ō-MĔG-ă-lē

SUFFIXES

Suffix	Meaning	Example	Pronunciation
-genesis	forming, producing, origin	path/o/genesis disease	păth-ō-JĔN-ĕ-sĭs
-gnosis	knowing	pro/gnosis before	prŏg-NŌ-sĭs
-gram	record, a writing	son/o/gram sound	SŌ-nō-grăm
-graph	instrument for recording	son/o/graph sound	SŌ-nō-grăf
-graphy	process of recording	myel/o/graphy spinal cord	mī-ĕ-LŎG-ră-fē
-pathy	disease	cyt/o/pathy cell	sī-TŎP-ĭ-thē

PREFIXES

Prefix	Meaning	Example	Pronunciation
ab-	from, away from	ab/axi/al axis pertaining to	ăb-ĂK-sē-ăl
ad-	toward	ad/duction movement	ă-DŬK-shŭn
infra-	below, under	infra/cost/al rib pertaining to	ĭn-fră-KŎS-tăl
peri-	around	peri/cardi/um heart noun ending	pĕr-ĭ-KĂR-dē-ŭm
trans-	across, through	trans/ocul/ar eye pertaining to	trăns-ŎK-ū-lăr
ultra-	excess, beyond	ultra/sound sound	ŬL-tră-sound

ABBREVIATIONS

Abbreviation	Meaning
AP	anteroposterior
CNS	central nervous system
CT scan	computed tomography scan
CV	cardiovascular
Dx	diagnosis
GI	gastrointestinal
GU	genitourinary
lat	lateral
LLQ	left lower quadrant
LUQ	left upper quadrant
MRI	magnetic resonance imaging
MS	musculoskeletal
PA	posteroanterior
RLQ	right lower quadrant
ROM	range of motion
RUQ	right upper quadrant
sono	sonogram, sonography
U & L, U/L	upper and lower

Case Study

Radiology Report of Cervical and Lumbar Spine

AP, lateral, and **odontoid** views of the cervical spine demonstrate some reversal of normal **cervical** curvature, as seen on lateral projection. There is some right lateral **scoliosis** of the cervical spine. The **vertebral** bodies, however, appear to be well maintained in height; the **intervertebral spaces** are well maintained. The odontoid is visualized and appears to be intact. The **atlantoaxial joint** appears symmetrical.

Impression. Films of the cervical spine demonstrate some reversal of normal cervical curvature and a minimal scoliosis, possibly secondary to muscle **spasm,** without evidence of recent bony disease or injury.

AP and lateral films of the **lumbar spine,** with spots of the **lumbosacral** junction, demonstrate an apparent minimal **spina bifida occulta** of the first sacral segment. The vertebral bodies, however, are well maintained in height; the intervertebral spaces appear well maintained.

Worksheet 4 provides a dictionary and reading application and an analysis of this case study.

Worksheet 1

Match the following elements with the definitions in the numbered list.

hist/o	-gram
home/o	-graphy
later/o	infra-
nucle/o	mono-
ventr/o	peri-
-cyte	ultra-

1. _____ tissue

2. _____ record, a writing

3. _____ excess, beyond

4. _____ belly side

5. _____ same

6. _____ cell

7. _____ below, under

8. _____ process of recording

9. _____ around

10. _____ to one side

Worksheet 2

Match the following directional terms with the definitions in the numbered list.

abduction	inferior	proximal
adduction	inversion	superior
anterior	lateral	supine
digital	medial	umbilical
distal	posterior	
eversion	prone	

1. _____ pertaining to the side

2. _____ pertaining to the midline of the body or structure

3. _____ farther from the attachment of an extremity to the trunk or structure

4. _____ near the attachment of an extremity to the trunk or a structure

5. _____ lying on the back with the face upward

6. _____ lying horizontal with the face downward

7. _____ movement toward the median plane

8. _____ movement away from the median plane

9. _____ toward the head or upper portion of the body or structure

10. _____ away from the head or toward the tail or lower part of a structure

11. _____ near the front of the body (ventral)

12. _____ near the back of the body (dorsal)

13. _____ turning inward or inside out

14. _____ turning outward

Worksheet 3

Match the following medical words with the definitions in the numbered list.

diagnosis   morbid   radiography   symptom
etiology   pathogenesis   radiologist   tomography
homeostasis   pathologist   radiopaque material ultrasonography
magnetic resonance prognosis   sign   x-ray
  imaging

1. _____ study of the cause of disease

2. _____ specialist in the study of radiography

3. _____ specialist in study of disease

4. _____ diseased or pathologic

5. _____ origin or development of a disease

6. _____ objective indicator of a disease

7. _____ a subjective experience such as pain or dizziness

8. _____ the probable outcome of a disease

9. _____ the determination of the cause and nature of a disease

10. _____ a stable internal environment

11. _____ substance that absorbs x-rays, used to visualize soft tissue

12. _____ literally means a "record of a slice"

13. _____ uses a magnetic field rather than an x-ray beam to produce an image

14. _____ a technique that reflects high-frequency sound waves off internal tissues to produce an image

15. _____ the beam of radiation used to produce a radiographic image

Worksheet 4

RADIOLOGY REPORT OF CERVICAL AND LUMBAR SPINE DICTIONARY
EXERCISE

Use a medical dictionary or other resource to define the following terms and determine their pronunciation; then practice reading the case study aloud (see p. 54).

AP _____

atlantoaxial joint _____

cervical _____

intervertebral spaces _____

lateral _____

lumbar spine _____

lumbosacral _____

odontoid _____

scoliosis _____

spasm _____

spina bifida occulta _____

vertebral _____

ANALYSIS OF RADIOLOGY REPORT OF CERVICAL AND LUMBAR SPINE

1. Why was an x-ray film taken of the cervical spine?

2. Did the patient appear to have experienced any type of recent injury to the spine?

3. What cervical vertebrae form the atlantoaxial joint?

4. Was the odontoid process fractured?

5. What did the radiologist believe was the possible cause of the minimal scoliosis?

Worksheet 5

On the following diagram, label the body planes and compare your answers with Figure 5–1.

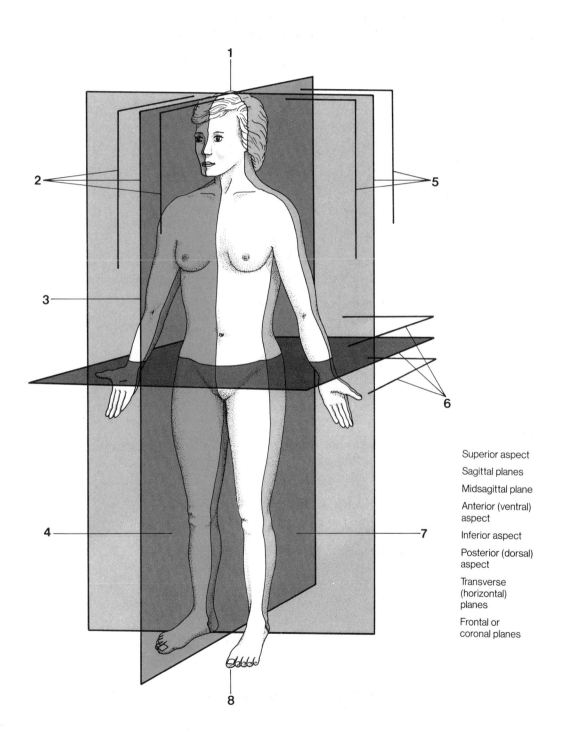

Superior aspect

Sagittal planes

Midsagittal plane

Anterior (ventral) aspect

Inferior aspect

Posterior (dorsal) aspect

Transverse (horizontal) planes

Frontal or coronal planes

Worksheet 6

Label the abdominopelvic regions on the following diagram and compare your answers with Figure 5–3.

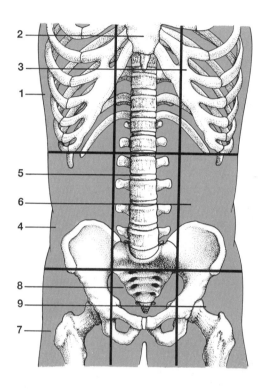

Right
hypochondriac
region

Right
lumbar
region

Right
inguinal
region

Hypogastric
region

Left
inguinal
region

Left
lumbar
region

Left
hypochondriac
region

Epigastric
region

Umbilical
region

Worksheet 7

On the following diagram, label the quadrants and compare your answers with Figure 5–4.

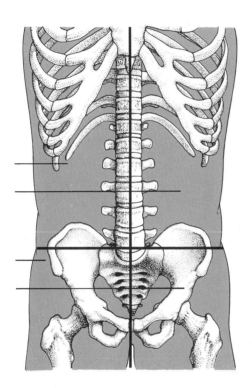

Right
upper
quadrant
(RUQ)

Right
lower
quadrant
(RLQ)

Left
upper
quadrant
(LUQ)

Left
lower
quadrant
(LLQ)

Chapter 6

Integumentary System

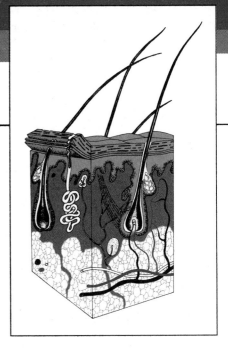

Chapter Outline

Student Objectives

Upon completion of this chapter, you will be able to do the following:

Define the main functions of the integumentary system and its appendages.

List the appendages of the integumentary system.

63

Student Objectives (Continued)

Identify combining forms, suffixes, and prefixes related to the integumentary system.

Identify several primary and secondary skin lesions.

Explain and identify major skin problems caused by exposure.

Identify surgical, diagnostic imaging, and laboratory procedures and abbreviations related to the integumentary system.

Explain pharmacology related to the treatment of integumentary disorders.

Demonstrate your knowledge by completing the worksheets.

Anatomy and Physiology

The largest organ in the body is the skin **(integument).** Together with the hair, nails, glands, and breasts, the skin constitutes the **integumentary system.**

SKIN

The skin covers all outer surfaces of the body and performs many important functions. It protects against injuries and bacterial invasion, aids in regulation of body temperature, and prevents dehydration. The skin also acts as a reservoir for food and water, works as a sensory receptor, and is responsible for the synthesis of vitamin D when exposed to sunlight. The skin is composed of two layers, the epidermis and the dermis, as shown in Figure 6–1.

The (1) **epidermis,** a layer of tissue with no blood or nerve supply, is the outermost layer of skin. It is made up of cells in several **strata** or sublayers called **stratified squamous epithelium.** The most important of these four or five sublayers are the (2) **stratum corneum** and the (3) **stratum germinativum.**

The stratum germinativum includes a basal layer where new cells are continually being produced, pushing the older cells toward the outer skin surface. As the cells move toward the stratum corneum, the outermost layer of the epidermis, they die and become filled with a hard protein material called **keratin.** The relatively waterproof characteristic of keratin prevents body fluids from evaporating and atmospheric moisture from entering the body. Keratin also acts as a barrier to pathogens and chemicals because most bacteria and other microorganisms cannot penetrate unbroken skin. One exception is the sap of poison ivy, the resin of which penetrates the skin and initiates an allergic reaction in susceptible people. The importance of the stratum corneum becomes especially apparent when it is lost (see Fig. 6–3).

The (4) **dermis,** or **corium,** is the layer of skin lying immediately under the epidermis. It is composed of living tissue that consists of numerous capillaries, lymphatics, and nerve endings. Hair follicles, sebaceous (oil) glands, and sweat glands are also located in the dermis. The (5) **subcutaneous tissue,** or **hypodermis,** is an underlying connective tissue layer that contains fat or adipose tissue and connects the skin to underlying organs.

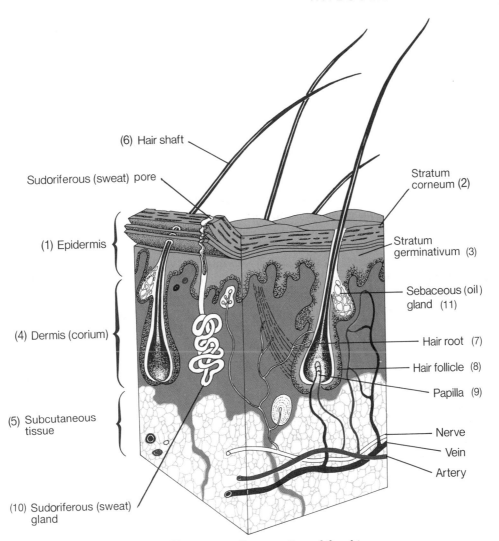

Figure 6–1 Cross section of the skin.

APPENDAGES OF THE SKIN

Hair

The visible part of the hair is referred to as the (6) **hair shaft** whereas that which is embedded in the dermis is called the (7) **hair root.** The root, together with its coverings, forms the (8) **hair follicle.** At the bottom of the follicle is a loop of capillaries enclosed in a covering called the (9) **papilla.** The cluster of epithelial cells lying over the papilla reproduces and is responsible for the eventual formation of the hair shaft. As long as these cells remain alive, hair will regenerate even if it is cut, plucked, or otherwise removed. Baldness (**alopecia**) occurs when the hairs of the scalp are not replaced owing to death of these cells.

Glands

Two important glands in the skin that produce secretions are the (10) **sudoriferous (sweat) glands** and the (11) **sebaceous (oil) glands.**

The sudoriferous glands are small structures that open as **pores** on the surface of the skin. They are found on the palms, soles, forehead, and armpits (axillae). The main functions of the sudoriferous glands are to cool the body by evaporation, to excrete waste products through the pores of the skin, and to moisten surface cells.

The sebaceous glands are the oil-secreting glands of the skin. These glands are filled with cells, the centers of which are saturated with fatty droplets. As these cells disintegrate, they yield an oily secretion called **sebum.** The acidic nature of sebum helps to destroy harmful organisms on the skin's surface and thus to prevent infection. Sebaceous glands are present over the entire body, except on the soles of the feet and the palms of the hands. They are especially prevalent on the scalp and face; around openings such as the nose, mouth, external ear, and anus; and on the upper back and scrotum.

Nails

The major function of the nails is to protect the tips of the fingers and toes from bruises and other kinds of injuries. The nailbed covers the dorsal surface of the last bone of each finger and toe. Most of the nail body appears pink because of the underlying vascular tissue. The crescent-shaped white area near the root of the nailbed is the **lunula.** It has a whitish appearance because the vascular tissue underneath does not show through. The lunula is the area in which new growth occurs.

Breasts

The breasts (Fig. 6–2), or mammary glands, are located in the upper anterior aspect of the chest. During puberty, the woman's breasts develop as a result of periodic stimulation of ovarian hormones estrogen and progesterone. Estrogen is responsible for (1) **adipose tissue** and increased size of the breasts as they reach full maturity. The size of the breast is basically determined by the amount of fat around the glandular tissue, but breast size is not indicative of functional ability. The other ovarian hormone, progesterone, forms the lobules that are present in the breast. Each breast has approximately 20 lobes of (2) **glandular tissue.** Milk in these lobes is drained by a (3) **lactiferous duct** that opens on the tip of the raised (4) **nipple.** Circling the nipple is a border of slightly darker skin called the (5) **areola.**

The main purpose of the breasts is to secrete milk for the nourishment of newborn infants. Thus, pregnancy causes the breasts to enlarge for this function. In women, breasts fully develop by age 16. At menopause, breast tissue begins to atrophy.

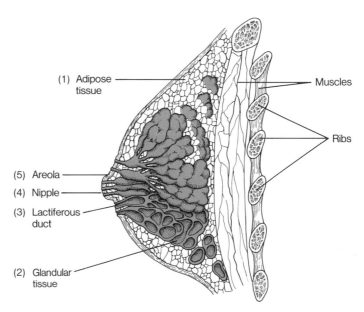

Figure 6–2 Cross section of the breast.

COMBINING FORMS

Combining Form	Meaning	Example	Pronunciation
aden/o	gland	aden/o/pathy disease	ăd-ĕ-NŎP-ăh-thē
adip/o		adip/oma tumor	ă-dĭ-PŌ-mă
lip/o	fat	lip/oid resembling	LĬP-oid
steat/o		steat/oma tumor	stē-ă-TŌ-mă
crypt/o	hidden	onych/o/crypt/osis nail abnormal condition	ŏn-ĭ-kō-krĭp-TŌ-sĭs
cutane/o		sub/cutane/ous under pertaining to	sŭb-kū-TĀ-nē-ŭs
dermat/o	skin	dermat/o/logy study of	dĕr-mă-TŎL-ō-jē
derm/o		derm/is noun ending	DĔR-mĭs
hidr/o	sweat	hidr/ aden/oma gland tumor	hī-drăd-ĕ-NŌ-mă
ichthy/o	dry, scaly	ichthy/osis abnormal condition	ĭk-thē-Ō-sĭs
kerat/o	horny tissue, hard, cornea	kerat/osis abnormal condition	kĕr-ă-TŌ-sĭs

COMBINING FORMS (Continued)

Combining Form	Meaning	Example	Pronunciation
lact/o	milk	lact/ic pertaining to	LĂK-tĭk
mamm/o	breast	mamm/o/plasty surgical repair	MĂM-ō-plăs-tē
mast/o	breast	mast/ectomy excision	măs-TĔK-tŏ-mē
myc/o	fungus	dermat/o/myc/osis skin abnormal condition	dĕr-mă-tō-mī-KŌ-sĭs
onych/o	nail	onych/o/malacia softening	ŏn-ĭ-kō-mă-LĀ-sē-āh
ungu/o	nail	ungu/al pertaining to	ŬNG-gwăl
pil/o	hair	pil/o/nid/al nest pertaining to	pī-lō-NĪ-dăl
trich/o	hair	trich/o/pathy disease	trĭk-ŎP-ă-thē
scler/o	hardening	scler/osis abnormal condition	sklĕ-RŌ-sĭs
squam/o	scaly	squam/ous pertaining to	SKWĀ-mŭs
thel/o	nipple	thel/itis inflammation	thē-LĪ-tĭs
xer/o	dry	xer/o/derma skin	zē-rō-DĔR-mă

COMBINING FORMS OF COLOR

Combining Form	Meaning	Example	Pronunciation
albin/o	white	albin/ism condition	ĂL-bĭn-ĭzm
leuk/o	white	leuk/o/derma skin	loo-kō-DĔR-mă
leuc/o	white	leuc/o/cyte cell	LOO-kō-sīt
anthrac/o	charcoal (coal dust)	anthrac/osis abnormal condition	ăn-thră-KŌ-sĭs

COMBINING FORMS OF COLOR (Continued)

Combining Form	Meaning	Example	Pronunciation
chlor/o	green	chlor/o/cyte 　　　　cell	KLŌ-rō-sīt
cirrh/o		cirrh/osis 　　　abnormal condition	sĭr-RŌ-sĭs
jaund/o	yellow	jaund/ice 　　　noun ending	JAWN-dĭs
xanth/o		xanth/emia 　　　blood	zăn-THĒ-mē-ăh
cyan/o	blue	cyan/o/derma 　　　　skin	sī-ă-nō-DĔR-mă
erythem/o		erythem/a 　　　noun ending	ĕr-ĭ-THĒ-mă
erythr/o	red	erythr/o/cyte 　　　cell	ĕ-RĬTH-rō-sīt
rube/o		rube/osis 　　　abnormal condition	roo-bē-Ō-sĭs
melan/o	black	melan/oma 　　　tumor	mĕl-ăh-NŌ-măh

SUFFIXES

Suffix	Meaning	Example	Pronunciation
-cyte	cell	lip/o/cyte fat	LĬP-ō-sīt
-derma	skin	scler/o/derma hardening	sklĕr-ă-DĔR-mă
-gram	record	mamm/o/gram breast	MĂM-ō-grăm
-graph	instrument for recording	mamm/o/graph breast	MĂM-ō-grăf
-graphy	process of recording	mamm/o/graphy breast	măm-ŎG-ră-fē
-logist	specialist in the study of	dermat/o/logist skin	dĕr-mă-TŎL-ō-jĭst
-logy	study of	dermat/o/logy skin	dĕr-mă-TŎL-ō-jē
-therapy	treatment	dermat/o/therapy skin	dĕr-mă-tō-THĔR-ă-pē

PREFIXES

Prefix	Meaning	Example	Pronunciation
epi-	above, upon	epi/derm/is skin noun ending	ĕp-ĭ-DĔR-mĭs
hyper-	excessive	hyper/hidro/ osis sweat abnormal condition	hī-pĕr-hī-DRŌ-sĭs
hypo- sub-	under, below	hypo/derm/ic skin pertaining to sub/cutane/ous skin pertaining to	hī-pō-DĔR-mĭk sŭb-kū-TĀ-nē-ŭs

Pathology

PRIMARY SKIN LESIONS

Areas of pathologically altered tissue are called **lesions.** Figure 6–3 illustrates and Table 6–1 describes several primary skin lesions.

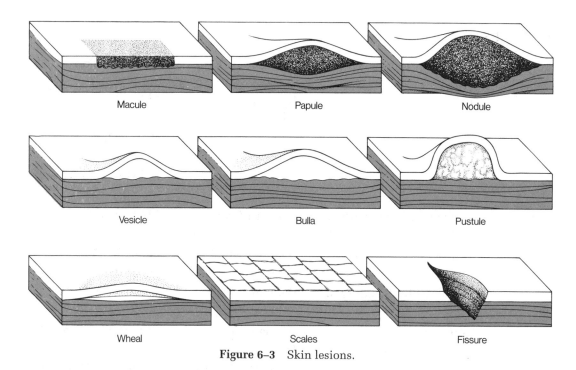

Macule   Papule   Nodule

Vesicle   Bulla   Pustule

Wheal   Scales   Fissure

Figure 6–3   Skin lesions.

Table 6–1 **Skin Lesions**

Type	Characteristics	Example
FLAT LESION		
Macule	Flat, discolored circumscribed lesion of any size	Freckle, flat mole, hyperpigmentation
ELEVATED LESION		
Papule	Solid elevated lesion, <1 cm in diameter	Nevus, warts, pimples
Nodule	Palpable circumscribed lesion, larger than a papule, 1–2 cm in diameter	Benign or malignant tumor
Wheal	Dome-shaped or flat-topped elevated lesion, slightly reddened and often changing in size and shape, usually accompanied by intense itching	Hives
Vesicle and bulla	Elevated lesion that contains fluid; a bulla is a vesicle >0.5 cm	Blister, Herpes zoster, second-degree burn
Pustule	Elevated lesion containing pus that may be sterile or contaminated with bacteria; small abscess on the skin	Acne, pustular psoriasis
Scale	Excessive dry exfoliation shed from upper layers of the skin	Psoriasis, ichthyosis
Cyst	Elevated, encapsulated mass of dermis or subcutaneous layers, solid or fluid-filled	Sebaceous cyst
Tumor	Swelling; well-demarcated, elevated lesion >2 cm in diameter	Fibroma, lipoma, steatoma, melanoma, hemangioma
DEPRESSED LESION		
Fissure	Small cracklike sore or break exposing the dermis; usually red	Athlete's foot, cheilosis
Ulcer	Loss of epidermis and dermis within a distinct border	Pressure sore, basal cell carcinoma

SECONDARY SKIN LESIONS

Secondary skin lesions are pathological skin alterations that are a result of a primary skin lesion. During the healing process, scabs **(crustations)** form over sores and wounds. The crusts are composed of dry pus, lymph, or blood and may vary in color and thickness.

When trauma, chemicals, or burns cause a superficial loss of tissue, the resulting skin lesion is called an **excoriation.** Excoriation is often caused by a scraping or rubbing away **(abrasion)** of epidermal tissue. When tissue injury exists without skin breakage, it is called a bruise **(contusion).** A more serious injury results when a wound is produced by the tearing of body tissue **(laceration),** as distinguished from a cut or incision. A laceration may be small or large and may be caused in many ways. Some common causes are a blow from a blunt instrument, a fall against a rough surface, and an accident with machinery.

Ulcers are open wounds. As they heal, a scar **(cicatrix)** often develops. Excessive scarring may produce an enlarged thickened scar **(keloid)** that may grow for a prolonged period of time. A predisposition to keloid formation is thought to be hereditary and occurs more often in dark-skinned people. Although this complication can have serious cosmetic implications, it is not life threatening.

BURNS

Burns are thermal injuries to the outer surfaces of the body. They can be classified according to three major categories, depending on the degree of severity (Fig. 6–4).

First-degree burns are superficial burns. The skin damage is limited to the top layers of the epidermis. These burns are distinguished by redness of the skin **(erythema)** and extreme sensitivity **(hyperesthesia)** to sensory stimuli, especially touch.

Second-degree burns are characterized by the formation of fluid-filled blisters **(vesicles** or **bullae),** caused by deeper penetration of heat. In most instances, a second-degree burn will not result in the formation of scar tissue.

Third-degree burns, which penetrate both the epidermis and the dermis, cause complete destruction of skin tissue and represent the most serious type of burn. This type of burn usually results in scar formation, which can be altered only by the process of skin grafting **(dermatoplasty).** When more than two thirds of the body's skin is destroyed, death usually results owing to excessive loss of body fluids. Without the proper amount of body fluids, the brain, heart, and other organs cannot perform their normal functions.

FROSTBITE

Frostbite causes a local destruction of the skin, as a result of freezing. Like burns, frostbite is classified according to its degree of severity: first-, second-, and third-degree.

ONCOLOGY

New autonomous growths **(neoplasms)** must be **microscopically** examined to determine if they are **malignant** or **benign.** Tumors are considered malignant when they invade normal tissue and eventually establish additional malignancies in other parts of the body **(metastasize).** Malignant neoplasms constitute the disease known as cancer. The spread of cancer through the body is influenced by the location **(site)** and type of malignancy.

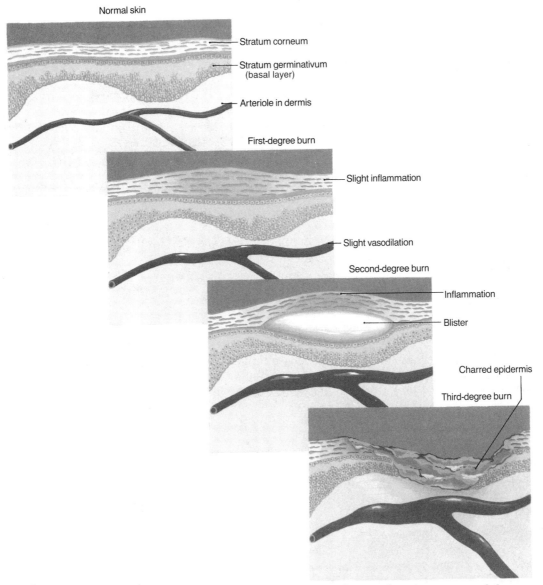

Figure 6–4   Normal skin section and representative sections showing first-degree, second-degree, and third-degree burns. (Adapted from Scanlon, VC and Sanders, T: Essentials of Anatomy and Physiology, ed 2. FA Davis, Philadelphia, 1995, Box Figure 5–A, with permission.)

Pathologists **grade** and **stage** tumors to help in diagnosis and treatment of the disease. Tumor grading (Table 6–2) is an evaluation of the degree of malignancy in a tumor. The TNM System of Staging (Table 6–3) determines the extent to which a tumor has spread through the body. **T** refers to size and extent of primary **tumor**. **N** indicates number of area lymph **nodes** involved. **M** refers to any **metastases** of the primary tumor.

The treatment of cancer involves chemotherapy and radiation, both of which can cause hair loss **(alopecia).** These treatments cause alopecia by damaging stem cells and hair follicles. The hair becomes brittle and may fall out or break off at the surface of the

Table 6–2 **Tumor Grading**

Grading		Characteristics of Tumor
Grade I:	Tumor cells well differentiated	Closely resembles normal parent tissue; thus retains some specialized functions
Grade II:	Tumor cells moderately differentiated	Less resemblance to tissue of origin; more variation in size and shape of tumor cells; increased mitoses
Grade III:	Tumor cells poorly to very poorly differentiated	Does not closely resemble tissue to origin; much variation in shape and size of tumor cells; greatly increased mitoses
Grade IV:	Tumor cells very poorly differentiated	No resemblance to tissue of origin; great variation in size and shape of tumor cells

scalp. Loss of other body hair is less common. Hair loss is a minor problem compared with the potentially life-threatening consequences of malignancy.

Basal Cell Carcinoma

Basal cell carcinoma, the most common type of skin cancer, which is often caused by overexposure to sunlight, is a malignancy of the basal cell layer of the epidermis (the stratum germinativum; see Fig. 6–1). These tumors grow slowly, but as they increase in size they often ulcerate and develop crusting that is firm to the touch. Although metastases occur infrequently with this type of cancer, the disease can invade the tissue sufficiently to destroy an ear, nose, or eyelid.

Squamous Cell Carcinoma

Squamous cell carcinoma is a tumor of the epidermis. There are two types: **in situ** (in position) and **invasive.** Because of its ability to invade and spread, this type of malignancy must be treated.

Table 6–3 **TNM System of Staging**

T_0	No evidence of primary tumor
T_{IS}	Carcinoma in situ
T_1, T_2, T_3, T_4	Progressive increase in tumor size and involvement
T_x	Tumor cannot be assessed
N_0	Regional lymph nodes not demonstrably abnormal
N_1, N_2, N_3, N_4	Increasing degrees of demonstrable abnormality and increasingly distant location of spread
N_x	Regional lymph nodes cannot be assessed
M_0	No evidence of distant metastasis
M_1, M_2, M_3	Ascending degrees of distant metastasis

Adapted from Classification and Staging of Cancer by Site: A Preliminary Handbook. American Joint Committee for Cancer Staging and End Results Reporting, 1976.

Malignant Melanoma

Malignant melanoma is a cancerous tumor of the skin originating from pigment cells **(melanocytes)** in the epidermis and dermis. The incidence of melanoma is doubling every 10 to 20 years. There is strong evidence that sunlight exposure is an important contributing factor for this disease. Avoiding the sun and using sunscreen have proved effective in preventing the disease.

Melanoma is diagnosed by biopsy. The primary mode of treatment at this time is excision. The extent of surgery is determined by staging the disease (Table 6–3).

Kaposi's Sarcoma

Kaposi's sarcoma, a tumor associated with **acquired immunodeficiency syndrome (AIDS),** is often fatal because the tumors metastasize to various organs. The lesions emerge as purplish-brown macules and develop into plaques and nodules. The lesions initially appear over the lower extremities and tend to spread symmetrically over the upper body, particularly the face and oral mucosa.

DIAGNOSTIC, SYMPTOMATIC, AND RELATED TERMS

Term	Meaning
chloasma klō-ĂZ-măh	hyperpigmentation of the skin characterized by yellowish-brown patches or spots
comedo KŎM-ē-dō	blackhead; discolored dried sebum plugging an excretory duct of the skin
decubitus ulcer dē-KŪ-bĭ-tŭs ŬL-sĕr	lesion due to impaired circulation in a portion of the body surface caused by prolonged pressure especially from a bed or chair; most frequently found in skin overlying a bony projection such as the hip, ankle, heel, shoulder, or elbow; also known as a bedsore
dermatitis dĕr-mă-TĪ-tĭs	inflammation of skin characterized by itching, redness, and various skin lesions
ecchymosis ĕk-ĭ-MŌ-sĭs	skin discoloration consisting of large, irregularly formed hemorrhagic area, with color changing from blue-black to greenish-brown or yellow
eczema ĔK-zĕ-mă	inflammatory skin disease with erythema, papules, vesicles, pustules, scales, crusts, and scabs, either alone or in combination
hirsutism HĔR-soot-ĭzm	condition characterized by the excessive growth of hair or presence of hair in unusual places, especially in women
impetigo ĭm-pĕ-TĪ-gō	inflammatory skin disease characterized by isolated pustules that become crusted and rupture

DIAGNOSTIC, SYMPTOMATIC, AND RELATED TERMS
(Continued)

Term	Meaning
pallor PĂL-ŏr	unnatural paleness or absence of color in the skin
pediculosis pē-dĭk-ū-LŌ-sĭs	infestation with lice, transmitted by personal contact or common use of brushes, combs, or headgear
pemphigus PĔM-fĭ-gŭs	acute or chronic adult disease characterized by the occurrence of successive crops of vesicles (bullae) that appear suddenly on apparently normal skin and then disappear, leaving pigmented spots
petechia, petechiae (pl.) pe-TĒ-kē-ăh, pē-TĒ-kē-ē	minute or small hemorrhagic spots on the skin (petechia is a smaller version of ecchymosis)
psoriasis sō-RĪ-ă-sĭs	chronic skin disease characterized by itching, red macules, papules, or plaques covered with silvery scales
purpura PŬR-pū-ră	any of several bleeding disorders characterized by hemorrhage into the tissues, particularly beneath the skin or mucous membranes, producing ecchymoses or petechiae
scabies SKĀ-bēz	contagious skin disease transmitted by the itch mite
tinea TIN-ē-ăh	any fungal skin disease, frequently caused by ringworm, whose name indicates the body part affected (e.g., tinea barbae [beard], tinea corporis [body], tinea pedis [athlete's foot]
urticaria ŭr-tĭ-KĀ-rē-ă	allergic reaction of the skin characterized by the eruption of pale red elevated patches called wheals (hives)
vitiligo vĭt-ĭl-Ī-gō	localized loss of skin pigmentation characterized by milk-white patches
wart wort	rounded epidermal growth caused by a virus, which include plantar warts, juvenile warts, and venereal warts; removable by cryosurgery, electrocautery, or acids; able to regrow if virus remains in the skin

Special Procedures

DIAGNOSTIC IMAGING PROCEDURES

Term	Description
mammography, mammogram măm-ŎG-ră-fē, MĂM-ō-grăm	radiographic examination of the breast to detect abnormalities of breast tissue
xeromammography, xeromammogram zē-rō-măm-MŎG-ră-fē, zē-rō-MĂM-mō-grăm	xeroradiography of the breast
xeroradiography zē-rō-rā-dē-ŎG-ră-fē	process to produce x-ray images on paper rather than on x-ray film; especially beneficial in diagnosis of breast tumors and minute breast calcifications

SURGICAL PROCEDURES

Term	Description
allograft ĂL-ō-grăft	transplant tissue obtained from the same species
biopsy BĪ-ŏp-sē	excision of a small piece of tissue by use of a syringe and needle or through a surgical procedure for microscopic examination; usually performed to establish a diagnosis
dermabrasion DĚRM-ă-brā-zhŭn	removal of acne scars, nevi, tattoos, or fine wrinkles on the skin through the use of sandpaper, wire brushes, or other abrasive materials on the anesthesized epidermis
electrodesiccation ē-lěk-trō-děs-ĭ-KĀ-shŭn	tissue destruction by dehydration (desiccation) using a high-frequency electric current
frozen section	thin slice of tissue cut from a frozen specimen, often used for rapid microscopic diagnosis
fulguration fŭl-gū-RĀ-shŭn	tissue destruction by means of high-frequency electric sparks
incision and drainage (I & D) ĭn-SĬZH-ŭn, DRĀN-ĭj	incising (cutting open) a lesion (e.g., abscess) and draining the contents
lumpectomy lŭm-PĚK-tō-mē	excision of a small primary breast tumor, leaving the remainder of the breast intact

SURGICAL PROCEDURES (Continued)

Term	Description
mammoplasty, mastoplasty MĂM-ăh-plăs-tē, MĂS-tō-plăs-tē	surgical reconstruction of the breast(s), sometimes augmented by substances such as fat tissue or silicone to alter the size and shape
radical mastectomy măs-TĔK-tō-mē	removing the breast and any involved skin, pectoral muscles, axillary lymph nodes, and subcutaneous fat
skin graft	using the skin from another part of the body, or from a donor, to repair a defect or trauma of the skin
xenograft	transplant tissue obtained from a different species

LABORATORY PROCEDURES

Skin Test	Description
patch test	used in testing for skin allergies, especially contact dermatitis. A small piece of gauze or filter paper, impregnated with a minute quantity of the substance to be tested (e.g., food, pollen, animal fur), is applied to the skin, usually on the forearm. After the patch is removed, a lack of noticeable reaction indicates a negative result; skin reddening or swelling indicates a positive result
scratch test	used in testing for allergies. A small quantity of a solution containing a suspected allergen is placed on a lightly scratched area of the skin. Redness or swelling at the scratch sites within 15 minutes indicates allergy to the substance and a positive result. If no reaction has occurred after 30 minutes, the test result is negative
Schick test	one of the best known intradermal tests used to determine immunity to diphtheria, in which diphtheria toxin is injected interdermally. A positive reaction, indicating susceptibility, is marked by redness and swelling at the site of injection. A negative reaction, indicating immunity, is marked by absence of redness or swelling
tuberculin test	used to determine past or present tuberculosis infection, using one of several methods. A purified protein derivative (PPD) of tubercle bacilli (tuberculin) is introduced into the skin by scratch, puncture (Heaf's and tine tests), or intradermal injection (Mantoux test). In all tests local inflammation is considered a positive result indicating past or present tuberculosis infection but does not reveal whether infection is active or inactive

PHARMACOLOGY

Medication	Action
astringents	topical agents that shrink the blood vessels locally, dry up secretions from seeping lesions, decrease sweating, and lessen skin sensitivity
anti-infectives, antibacterials, antifungals	agents that eliminate epidermal infections, which can be administered either topically or systemically. Topical medications create a skin environment that is lethal to microbes. Generally, a specific fungicide must be prescribed for a given fungus strain, whereas one antibiotic effectively eliminates several types of bacteria
anti-inflammatory drugs, topical corticosteroids	these topically applied drugs relieve three common symptoms of skin disorders: pruritus (itching); vasodilation, and inflammation
antipruritics	agents that prevent or relieve itching
antiseptics	topically applied agents that destroy bacteria, thus preventing the development of infections in cuts, scratches, and surgical incisions
keratolytics	agents that destroy and soften the outer layer of skin so that it is sloughed off or shed. The strong keratolytics are effective for removing warts and corns and aid in penetration of antifungal drugs. Milder preparations are used to promote shedding of scales and crusts in eczema, psoriasis, seborrheic dermatitis, and other dry, scaly conditions. Very weak keratolytics irritate inflamed skin, acting as tonics to speed up healing
parasiticides	used to destroy insect parasites that infest the skin. Scabicides kill mites and their eggs. Pediculicides destroy lice and their eggs
protectives	function by covering, cooling, drying, or soothing inflamed skin. Protectives do not penetrate the skin or soften it, but form a long-lasting film, which protects the skin from air, water, and clothing during the natural healing process
topical anesthetics	prescribed for pain on skin surfaces or mucous membranes caused by wounds, hemorrhoids, or sunburn. They relieve pain and itching by numbing the skin layers and mucous membranes and are applied directly by means of sprays, creams, gargles, suppositories, and other preparations

ABBREVIATIONS

Abbreviation	Meaning
Bx	biopsy
decub.	decubitus
derm.	dermatology
FS	frozen section
ID	intradermal
I & D	incision and drainage
SC	subcutaneous
ung	ointment

Case Study
Pathology Report of Skin Lesion

Specimen. Skin on (a) **dorsum** left wrist and (b) left forearm, **ulnar,** near elbow

Clinical Diagnosis. Bowen's disease versus **basal cell carcinoma** versus **dermatitis**

Microscopic Description. (a) There is mild **hyperkeratosis** and moderate **epidermal hyperplasia** with full-thickness **atypia** of **squamous-keratinocytes.** Squamatization of the basal cell layer exists. A lymphocytic inflammatory infiltrate is present in the **papillary dermis. Solar elastosis** is present. (b) Nests, strands, and columns of atypical **neoplastic** basaloid keratinocytes grow down from the epidermis into the underlying dermis. Fibroplasia is present. Solar elastosis is noted.

Pathological Diagnosis. (a) Bowen's disease of left wrist; (b) nodular and infiltrating basal cell carcinoma skin left forearm, near elbow.

   Worksheet 5 provides a dictionary and reading application and an analysis of this case study.

Worksheet 1

Use mast/o (breast) to build medical words meaning:

1. pain in the breast _____

2. inflammation of a breast _____

3. any disease of the breast _____

4. without or lack of a breast (development) _____

Use mamm/o (breast) to build medical words meaning:

5. record (x-ray film) of the breast _____

6. pertaining to the breast _____

Use adip/o or lip/o (fat) to build medical words meaning:

7. tumor consisting of fat _____

8. hernia containing fat _____

9. resembling fat _____

10. fat cell _____

Use dermat/o (skin) to build medical words meaning:

11. inflammation of the skin _____

12. specialist in skin (diseases) _____

Use onych/o (nail, nailbed) to build medical words meaning:

13. inflammation of the nailbed _____

14. tumor of the nailbed _____

15. disease of the nails _____

16. abnormal condition of the nails caused by a fungus _____

17. softening of the nails _____

18. abnormal condition of a hidden (ingrown) nail _____

Use trich/o (hair) to build medical words meaning:

19. disease of the hair _____

20. abnormal condition of hair caused by a fungus _____

Worksheet 2
Build a surgical term meaning:

1. excision of a breast _____

2. surgical repair or reconstruction of a breast _____

3. excision of fat (adipose tissue) _____

4. removal of the nail _____

5. incision of a nail _____

6. surgical repair (plastic surgery) of the skin _____

Worksheet 3
Match the following medical words with the definitions in the numbered list.

alopecia   petechiae
chloasma   scabies
ecchymosis   tinea
impetigo   urticaria
pediculosis   vitiligo
pedicturus   wart

1. _____ infestation with lice

2. _____ depigmentation in areas of the skin characterized by milk-white patches

3. _____ any fungal skin disease, especially ringworm

4. _____ a contagious skin disease transmitted by the itch mite

5. _____ a skin infection characterized by vesicles that become pustular and crusted and then rupture

6. _____ severe itching of the skin, also known as hives

7. _____ hyperpigmentation of the skin, characterized by yellowish-brown patches or spots

8. _____ hemorrhagic spot or bruise on the skin

9. _____ minute or small hemorrhagic spots on the skin

10. _____ loss or absence of hair

Worksheet 4

SPECIAL PROCEDURES, PHARMACOLOGY, AND ABBREVIATIONS

Match the following words or abbreviations with the definitions in the numbered list.

antibacterials

antipruritics

antiseptics

astringents

Bx

dermabrasion

electrodesiccation

fulguration

keratolytics

mammography

parasiticides

protectives

Schick test

ung

1. _____ agents that prevent or relieve itching

2. _____ topically applied agents that destroy bacteria

3. _____ agents used to shrink the blood vessels locally, dry up seeping lesions secretions, and lessen skin sensitivity

4. _____ use of sandpaper, wire brushes, or other abrasive materials to remove acne scars, nevi, tattoos, or fine wrinkles

5. _____ agents that kill parasitic skin infestations

6. _____ agents that soften the outer layer of skin so that it sloughs off

7. _____ excision of a small piece of tissue for microscopic examination

8. _____ used to determine immunity to diphtheria by injecting diphtheria toxin intradermally

9. _____ agents that cool, dry, and soothe inflamed skin

10. _____ ointment

Worksheet 5

PATHOLOGY REPORT OF SKIN LESION DICTIONARY EXERCISE

Use a medical dictionary or other resource to define the terms and determine their pronunciation; then practice reading the case study aloud (page 80).

atypia _____

basal cell carcinoma _____

Bowen's disease _____

dermatits _____

dermis _____

dorsum _____

epidermal hyperplasia _____

fibroplasia _____

hyperkeratosis _____

keratinocytes _____

neoplastic _____

papillary _____

pathology _____

solar elastosis _____

squamous _____

ulnar _____

ANALYSIS OF PATHOLOGY REPORT OF SKIN LESION

1. What is the basal cell layer in Figure 6–4 referred to as?

2. What was the inflammatory infiltrate?

3. What was the pathologist's diagnosis for the left forearm?

4. What was the pathologist's diagnosis for the left wrist?

Worksheet 6

Identify the skin lesions depicted here. To check your answers, refer to Figure 6–3.

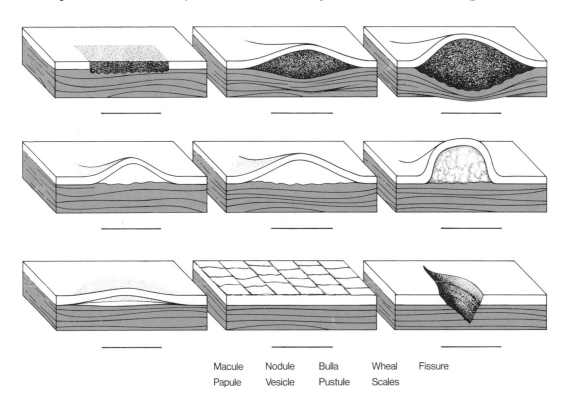

Macule   Nodule   Bulla   Wheal   Fissure
Papule   Vesicle   Pustule Scales

Worksheet 7

Label the following illustration. Check your answers by referring to Figure 6–1.

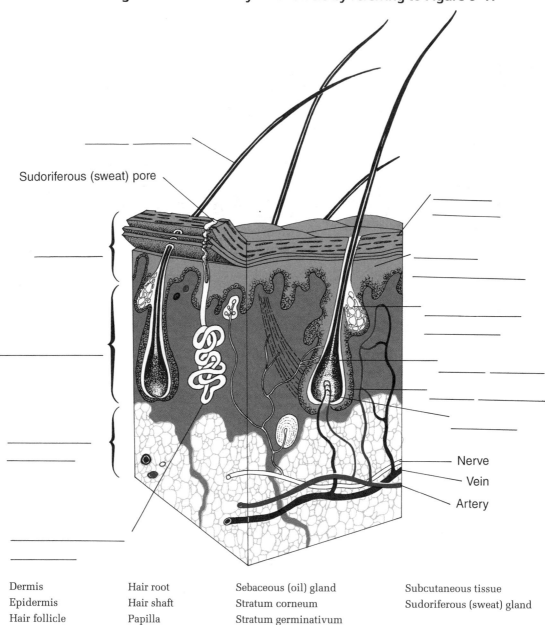

Sudoriferous (sweat) pore

Nerve

Vein

Artery

Dermis	Hair root	Sebaceous (oil) gland	Subcutaneous tissue
Epidermis	Hair shaft	Stratum corneum	Sudoriferous (sweat) gland
Hair follicle	Papilla	Stratum germinativum	

Chapter 7

Gastrointestinal System

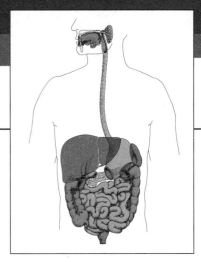

Chapter Outline

Student Objectives
Upon completion of this chapter, you will be able to do the following:

Explain the main functions of the gastrointestinal system.

Identify the organs of the alimentary canal.

Identify accessory organs of digestion.

Explain the role of the liver and gallbladder in digestion.

87

Student Objectives (Continued)

Identify combining forms, suffixes, and prefixes related to the gastrointestinal system.

Identify and discuss pathology related to the gastrointestinal system.

Identify diagnostic, symptomatic, diagnostic imaging, endoscopic, surgical, and laboratory procedures and abbreviations related to the gastrointestinal system.

Explain pharmacology related to treatment of gastrointestinal disorders.

Demonstrate your knowledge of the chapter by completing the worksheets.

Anatomy and Physiology

The purpose of the gastrointestinal (GI) system is to break down food, prepare it for absorption, and eliminate waste. This system consists of the GI tract, a tube extending from the mouth to the anus. The accessory digestive organs include the teeth, tongue, salivary glands, liver, gallbladder, and pancreas. As you read the following material, refer to Figure 7–1.

MOUTH (ORAL OR BUCCAL CAVITY)

The GI tract begins at the mouth or (1) **oral cavity.** The structures within the oral cavity are the cheeks, or **bucca,** and the (2) **tongue.** The main functions of the tongue are food manipulation during the chewing process, deglutition (swallowing), speech production, and taste. On the upper surface of the tongue are small elevations called **papillae.** These sense organs are capable of perceiving four distinct stimuli found in foods: bitterness, sweetness, saltiness, and sourness.

The (3) **teeth,** also found in the oral cavity, play an important role in initial stages of digestion. The chewing process of the teeth, known as **mastication,** mechanically breaks down food into smaller pieces and mixes it with saliva. Teeth are covered by a hard enamel, giving them a white and smooth appearance. Beneath the enamel is the main structure of the tooth, the **dentin.** In the innermost part of the tooth is the **pulp,** which contains nerves and blood vessels. The teeth are imbedded in pink fleshy tissue known as gums, or **gingiva.**

The two structures forming the roof of the mouth are the (4) **hard palate** (the anterior portion) and the (5) **soft palate** (the posterior portion). The soft palate, which forms a partition between the mouth and the nasopharynx, is continuous with the hard palate. The entire oral cavity, like the rest of the digestive tract, is lined with mucous membranes.

After food is chewed, it is formed into a round, sticky mass called a **bolus,** which is pushed by the tongue from the mouth into the (6) **pharynx,** or throat. Its downward movement is guided into the pharynx by the soft, fleshy, V-shaped tissue called the (7) **uvula.**

The pharynx serves as a passageway for air and food. It provides a resonating chamber for speech sounds and has both respiratory and digestive functions.

The funnel-shaped pharynx connects the oral and nasal cavities to the esophagus and trachea. The lowest portion of the pharynx further divides into two tubes: one that leads to the lungs, called the (8) **trachea,** and one that leads to the stomach, called the (9) **esophagus.**

A small flap of tissue, the (10) **epiglottis,** covers the trachea. The main function of the epiglottis is to prevent food from entering the trachea, by channeling it to the stomach through the esophagus.

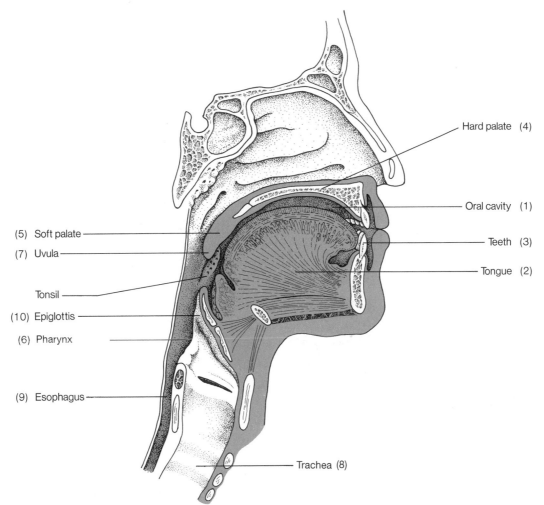

Hard palate (4)

Oral cavity (1)

(5) Soft palate

Teeth (3)

(7) Uvula

Tongue (2)

Tonsil

(10) Epiglottis

(6) Pharynx

(9) Esophagus

Trachea (8)

Figure 7–1 Sagittal view of the head showing oral nasal, and pharyngeal components of the digestive system.

STOMACH

The **stomach** (Fig. 7–2) is a saclike structure located in the left upper quadrant (LUQ) of the abdominal cavity. It extends from the (1) **esophagus** to the first part of the small intestine, the (2) **duodenum.**

Mechanical and chemical digestion of food takes place in the stomach, entering the small intestine as a pasty material called **chyme.** The terminal portion of the esophagus is referred to as the (3) **lower esophageal (gastroesophageal) sphincter,** or cardiac sphincter. The muscle fibers of this region constrict after food passes into the stomach, to prevent the stomach contents from being regurgitated into the esophagus. The (4) **body** of the stomach, the large central portion, together with the (5) **fundus,** the upper portion, are mainly storage areas. Most digestion takes place in the funnel-shaped terminal portion, the (6) **pylorus.** The interior lining of the stomach is composed of mucous membranes (mucosa). They are shaped into numerous macroscopic longitudinal folds, called (7) **rugae,** which permit stomach distension. The rugae gradually smooth out as the stomach

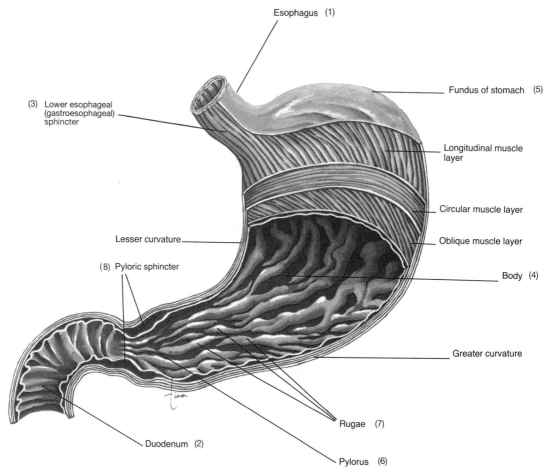

Figure 7–2 Anterior view of the stomach. The stomach wall has been sectioned to show the muscle layers and the rugae of the mucosa. (Adapted from Scanlon, VC and Sanders, T: Essentials of Anatomy and Physiology, ed 2. FA Davis, Philadelphia, 1995, p 373.)

fills. Located within the rugae are digestive glands, producing hydrochloric acid (HCl) and enzymes. The pylorus narrows to form the duodenal portion of the small intestine at the (8) **pyloric sphincter.** This junction regulates the movement of chyme into the small intestine and prohibits backflow.

SMALL INTESTINE (SMALL BOWEL)

The small intestine, a continuation of the GI tract, is about 21 feet long (Fig. 7–3). Digestion is completed in the small intestine, and the end products of digestion are absorbed into the blood and lymph. The small intestine consists of three parts:

- The (1) **duodenum,** the uppermost division, which is about 10 inches long
- The (2) **jejunum,** which is approximately 8 feet long
- The (3) **ileum,** which is about 12 feet long

Most of the absorption of food takes place in the ileum through tiny fingerlike projections called **villi.** Inside the villi are a network of fine capillaries, veins, and arterioles that

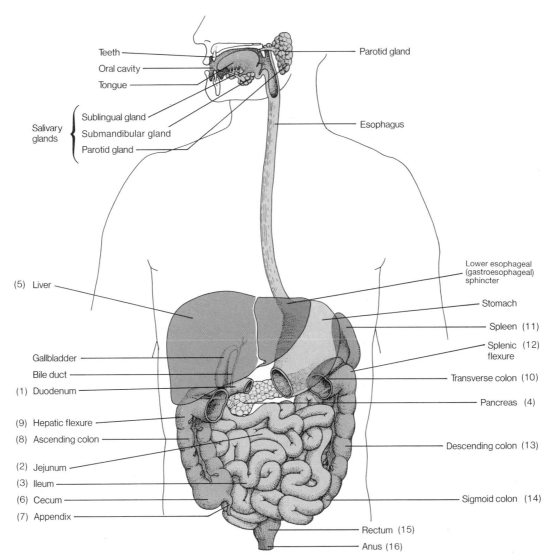

Figure 7–3   The digestive system.

allows food to be absorbed into the bloodstream. Other glands, such as the (4) **pancreas** and (5) **liver,** also produce digestive secretions that combine with chyme in the duodenum.

LARGE INTESTINE (LARGE BOWEL)

The large intestine, which is about 5 feet long, extends from the ileum to the anus. It is divided into four major regions: cecum, colon, rectum, and anus (Fig. 7–3).

The (6) **cecum** is the first 2 or 3 inches of the large intestine. A wormlike projection, the (7) **appendix,** hangs from the cecum. Its function in the digestive system is unknown, but problems arise if it becomes infected or inflamed.

The cecum merges with the colon. The colon is divided into ascending, transverse, descending, and sigmoid portions.

- The (8) **ascending colon** extends from the cecum to the lower border of the liver and turns abruptly to form the (9) **hepatic flexure.**
- The colon continues across the abdomen to the left side as the (10) **transverse colon,** curving beneath the lower end of the (11) **spleen** to form the (12) **splenic flexure.**
- The transverse colon turns downward as the (13) **descending colon** and continues until it forms the (14) **sigmoid colon** and the (15) **rectum.** The rectum, which is the last part of the gastrointestinal tract terminates at the (16) **anus.**

The main functions of the colon are to absorb water and minerals and eliminate undigestible material. No digestion takes place in the large intestine. The only secretion of the colonic mucosa is mucus, which lubricates fecal material so it can pass from the body.

Accessory Organs of Digestion

Even though food does not pass through the liver, pancreas, and gallbladder, these organs play a vital role in the proper digestion and absorption of nutrients. Refer to Figure 7–4 as you read the following material.

LIVER

The (1) **liver,** the largest glandular organ in the body, weighs approximately 3 to 4 lb. It is located beneath the diaphragm in the right upper quadrant (RUQ) of the abdominal cavity. The liver performs many vital activities, and death occurs once its function is lost. Some important functions of the liver include the following:

1. Production of bile, used in the small intestine to emulsify and absorb fats
2. Removal of **glucose** (sugar) from blood, which it synthesizes and stores as **glycogen** (starch)
3. Storage of vitamins, such as B_{12}, A, D, E, and K
4. Destruction or transformation of some toxic products into less harmful compounds
5. Maintenance of normal glucose levels in the blood
6. Destruction of old erythrocytes and release of bilirubin
7. Production of various blood proteins such as prothrombin and fibrinogen, which aid in the clotting of blood

PANCREAS

The (2) **pancreas** is an elongated, somewhat flattened organ that lies posterior and slightly inferior to the stomach. In the digestive system, it provides digestive juice that passes through the (3) **pancreatic duct.** The pancreatic duct extends along the pancreas and, together with the bile duct from the liver, enters the (4) **duodenum.**

GALLBLADDER

The (5) **gallbladder** serves as a storage area for bile. When bile is needed for digestion, the gallbladder releases it into the duodenum through the (6) **common bile duct.** Bile is also drained from the liver through the (7) **hepatic duct.** The hepatic duct unites with the

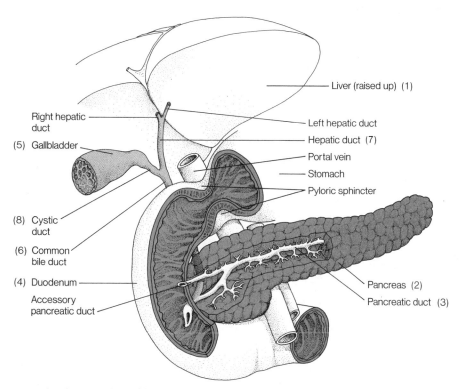

Figure 7–4 The liver, gallbladder, pancreas, and duodenum with associated ducts and blood vessels.

(8) **cystic duct** and pancreatic duct to form the common bile duct, which transports various digestive juices to the duodenum.

Combining Forms

MOUTH

Combining Form	Meaning	Example	Pronunciation
or/o		or/al _pertaining to_	ŎR-ăl
stomat/o	mouth	stomat/itis _inflammation_	stō-mă-TĪ-tĭs
gloss/o		gloss/ectomy _excision_	glŏs-ĔK-tō-mē
lingu/o	tongue	lingu/al _pertaining to_	LĬNG-gwăl
bucc/o	cheek	bucc/al _pertaining to_	BŬK-ăl

MOUTH (Continued)

Combining Form	Meaning	Example	Pronunciation

cheil/o
labi/o
	lip	cheil/o/plasty
		    surgical repair
		labi/al
		    pertaining to
			KĪ-lō-plăs-tē
			
			LĀ-bē-ăl

dent/o odont/o	teeth	dent/ist specialist orth/odont/ist straight specialist	DĔN-tĭst ŏr-thō-DŎN-tĭst
gingiv/o	gum(s)	gingiv/itis inflammation	jĭn-jĭ-VĪ-tĭs

PHARYNX, STOMACH, AND ESOPHAGUS

Combining Form	Meaning	Example	Pronunciation
esophag/o	esophagus	esophag/o/scope instrument to examine	ē-SŎF-ă-gō-skōp
gastr/o	stomach	gastr/o/scopy visual examination	găs-TRŎS-kō-pē
pharyng/o	pharynx	pharyng/itis inflammation	făr-in-JĪ-tĭs
pylor/o	pylorus	pylor/o/tomy incision, cut into	pī-lor-ŎT-ō-mē

SMALL INTESTINE AND COLON (LARGE INTESTINE)

Combining Form	Meaning	Example	Pronunciation
an/o	anus	an/al pertaining to	Ā-năl

append/o
appendic/o
	appendix	append/ectomy
		    excision
		appendic/itis
		    inflammation
			ăp-ĕn-DĔK-tō-mē
			
			ă-pĕn-dĭ-SĪ-tĭs

SMALL INTESTINE AND COLON (LARGE INTESTINE) (Continued)

Combining Form	Meaning	Example	Pronunciation

col/o
colon/o
	colon	col/o/centesis
		    puncture
		colon/o/scope
		    instrument to
		    examine
			kō-lō-sĕn-TĒ-sĭs
			
			kō-LŎN-ō-skōp

duoden/o	duodenum	duoden/o/stomy
		    forming an opening
		    (mouth)
			dū-ŏd-ĕ-NŎS-tō-mē

enter/o	intestines (usually small intestine)	enter/o/pathy disease	ĕn-tĕr-ŎP-ă-thē

ile/o	ileum	ile/o/stomy
		    forming an opening
		    (mouth)
			ĭl-ē-ŎS-tō-mē

jejun/o	jejunum	jejun/o/rrhaphy suture	jĕ-joo-NOR-ă-fē

proct/o	anus, rectum	proct/o/logist
		    specialist in the study
		    of
			prŏk-TŎL-ō-jĭst

rect/o	rectum	rect/o/cele hernia, swelling	RĔK-tō-sēl
sigmoid/o	sigmoid colon	sigmoid/o/scopy visual examination	sĭg-moi-DŎS-kō-pē

ACCESSORY ORGANS OF DIGESTION: LIVER, PANCREAS, AND BILIARY SYSTEM

Combining Form	Meaning	Example	Pronunciation
cholangi/o	bile vessel	cholangi/ole small	kō-LĂN-jē-ō
cholecyst/o	gallbladder	cholecyst/o/gram record	kō-lē-SĬS-tō-grăm
chol/e	bile, gall	chol/emia blood	kō-LĒ-mē-ăh

ACCESSORY ORGANS OF DIGESTION: LIVER, PANCREAS, AND BILIARY SYSTEM (Continued)

Combining Form	Meaning	Example	Pronunciation
choledoch/o	bile duct	choledoch/o/lith stone, calculus	kō-LĔD-ō-kō-lĭth
hepat/o	liver	hepat/oma tumor	hĕp-ă-TŌ-mă
pancreat/o	pancreas	pancreat/itis inflammation	păn-krē-ă-TĪ-tĭs
sial/o	saliva, salivary glands	sial/o/lith stone, calculus	sī-ĂL-ō-lĭth

SUFFIXES

Suffix	Meaning	Example	Pronunciation
-emesis	vomiting	hemat/emesis blood	hĕm-ăt-ĔM-ĕ-sĭs
-iasis	abnormal condition (produced by something specified)	chol/e/lith/iasis gall stone	kō-lē-lĭ-THĪ-ă-sĭs
-lith	stone, calculus	chol/e/lith gall, bile	KŌ-lē-lĭth
-megaly	enlargement	hepat/o/megaly liver	hĕp-ă-tō-MĔG-ă-lē
-pepsia	digestion	dys/pepsia difficult, painful	dĭs-PĔP-sē-ăh
-phagia	swallowing, eating	dys/phagia difficult, painful	dĭs-FĀ-jē-ăh
-plasty	surgical repair	herni/o/plasty hernia	HĔR-nē-ō-plăs-tē
-prandial	meal	post/prandial after	pōst-PRĂN-dē-ăl

PREFIXES

Prefix	Meaning	Example	Pronunciation
dia-	through	<u>dia</u>/rrhea flow	dī-ăh-RE-ăh
dys-	bad, painful, difficult	<u>dys</u>/trophy nourishment, development	DĬS-trō-fē
hyper-	excessive	<u>hyper</u>/emesis vomiting	hī-pĕr-ĔM-ĕ-sĭs
peri-	around	<u>peri</u>/an/ al anus pertaining to	pĕr-ē-Ā-năl
sub-	under, below	<u>sub</u>/ling/ ual tongue pertaining to	sŭb-LING-gwăl

Pathology

ULCERS

An **ulcer** is an open sore **(lesion)** of the skin or mucous membrane. Most ulcers occur in the stomach or duodenum. It is not uncommon for ulcers to be accompanied by formation of pus. Ulcers in the stomach or duodenum may be due to excess acid in gastric juice, which breaks down mucous membranes causing underlying tissue destruction, by an inherent defect in the mucosal lining of the stomach or bacteria in the stomach. If left untreated, the tissue destruction eventually leads to a hole **(perforation).** When this occurs, food and enzymes enter the abdominal cavity through the **perforated ulcer,** causing contamination of other organs. In the past, usual treatment included drugs that inhibit the secretion of stomach acids **(antacids).** Current treatment involves using antibiotics to destroy bacteria that cause the ulcers.

    Peptic ulcers (named for the enzyme pepsin) are erosions of the mucous membranes of the stomach or duodenum. Generally, an ulcer may develop any place in which gastric juice and acid digest the damaged mucous membrane. Ulcers develop most commonly in the duodenum, next most frequently in the stomach, and rarely in the lower portion of the esophagus. They may be of long duration **(chronic)** or arise suddenly **(acute).**

    Agents that weaken the mucosal lining of the stomach, such as alcohol, smoking, aspirin, and abnormally high secretions of HCl, increase the likelihood of developing peptic ulcers. Many people between the ages of 20 and 45 tend to develop duodenal ulcers rather than other types of ulcers.

    Inflammation of the colon with formation of ulcers in the lining of the intestine **(ulcerative colitis)** can occur at any age but is most common in young adults. Anxiety and nervous tension may be the cause **(etiology)** of the disease. The chief symptom of ulcerative colitis is frequent passage of watery bowel movements **(diarrhea).** Patients may feel very weak, lose weight, and sometimes experience anemia. They may also suffer from pain in

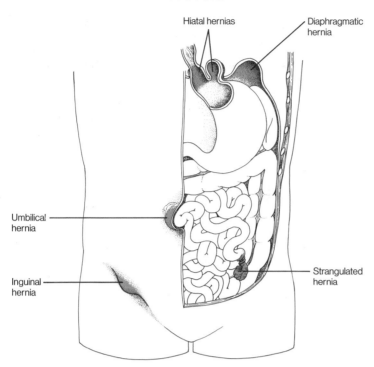

Hiatal hernias

Diaphragmatic hernia

Umbilical hernia

Inguinal hernia

Strangulated hernia

Figure 7–5 Types of abdominal hernias.

the joints **(arthralgia).** In severe cases, it may be necessary to create an opening **(stoma)** surgically for bowel evacuation to a bag worn on the abdomen.

HERNIAS

A **hernia** is a protrusion of an organ, tissue, or structure through the wall of the cavity in which it is naturally contained (Fig. 7–5). This definition may apply to any part of the body (e.g., the protrusion of the brain through a cranial fissure **[encephalocele]**). In general, though, the term is applied to the protrusion of an abdominal organ **(viscus)** through an opening in the abdominal wall.

Hernias are found most commonly in the abdominal region, but they may develop in the diaphragm **(diaphragmatic hernia)** or in the opening where the esophagus passes through the diaphragm **(hiatal hernia).** With this condition, the lower end of the esophagus and the adjacent part of the stomach herniate into the thorax **(gastroesophageal hernia).** This results in gastroesophageal reflux, a condition in which stomach acid backs up into the esophagus.

The **inguinal hernia** develops in the groin where the abdominal folds of flesh meet the thighs. In initial stages, it may hardly be noticeable and appears as a soft lump under the skin, no larger than a marble. In early stages. an inguinal hernia is usually reducible; that is, it can be pushed gently back into its normal place. With this type of hernia, pain may be minimal. As time passes, pressure of the abdomen against the weak abdominal wall may increase the size of the opening as well as the size of the hernia lump. If the blood supply to the hernia is cut off because of pressure **(strangulation),** gangrene **(necrosis)** may develop.

The protrusion of part of the intestine at the navel **(umbilical hernia)** occurs more frequently in obese women and among those who had several pregnancies.

Hernias also occur in newborn infants **(congenital)** or during early childhood. If the defect has not corrected itself by 2 years of age, the deformity can be surgically corrected. Treatment consists of surgical repair of the hernia **(hernioplasty),** with suture of the abdominal wall **(herniorrhaphy).**

BOWEL OBSTRUCTIONS

A life-threatening obstruction in which the bowel twists on itself **(volvulus)** with occlusion of the blood supply occurs most frequently in middle-aged and elderly men. The accumulation of gas and fluid coupled with loss of blood supply **(ischemia)** in the trapped bowel eventually leads to tissue death **(necrosis),** perforation, and an inflammation of the peritoneum **(peritonitis).** Surgery is required to untwist the bowel.

Telescoping of the intestine within itself **(intussusception)** occurs when one part of the intestine slips into another part located below it, much as a telescope is shortened by pushing one section into the next. This is a rare type of intestinal obstruction more common in infants 10 to 15 months of age than in adults. Surgery is usually necessary to correct this obstruction.

HEMORRHOIDS

Enlargement of the veins in the mucous membrane of the anal canal causes hemorrhoids, which may occur inside **(internal)** or outside **(external)** the rectal area.

Hemorrhoids are usually caused by straining to evacuate a fecal concretion or stone **(fecalith).** They sometimes develop during pregnancy because of pressure on the veins from the enlarged uterus. They may also result from pressure on the veins caused by a disorder of the liver or the heart, or may be symptomatic of a tumor that exerts pressure against the veins.

Temporary relief from hemorrhoids can usually be obtained by cold compresses, sitz baths, stool softeners, or an analgesic ointment. Treatment of an advanced hemorrhoidal condition is by surgical removal **(hemorrhoidectomy).**

LIVER DISORDERS

One of the symptoms of many liver disorders is a yellowing of the skin **(jaundice).** This condition, also known as **icterus,** may result when the bile duct is blocked, causing bile to enter the bloodstream. Jaundice is noted in patients who suffer from cirrhosis of the liver and often is related to poor nutrition and excessive alcohol consumption. Icterus may also be exhibited in patients who suffer from **hepatitis.**

A growing public health concern is the increasing incidence of **viral hepatitis.** Even though its mortality rate is low, the disease is easily transmitted and can cause significant morbidity and prolonged loss of time from school or employment. Viral hepatitis includes several forms, the two most common being hepatitis A, also called infectious hepatitis, and hepatitis B, also called serum hepatitis. The most common causes of hepatitis A are ingestion of contaminated food, water, or milk. Hepatitis B is usually transmitted by routes other than the mouth **(parenteral)** (e.g., blood transfusions, semen, and so forth). Owing to patient exposure, health care personnel are at increased risk of contracting hepatitis B, but a vaccine that provides immunity to this type is available.

DIVERTICULOSIS

Diverticulosis is a condition in which small, blisterlike pockets develop in the walls of the large intestine and may balloon out from the large intestine. These pouchlike areas usually do not cause any problem unless they become inflamed **(diverticulitis).** Pain, usually in the left lower quadrant (LLQ) of the abdomen, extreme constipation **(obstipation)** or diarrhea, fever, abdominal swelling, and occasional blood in the bowel movement are some of the symptoms of diverticulitis. The usual treatment for diverticulitis consists of bed rest, antibiotics, and a soft diet. In severe cases, however, excision of the diverticulum **(diverticulectomy)** may be advised.

ONCOLOGY

Although stomach cancer is rare in the United States, it is common in many parts of the world where food preservation is questionable. It is significant because of its high mortality rate. Men are more susceptible to stomach cancer than women. The neoplasm nearly always develops from the epithelial or mucosal lining of the stomach in the form of a cancerous glandular tumor **(gastric adenocarcinoma).** Persistent indigestion is one of the important warning signs of stomach cancer. Other types of GI carcinomas include **esophageal carcinomas, hepatocellular carcinomas, pancreatic carcinomas,** and **adenocarcinomas of the colon.**

DIAGNOSTIC, SYMPTOMATIC, AND RELATED TERMS

Term	Meaning
absorption ăb-SORP-shŭn	passage of simple nutrients into the bloodstream
aerophagia ā-ĕr-ō-FĀ-jē-ăh	swallowing air
anorexia ăn-ō-RĔK-sē-ăh	loss of appetite
anorexia nervosa an-ō-RĔK-sē-ăh nĕr-VŌ-să	eating disorder characterized by a refusal to maintain body weight appropriate for age and height; intense fear of gaining weight or becoming obese, this fear does not diminish as weight loss progresses and patient becomes emaciated. Psychiatric therapy is usually required if patient refuses to eat
ascites ăh-SĪ-tēz	accumulation of serous fluid in the peritoneal cavity

DIAGNOSTIC, SYMPTOMATIC, AND RELATED TERMS
(Continued)

Term	Meaning
borborygmus bŏr-bō-RĬG-mŭs	gurgling or splashing sound normally heard over the large intestine, caused by passage of gas through the liquid contents of the intestine
bulimia bū-LĬM-ē-ăh	eating disorder characterized by binge eating followed by purging; use of laxatives or diuretics; strict dieting or fasting, or vigorous exercise in order to prevent weight gain; and persistent overconcern with body shape and weight
Crohn's disease, granulomatous colitis, regional enteritis krōnz	inflammatory condition of the intestinal tract, most commonly the ileum; distinguished from closely related bowel disorders by its inflammatory pattern
cirrhosis sĭr-RŌ-sĭs	liver disease with degeneration of liver cells
colic KŎL-ĭk	spasm in any hollow or tubular soft organ accompanied by pain, especially in the colon
deglutition dĕg-loo-TĬSH-ŭn	the act of swallowing
dyspepsia dĭs-PĔP-sē-ăh	gastric indigestion or ''upset stomach,'' usually referring to epigastric discomfort following meals
dysphagia dĭs-FĀ-jē-ăh	inability or difficulty in swallowing
emesis ĔM-ĕ-sĭs	vomiting
eructation ĕ-rŭk-TĀ-shŭn	the act of belching; the raising of gas or a small quantity of acid from the stomach
fecalith FĒ-kăh-lĭth	fecal concretion
flatus FLĀ-tŭs	gas or air expelled through the anus
halitosis hăl-ĭ-TŌ-sĭs	offensive or ''bad'' breath
hematemesis hĕm-ăh-TĔM-ĕ-sĭs	vomiting blood
leukoplakia loo-kō-PLĀ-kē-ăh	white patches on the mucous membrane of the tongue or cheek, common in smokers and possibly a forerunner to cancer

DIAGNOSTIC, SYMPTOMATIC, AND RELATED TERMS (Continued)

Term	Meaning
melena MĔL-ĕ-nă	black, tarry feces due to action of intestinal secretions on free blood
obstipation ŏb-stĭ-PĀ-shŭn	extreme constipation
peristalsis pĕr-ĭ-STĂL-sĭs	a progressive wavelike movement that occurs involuntarily in hollow tubes of the body, especially the alimentary canal
polyphagia pŏl-ē-FĀ-jē-ăh	excessive eating
pyloric stenosis pī-LŎR-ĭk stĕ-NŌ-sĭs	narrowing of the gastric pylorus; may be due to excessive thickening of the circular muscle of the pylorus
regurgitation rē-gŭr-jĭ-TĀ-shŭn	a backward flowing, as in the return of solids or fluids to the mouth from the stomach or the backward flow of blood through a defective heart valve
steatorrhea stē-ăh-tō-RĒ-ăh	excessive amount of fat in the feces due to improper fat digestion (malabsorption)
visceroptosis vĭs-ĕr-ŏp-TŌ-sĭs	downward displacement of the viscera (internal organs enclosed within a cavity), especially the abdominal organs

Special Procedures

DIAGNOSTIC IMAGING PROCEDURES

Term	Description
barium enema, lower GI BĂ-rē-ŭm ĔN-ĕ-mă	enema using a liquid contrast medium, barium sulfate; retained in the lower GI tract during fluoroscopic and radiographic studies for diagnosing obstructions or other abnormalities of the colon
esophagram ē-SŎF-ă-grăm	radiologic evaluation of the esophagus while administering a barium sulfate suspension under fluoroscopic guidance (also known as barium swallow)
upper GI	radiographic examination of the upper GI tract after barium sulfate, a liquid contrast medium, is swallowed; used for diagnosing obstructions or other abnormalities of the esophagus, duodenum, and stomach

DIAGNOSTIC IMAGING PROCEDURES (Continued)

Term	Description
cholecystography, gallbladder series kō-lē-sĭs-TŎG-ră-fē	radiographic images of the gallbladder after administration of a radiopaque contrast medium; used to evaluate the functioning of the gallbladder and determine the presence of disease or gallstones
CT scan (liver, spleen)	visualization of the liver after a radioactive substance is injected intravenously (IV) and absorbed by the liver cells; used for diagnosing cysts, ruptures, tumors, abscesses, and other abnormalities
endoscopic retrograde cholangiopancreatography (ERCP) ĕn-do-SKŎ-pĭk RĔT-rō-grād ko-lăn-jē-o-păn-krē-ā-TŎG-ră-fē	radiographic images of pancreas and bile ducts after IV injection of a radiopaque contrast medium
percutaneous transhepatic cholangiography pĕr-kū-TĀ-nē-ŭs trăns-hĕp-ĂT-ĭc kō-lăn-jē-ŎG-ră-fē	radiographs of bile vessels after injection of a radiopaque contrast medium through the skin into the liver
sialography sī-ă-LŎG-ră-fē	radiologic examination of the salivary glands and ducts following injection of a radiopaque contrast agent
T-tube cholangiogram kō-LĂN-jē-ō-grăm	radiographic examination of the hepatic and biliary ducts, following introduction of a radiopaque contrast medium through a surgically placed T-shaped drainage tube

ENDOSCOPIC PROCEDURES

Term	Description
colonoscopy kō-lŏn-ŎS-kō-pē	visual examination of the colon using a colonoscope; may permit the removal of polyps, tissue for biopsy; used to confirm or establish a diagnosis
esophagogastroduodenoscopy (EGD) ē-sŏf-ă-gō-găs-trō-dū-ŏd-ĕ-NŎS-kō-pē	visual examination of the esophagus, stomach, and duodenum using an endoscope
esophagoscopy ē-sŏf-ă-GŎS-kō-pē	use of an esophagoscope for visual examination of or removal of a foreign object from the esophagus
gastroscopy găs-TRŎS-kō-pē	visual examination of the interior of the stomach using a gastroscope inserted through the mouth and esophagus

ENDOSCOPIC PROCEDURES (Continued)

Term	Description
proctosigmoidoscopy, sigmoidoscopy prŏk-tō-sĭg-moy-DŎS-kō-pē, sĭg-moy-DŎS-kō-pē	visual examination of the rectum and sigmoid colon using a sigmoidoscope or proctoscope; may permit the removal of polyps, tissue for biopsy; used to confirm or establish a diagnosis

SURGICAL PROCEDURES

Term	Description
anastomosis ăh-năs-tō-mō-sĭs	surgical connection of two tubular structures
biliary lithotripsy BĬL-ē-ār-ē LĬTH-ō-trĭp-sē	procedure that destroys gallstones using shock waves; gallstones pass out of the body painlessly in pulverized form
cecectomy sē-SĔK-tō-mē	excision of cecum
cholecystectomy kō-lē-sĭs-TĔK-tō-mē	excision of the gallbladder
choledochoplasty kō-lĕd-ō-kō-PLĂS-tē	reconstruction of a bile duct
colostomy kō-LŎS-tō-mē	creation of an opening (mouth) of some portion of the colon through the abdominal wall to its outside surface, to divert fecal flow to a colostomy bag
hepatic lobectomy hĕ-PĂT-ĭk lō-BĔK-tō-mē	excision of a lobe of the liver
ileostomy ĭl-ē-ŎS-tō-mē	creating a surgical passage through the abdominal wall into the ileum. The fecal material drains into a bag worn on the abdomen
liver biopsy BĪ-ŏp-sē	a large-bore needle removes a core of liver tissue for microscopic examination. Used to confirm or establish a diagnosis
proctoplasty PRŎK-tō-plăs-tē	surgical repair or reconstruction of the rectum or colon
pyloromyotomy pī-lō-rō-mī-OT-ō-mē	incision of the longitudinal and circular muscles of the pylorus, to treat hypertrophic pyloric stenosis
stomatoplasty STŌ-măh-tō-plăs-tē	surgical repair of the mouth

LABORATORY PROCEDURES

Test	Description
alkaline phosphatase ĂL-kă-līn FŎS-fă-tās	used to determine blood levels of this enzyme (diseased liver excretes elevated levels of this enzyme)
aspiration biopsy cytology (ABC) ăs-pĭ-RĀ-shŭn BI-ŏp-sē sī-TŎL-ō-jē	microscopic study of cells obtained from superficial or internal lesions by suction through a fine needle; used primarily as a diagnostic procedure, usually to detect nuclear and cytoplasmic changes in tissue
fasting blood sugar (FBS)	measures blood glucose level after a 12-hour fast
glucose tolerance test (GTT) GLOO-kōs	performed by giving glucose (sugar) to a patient orally or intravenously, drawing blood samples at specified intervals, and determining the blood glucose level of each sample; most often used to assist in the diagnosis of diabetes or other disorders that affect carbohydrate metabolism
occult blood	a chemical test or microscopic examination for blood, especially in feces, that is not apparent on visual inspection; determines bleeding in GI disorders; helps detect colon cancer
stool culture	determines the presence of microorganisms after feces are placed in a special media that are conducive to their growth

PHARMACOLOGY

Medication	Action
antacids	neutralize excess stomach acid and relieve gastritis and ulcer pain; also used to relieve indigestion and reflux esophagitis (heartburn)
antidiarrheals	relieve diarrhea either by absorbing the excess fluids that cause diarrhea or by lessening intestinal motility (slowing the movement of fecal material through the intestine), allowing more time for absorption of water
antiemetics, antinauseants	suppress nausea and vomiting, mainly by acting on brain control centers to stop nerve impulses; also used to control motion sickness and dizziness associated with inner ear infections. Some antihistamines and tranquilizers have antiemetic properties

PHARMACOLOGY (Continued)

Medication	Action
antiflatulents	reduce the feeling of gassiness and bloating (flatulence) that accompany indigestion. These agents facilitate the passing of gas by breaking down gas bubbles to a smaller size and by mildly stimulating intestinal motility
antispasmodics	prevent or reduce smooth muscle spasms by acting on the automatic nervous system, thus relieving certain spastic conditions of the bowel
cathartics, laxatives, purgatives	promote bowel movement or defecation or both: in smaller doses, they relieve constipation and are called laxatives; in larger doses, they evacuate the entire GI tract and are called purgatives (used before surgery or intestinal radiological examinations)
emetics	used to induce vomiting, especially in cases of poisoning

ABBREVIATIONS*

Abbreviations Related to Medication Time Schedules	Meaning
ac	before meal
bid	twice a day
hs	at bedtime
npo	nothing by mouth
pc	after meals
po	orally; by mouth
pp	after meals (postprandial)
prn	as required
qam	every morning
qd	every day
qh	every hour
q2h	every 2 hours
qid	four times a day
qpm	every night
stat	immediately
tid	three times a day

ABBREVIATIONS (Continued)

Abbreviations Related to Diagnostic Tests	Meaning
ABC	aspiration biopsy cytology
Ba	barium
BaE	barium enema
CT scan, CAT scan	computerized tomography scan
Dx	diagnosis
EGD	esophagogastroduodenoscopy
ERCP	endoscopic retrograde cholangiopancreatography
GI	gastrointestinal
FBS	fasting blood sugar
GTT	glucose tolerance test
HCl	hydrochloric acid
IV	intravenous
IVC	intravenous cholangiography
SGOT, SGPT	liver function enzyme tests
UGI	upper gastrointestinal

Other Abbreviations Related to the GI System	Meaning
BM	bowel movement
HAV	hepatitis A virus
HBV	hepatitis B virus
LLQ	left lower quadrant
LUQ	left upper quadrant
PE	physical examination
PMH	past medical history
RUQ	right upper quadrant

*Because many of these abbreviations deal with pharmacology and the administration of medication, they are not unique to the GI system.

Case Study

GI Evaluation

The patient's abdominal pain began 2 years ago when she first had intermittent, sharp **epigastric** pain. Each episode lasted 2 to 4 hours. Eventually she was diagnosed as having **cholecystitis** with **cholelithiasis,** and underwent **cholecystectomy.** Three to five large calcified stones were found.

Her postoperative course was uneventful until 4 months ago, when she began having continuous deep right-sided pain. This pain followed a **crescendo** pattern and peaked several weeks ago, at a time when family stress was also at its climax. Since then, the pain has been following a **decrescendo** pattern. It does not cause any nausea or vomiting, does not trigger any urge to **defecate,** and was not alleviated by passage of **flatus.** Her **PMH** is significant only for **tonsillectomy, appendectomy,** and the cholecystectomy. Her PE findings indicate that there was no **hepatomegaly** or splenomegaly. The rectal examination confirmed normal **sphincter** tone and **heme**-negative **stool.**

Worksheet 5 provides a dictionary and reading application and an analysis of this case study.

Worksheet 1

Use esophag/o (esophagus) to build words meaning:

1. pain in the esophagus _____

2. spasm of the esophagus _____

3. stricture or narrowing of the esophagus _____

Use gastr/o (stomach) to build words meaning:

4. inflammation of the stomach _____

5. pain in the stomach _____

6. disease of the stomach _____

7. enlargement of the stomach _____

Use duoden/o (duodenum), jejun/o (jejunum), or ile/o (ileum) to build words meaning:

8. relating to the duodenum _____

9. inflammation of the ileum _____

10. concerning the jejunum and ileum _____

Use enter/o (small intestine) to build words meaning:

11. inflammation of the small intestine _____

12. disease of the small intestine _____

Use col/o (colon) to build words meaning:

13. inflammation of the colon _____

14. visual examination of the colon _____

15. inflammation of the small intestine and colon _____

16. prolapse or downward displacement of the colon _____

17. disease of the colon _____

Use proct/o (anus, rectum) or rect/o (rectum) to build words meaning:

18. narrowing or constriction of the rectum _____

19. herniation of the rectum _____

20. paralysis of the anus (anal muscles) _____

Use chol/e (bile, gall) to build words meaning:

21. inflammation of the gallbladder _____

22. abnormal condition of a gallstone _____

Use hepat/o (liver) or pancreat/o (pancreas) to build words meaning:

23. tumor of the liver _____

24. enlargement of the liver _____

25. inflammation of the pancreas _____

Worksheet 2

Build a surgical term meaning:

1. excision of gum tissue _____

2. partial or complete excision of the tongue _____

3. repair of the esophagus _____

4. removal of part or all of the stomach _____

5. forming an opening between the stomach and jejunum _____

6. excision of (part of) the esophagus _____

7. forming an opening between the stomach, small intestine, and colon _____

8. repair of the intestine _____

9. fixation of the small intestine (to the abdominal wall) _____

10. suture of the bile duct _____

11. forming an opening into the colon _____

12. fixation of a movable liver (to the abdominal wall) _____

13. repair of the anus and rectum _____

14. removal of the gallbladder _____

15. repair of a bile duct _____

Worksheet 3

Match the following words with the definitions in the numbered list.

anorexia   fecalith
bulimia   halitosis
cirrhosis   hematemesis
dyspepsia   melena
dyspnea   melagra
dysphagia   obstipation

1. _____ vomiting blood

2. _____ difficulty swallowing or inability to swallow

3. _____ fecal concretion

4. _____ "bad" breath

5. _____ loss of appetite

6. _____ poor digestion

7. _____ black stool

8. _____ liver disease frequently resulting in jaundice

9. _____ intractable constipation

10. _____ binging and purging

Worksheet 4

SPECIAL PROCEDURES, PHARMACOLOGY, AND ABBREVIATIONS

Match the following words with the definitions in the numbered list.

antiflatulents
anastomosis
antacids
antidiarrheals
bid
cathartics
choledochoplasty
emetics
FBS
gastroscopy
intravenous cholangiography

lower GI
occult blood
pc, pp
oral cholecystography
proctosigmoidoscopy
pyloromyotomy
qid
spleen scan
stat
stomatoplasty
upper GI

1. _____ after meals

2. _____ used to determine bleeding in GI disorders; helps detect colon cancer

3. _____ agents that produce vomiting

4. _____ twice a day

5. _____ surgical reconstruction of a bile duct

6. _____ an enema with a barium solution is administered while a series of radiographs are taken of the large intestine

7. _____ visual examination of the stomach

8. _____ surgical reconstruction of the mouth

9. _____ promote bowel movement and/or defecation

10. _____ surgical formation of a passage or opening between two hollow viscerae or vessels

11. _____ oral administration of dye precedes radiographs of the gallbladder

12. _____ a radioactive substance is injected IV in order to visualize the spleen

13. _____ reduce the feelings of gassiness and bloating caused by indigestion

14. _____ neutralize excess acid in the stomach and help relieve gastritis and ulcer pain

15. _____ used to detect abnormalities of glucose metabolism

16. _____ radiographs of bile vessels are taken after dye is injected in a vein

17. _____ four times a day

18. _____ immediately

19. _____ endoscopic procedure for visualization of the rectosigmoid colon

20. _____ barium solution swallowed for a radiographic examination of the esophagus, stomach, and duodenum

Worksheet 5

GI EVALUATION DICTIONARY EXERCISE

Use a medical dictionary or other resource to define the terms and determine their pronunciation; then practice reading the case study aloud (p. 108).

appendectomy _____

cholecystectomy _____

cholecystitis _____

cholelithiasis _____

crescendo _____

decrescendo _____

defecate _____

epigastric _____

flatus _____

heme _____

hepatomegaly _____

PMH _____

sphincter _____

stool _____

tonsillectomy _____

ANALYSIS OF GI EVALUATION

1. While referring to Figure 7–3, describe where the gallbladder is located in relation to the liver.

2. Has the patient had any other surgeries?

3. If so, what were they?

4. How does her most recent postoperative episode of discomfort (pain) differ from the initial pain she described?

Worksheet 6

Label the following illustration. Check your answers by referring to Figure 7–1.

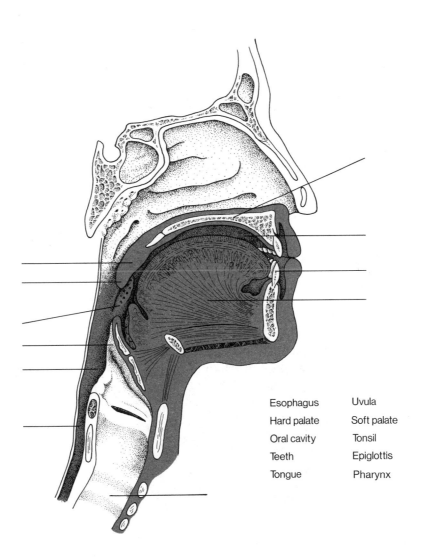

Esophagus	Uvula
Hard palate	Soft palate
Oral cavity	Tonsil
Teeth	Epiglottis
Tongue	Pharynx

Worksheet 7

Label the following illustration. Check your answers by referring to Figure 7–3.

Appendix
Parotid gland
Esophagus
Lower esophageal sphincter
Stomach
Spleen
Splenic flexure
Pancreas
Transverse colon
Descending colon
Sigmoid colon
Rectum
Anus
Ileum
Cecum

Tongue
Salivary glands
Sublingual gland
Submandibular gland
Liver
Gallbladder
Bile duct
Duodenum
Hepatic flexure
Ascending colon
Jejunum
Teeth
Oral cavity

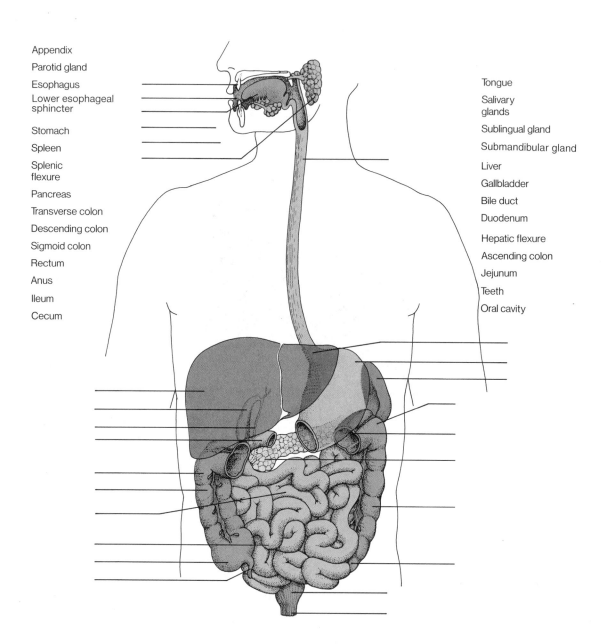

Chapter 8

Respiratory System

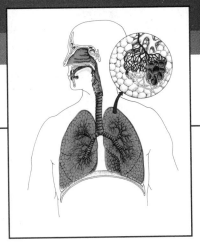

Chapter Outline

STUDENT OBJECTIVES

ANATOMY AND PHYSIOLOGY
Internal Respiration
External Respiration
Respiratory Structures

COMBINING FORMS

SUFFIXES

PREFIXES

PATHOLOGY
Chronic Obstructive Pulmonary Disease
Bronchiectasis
Pleural Effusions
Tuberculosis
Bronchopneumonia
Cystic Fibrosis
Respiratory Distress Syndrome

Oncology
  □ Primary Pulmonary Cancer

DIAGNOSTIC, SYMPTOMATIC, AND
  RELATED TERMS

SPECIAL PROCEDURES
Diagnostic Imaging Procedures
Clinical Procedures
Surgical Procedures
Laboratory Procedures

PHARMACOLOGY

ABBREVIATIONS

CASE STUDY
  □ Respiratory Evaluation

WORKSHEETS

Student Objectives
Upon completion of this chapter, you will be able to do the following:

List the major structures of the respiratory system and briefly describe the function of each.

Differentiate between external and internal respiration.

List the structures associated with the respiratory system and describe their function.

Describe the function of the diaphragm and intercostal muscles in the breathing process.

Identify combining forms, suffixes, and prefixes related to the respiratory system.

Identify and discuss pathology related to the respiratory system.

Student Objectives (Continued)

Identify diagnostic imaging, clinical, surgical, and laboratory procedures and abbreviations related to the respiratory system.

Discuss pharmacology related to the treatment of respiratory disorders.

Demonstrate your knowledge of the chapter by completing the worksheets.

Anatomy and Physiology

The respiratory system consists of the organs that are responsible for the breathing process. Along with the cardiovascular system, it exchanges oxygen (O_2) and carbon dioxide (CO_2) at the cellular level. The entire breathing process involves internal and external respiration.

INTERNAL RESPIRATION

All body cells require a continuous source of O_2 for metabolism and a means for removing CO_2, a waste product produced as part of the metabolic process. These two needs are satisfied during a process called **internal** or **cellular respiration.** Respiration involves an exchange of gases. In internal respiration, CO_2 leaves body cells and enters the blood in surrounding capillaries. Meanwhile, O_2 from the blood passes into cells. When the exchange is completed, blood flows from the capillaries, enters veins, and returns to the heart.

EXTERNAL RESPIRATION

External respiration consists of two separate, simultaneous activities:

- ventilation, with one breathing cycle consisting of one inhalation and one exhalation
- exchanging O_2 in the lungs with CO_2 in the pulmonary capillaries

Ventilation is the movement of air into and out of the lungs. It allows for the exchange of gases in the lungs with the gases found in the environment. During expiration (exhaling), CO_2 is expelled; during inspiration (inhaling), environmental air, rich in O_2, enters the lungs. Breathing is largely an involuntary activity brought about by nervous stimulation of the diaphragm and intercostal muscles.

Blood entering the pulmonary capillaries contains a high concentration of CO_2. As blood flows through the pulmonary capillaries, it gains O_2 from the lungs. Simultaneously, CO_2 diffuses from the blood and enters the lungs.

RESPIRATORY STRUCTURES

As you read the following paragraphs, refer to Figure 8–1, to help you understand the anatomy and physiology of the respiratory system.

During the breathing process, air is drawn into the (1) **nasal cavity.** The nasal cavity is divided into a right and left side by a vertical partition called the nasal **septum.** The interior portion of the nasal cavity warms, moistens, and filters incoming air.

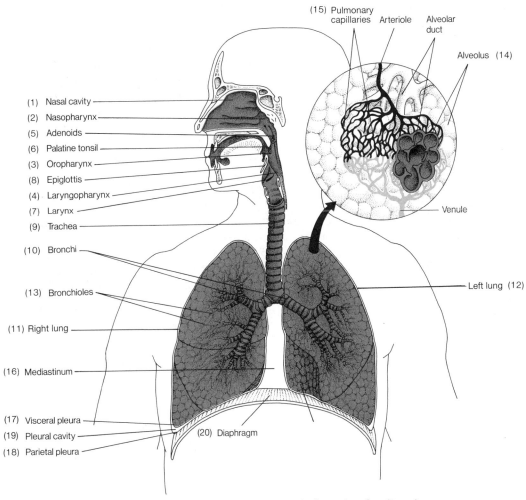

(15) Pulmonary capillaries
Arteriole
Alveolar duct
Alveolus (14)
Venule

(1) Nasal cavity
(2) Nasopharynx
(5) Adenoids
(6) Palatine tonsil
(3) Oropharynx
(8) Epiglottis
(4) Laryngopharynx
(7) Larynx
(9) Trachea
(10) Bronchi
(13) Bronchioles
(11) Right lung
(16) Mediastinum
(17) Visceral pleura
(19) Pleural cavity
(18) Parietal pleura
(20) Diaphragm
Left lung (12)

Figure 8–1 Respiratory system, including alveolus (*inset*).

The receptors for the sense of smell are located in the nasal cavity. These receptors, called the **olfactory** neurons, are found among the epithelial cells lining the nasal tract and are covered with a layer of mucus. Because these receptors are located higher in the nasal passage than that normally reached by inhaled air, a person must sniff or inhale deeply to identify weak odors.

Air passes from the nasal cavity to the pharynx, a muscular tube that serves as a passageway for food and air. It consists of three sections:

- the (2) **nasopharynx,** posterior to the nose
- the (3) **oropharynx,** posterior to the mouth
- the (4) **laryngopharynx,** superior to the larynx

Within the nasopharynx is a collection of lymphatic tissue known as (5) **adenoids,** or **pharyngeal tonsils.** The (6) **palatine tonsils,** more commonly known as tonsils, are located in the oropharynx. The (7) **larynx** ("voice box"), found in the laryngopharynx, is responsible for sound production, or phonation. A leaf-shaped structure on top of the larynx, the (8) **epiglottis,** seals off the air passage to the lungs during swallowing. This ensures that food or liquids do not obstruct the flow of air to the lungs. The larynx is a short passage that joins the pharynx with the (9) **trachea** (windpipe). The inner wall of the trachea is composed of a mucous membrane lining embedded with tiny hairs called cilia. This membrane traps incoming particles and the cilia move the entrapped material upward into the pharynx. The trachea is composed of smooth muscle embedded with C-shaped cartilage rings, which provide rigidity to keep the air passage open. The trachea divides into two branches called (10) **bronchi** (singular, **bronchus**). One branch leads to the (11) **right lung** and the other to the (12) **left lung.** Like the trachea, bronchi contain C-shaped cartilage rings.

Each bronchus divides into smaller and smaller branches, eventually forming (13) **bronchioles.** Where bronchioles terminate, tiny air sacs called (14) **alveoli** (singular, **alveolus**) are formed. An alveolus resembles a small balloon because it expands and contracts

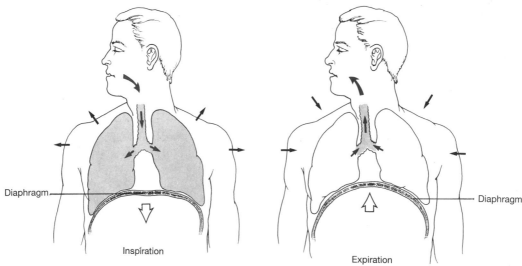

Figure 8–2   The diaphragm contracts and flattens during inhalation, then relaxes during exhalation.

with inflow and outflow of air. The (15) **pulmonary capillaries** lie adjacent to the thin tissue membranes of the alveoli. CO_2 diffuses from the blood within the pulmonary capillaries and enters the alveolar spaces. Simultaneously, O_2 from the alveoli diffuses into the blood. After the exchange of gases, blood returns to the heart, from which it is pumped to body tissues for internal respiration.

The lungs are divided into lobes: three lobes in the right lung and two lobes in the left lung. The space between the right and left lungs, called the (16) **mediastinum,** contains the heart, aorta, esophagus, and bronchi.

A serous membrane, the **pleura,** envelopes the lungs and folds over to line the walls of the thoracic cavity. The innermost membrane lying next to the lung is the (17) **visceral pleura;** the outermost membrane, lining the thoracic cavity, is the (18) **parietal pleura.** Between these two membranes is the (19) **pleural cavity.** It contains a small amount of lubricating fluid, which permits the visceral pleura to glide smoothly over the parietal pleura during breathing.

Ventilation depends on a pressure differential between the atmosphere and chest cavity. A large muscular partition, the (20) **diaphragm,** lies between the chest and abdominal cavities. The diaphragm assists in changing the volume of the thoracic cavity in order to produce the needed pressure differential for ventilation. When the diaphragm contracts, it partially descends into the abdominal cavity, thus decreasing the pressure within the chest and drawing air into the lungs. When the diaphragm relaxes, it slowly re-enters the thoracic cavity, thus increasing the pressure within the chest. As the pressure increases, air leaves the lungs (Fig. 8–2).

The **intercostal** muscles assist the diaphragm in changing the volume of the thoracic cavity by elevating and lowering the rib cage.

COMBINING FORMS

Combining Form	Meaning	Example	Pronunciation
nas/o	nose	nas/al — pertaining to	NĀ-zl
rhin/o		rhin/o/plasty — surgical repair	RĪ-nō-plăs-tē
adenoid/o	adenoid	adenoid/ectomy — excision, removal	ăd-ě-noid-ĔK-tō-mē
tonsill/o	tonsils	tonsill/o/tome — instrument to cut	tŏn-SĬL-ō-tōm
pharyng/o	pharynx, throat	pharyng/o/scope — instrument to view or examine	făr-ĬN-gō-skōp
laryng/o	larynx (voice box)	laryng/o/plegia — paralysis	lă-rĭng-gō-PLĒ-jē-ă
trache/o	trachea	trache/o/stomy — forming an opening (mouth)	trā-kē-ŎS-tō-mē

COMBINING FORMS (Continued)

Combining Form	Meaning	Example	Pronunciation

bronchi/o
bronch/o
	bronchus	bronchi/ectasis
		    expansion, dilation
		bronch/o/scope
		    instrument to view or
		    examine
			brŏng-kē-ĔK-tā-sĭs
			
			BRŎNG-kă-skōp

pneum/o
pneumat/o
	air, gas	pneum/o/cele
		    hernia, swelling
		pneumat/ic
		    pertaining to
			NŪ-mō-sēl
			
			nū-MĂT-ĭk

pneumon/o
pulmon/o
	lung	pneumon/o/lysis
		    separation, destruction,
		    loosening
		pulmon/ary
		    pertaining to
			nū-MŎL-ĭs-ĭs
			
			PŬL-mō-nĕ-rē

lob/o	lobe	lob/ar pertaining to	LŌ-băr
alveol/o	alveolus	alveol/ar pertaining to	ăl-VĒ-ō-lăr
pleur/o	pleura	pleur/algia pain	ploo-RĂL-jē-a
phren/o	diaphragm, mind	phren/ectomy excision	frĕ-NĔK-tō-mē

pector/o
steth/o
thorac/o
	chest	pector/al
		    pertaining to
		steth/o/scope
		    instrument to view or
		    examine
		thorac/o/centesis
		    puncture
			PĔK-tō-răl
			
			STĔTH-ō-skōp
			
			thō-răk-ō-sĕn-TĒ-sĭs

spir/o	breathe	spir/o/meter instrument for measuring	spĭ-RŎM-ĕt-ĕr
coni/o	dust	pneum/o/coni/osis lung abnormal condition	nū-mō-kō-nē-Ō-sĭs
anthrac/o	charcoal (coal dust)	anthrac/osis abnormal condition	ăn-thră-KŌ-sĭs
ox/o	oxygen	hyp/ ox/emia decrease blood	hī-pŏk-SĒ-mē-ăh

COMBINING FORMS (Continued)

Combining Form	Meaning	Example	Pronunciation
orth/o	straight	orth/o/pnea breathing	ŏr-thŏp-NĒ-ăh
atel/o	incomplete, imperfect	atel/ectasis dilation, expansion	ăt-ē-LĔK-tăh-sĭs

SUFFIXES

Suffix	Meaning	Example	Pronunciation
-capnia	carbon dioxide (CO_2)	hyper/capnia excessive	hī-pĕr-KĂP-nē-ăh
-osmia	smell	an/osmia lack of	ăn-ŎZ-mē-ăh
-phonia	voice	dys/phonia difficult, painful	dĭs-FŌ-nē-ăh
-pnea	breathing	eu/pnea good, normal	ūp-NĒ-ăh
-ptysis	spitting	hem/o/ptysis blood	hē-MŎP-tĭ-sĭs
-thorax	chest	pneum/o/thorax air	nū-mō-THŌ-răks

PREFIXES

Prefix	Meaning	Example	Pronunciation
brady-	slow	brady/pnea breathing	brăd-ĭp-NĒ-ăh
eu-	good, normal	eu/pnea breathing	ūp-NĒ-ăh
tachy-	rapid	tachy/pnea breathing	tăk-ĭp-NĒ-ăh

Pathology

CHRONIC OBSTRUCTIVE PULMONARY DISEASE

Chronic obstructive pulmonary disease (COPD), also called chronic obstructive lung disease (COLD), includes respiratory disorders characterized by a chronic partial obstruction of the air passages. The patient experiences difficulty in breathing **(dyspnea)** on exertion, and often exhibits a chronic cough. The three major disorders included in COPD are asthma, chronic bronchitis, and emphysema.

Asthma produces periods of spasms in the bronchial passages. One important cause of asthma is exposure to allergens or irritants. Other causes include stress, cold, and exercise. Bronchospasms associated with asthma are often sudden and violent **(paroxysmal)**, causing dyspnea. During recovery, coughing episodes produce large amounts of mucus **(productive cough).** Over a period of time, the epithelium of the bronchial passages thicken, making breathing difficult. Treatment includes agents that loosen and break down mucus **(mucolytics)** and medications that open up the bronchi **(bronchodilators)** by relaxing the smooth muscles of the bronchi.

Chronic bronchitis is an inflammation of the bronchi believed to be caused primarily by smoking and air pollution. Other agents such as viruses and bacteria, however, may also be responsible for the disorder. Owing to its chronic nature, this type of bronchitis is characterized by swelling of the mucosa and a heavy, productive cough, often accompanied by chest pain. Patients usually seek medical attention when they suffer exercise intolerance, wheezing, and shortness of breath. Bronchodilators and medications that facilitate the removal of mucus **(expectorants)** help to widen the air passages. Steroids are often needed as the disease progresses.

Emphysema is a disease that causes alveoli to lose elasticity. The air sacs expand **(dilate)** but are unable to contract to their initial size. Residual air becomes trapped in the alveoli, resulting in a characteristic "barrel chest" appearance. This disease is often found in combination with another respiratory disorder such as asthma, tuberculosis, or chronic bronchitis. It is also associated with long-term heavy smoking. Emphysema sufferers often find it easier to breathe when sitting or standing erect **(orthopnea).** As the disease progresses, however, orthopnea is no longer effectual. Treatment for emphysema is similar to that for chronic bronchitis.

BRONCHIECTASIS

The bronchial dilation found in bronchiectasis usually leads to secondary infections involving the lower portions of the lungs. Copious amounts of sputum mixed with pus **(mucopurulent sputum)** and bloody sputum **(hemoptysis)** are associated with this disorder. Mucolytics and bronchodilators provide temporary relief. Antibiotics and postural drainage often prove helpful for long-term treatment.

PLEURAL EFFUSIONS

Pleural effusion is an excess of fluid in the pleural cavity. The pleural cavity normally contains only a small amount of lubricating fluid, but in many disorders this amount increases. These conditions include failure of the heart to pump adequate amounts of blood to body tissues **(congestive heart failure),** liver diseases associated with an accu-

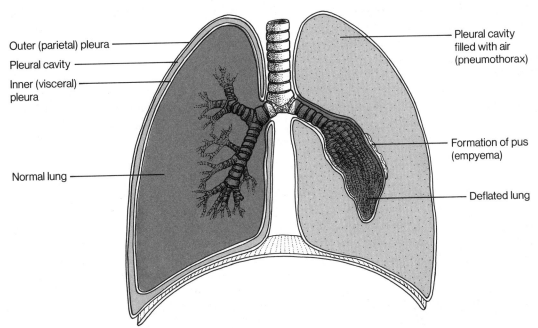

Outer (parietal) pleura

Pleural cavity

Inner (visceral) pleura

Normal lung

Pleural cavity filled with air (pneumothorax)

Formation of pus (empyema)

Deflated lung

Figure 8–3   *Pneumothorax* is the presence of air in the pleural cavity, which can cause a lung to collapse. *Empyema* is the accumulation of pus in the cavity between the pleura and the lung tissue.

mulation of fluid in the abdominal cavity **(ascites),** infectious lung diseases, and trauma. Two noninvasive techniques used in the diagnosis of pleural effusion are listening to the sounds of the chest cavity with a stethoscope **(auscultation)** and gently tapping the chest with the fingers to determine the position, size, or consistency of the underlying structures **(percussion).** Different types of pleural effusions include pus in the pleural space **(empyema),** serum in the pleural space **(hydrothorax),** blood in the pleural space **(hemothorax),** air in the pleural space **(pneumothorax),** and a mixture of pus and air in the pleural space **(pyopneumothorax)** (Fig. 8–3). Depending on the amount and type of fluid, treatment may include surgical puncture of the chest **(thoracocentesis, thoracentesis)** to remove excess fluid. Sometimes chest tubes are inserted to facilitate removal of the fluid.

TUBERCULOSIS

Tuberculosis (TB) is an infectious disease that afflicts more than 2.5 billion people worldwide. Although the number of US citizens with the disease decreased by about 6 percent per year since 1953, over the last several years the trend has reversed and a significant number of new cases are currently reported yearly. The increase in the disease is correlated with the increase of drug-resistant strains, the number of people with acquired immunodeficiency syndrome (AIDS), and those who are homeless or live in poverty.

Tuberculosis is spread by inhaling droplets of respiratory secretions **(aerosol transmission)** or particles of dry sputum containing the TB organism, which can remain alive **(viable)** and infectious for 6 to 8 months outside of the body. The first time the TB organism enters the body **(primary tuberculosis),** the disease develops slowly. It eventually produces focal lesions encased in small pockets called granulomas **(tubercles).** Usually the granulomas remain dormant for years, keeping the patient asymptomatic. When the immune system becomes impaired **(immunocompromised)** or when the patient is reintroduced to the bacterium, the full-blown disease develops.

Although primarily a lung disease, TB can infect the bones, genital tract, meninges, and peritoneum and is highly communicable. Many of the TB strains that infect AIDS patients are not responsive to standard medications **(drug resistant),** and treatment becomes a challenge.

BRONCHOPNEUMONIA

The term **bronchopneumonia** refers to any inflammatory disease of the lungs. It may be caused by a variety of agents, including bacteria, viruses, diseases, chemicals, and other substances. Infectious pneumonias are primarily attributed to bacteria or viruses. A sometimes-fatal type of pneumonia is associated with influenza or may result from food or liquid inhalation. Some pneumonias affect only a lobe of the lung **(lobar pneumonia),** whereas others affect both the right and left lungs **(bilateral** or **"double" pneumonia).** Chest pain, mucopurulent sputum, and spitting of blood **(hemoptysis)** are frequent symptoms of the disease. The lungs may undergo solidification **(consolidation)** owing to a pathological engorgement.

Pneumocystis carinii pneumonia (PCP) is a particularly important disease associated with AIDS. Recent evidence suggests that it is caused by a fungus that resides in or on most people **(normal flora)** but causes no harm as long as the individual remains healthy. When the immune system becomes compromised, however, this organism becomes infectious **(opportunistic).** Diagnosis relies on examination of biopsied lung tissue or bronchial washings **(lavage).**

CYSTIC FIBROSIS

Cystic fibrosis, a hereditary disorder, affects the exocrine glands. The disease causes widespread involvement **(systemic),** especially of the lungs, pancreas, and digestive tract. Mucus produced in an individual afflicted with cystic fibrosis is extremely thick **(viscous)** and blocks the bronchioles. Air becomes trapped in the lungs, but use of mists **(aerosols)** and postural drainage provides relief.

An important finding in cystic fibrosis is an increase in the amount of salt excreted in sweat. Although the disease is fatal, improved methods of treatment have extended life expectancy, and many children now survive to young adulthood.

RESPIRATORY DISTRESS SYNDROME

Respiratory distress syndrome (RDS) is most often caused by the absence or impairment in the production of a phospholipid substance of the lungs called surfactant. This substance aids in decreasing the surface tension of the alveoli. Lungs require surfactant in order to fill with air and expand **(compliance).** Lacking surfactant, the alveoli collapse and inhalation becomes extremely difficult.

When this condition is found in newborns infants, it is called **infant respiratory distress syndrome (IRDS)** or **hyaline membrane disease (HMD).** IRDS is most frequently seen in premature infants or infants born to diabetic mothers. Before birth, lung tissue normally develops surfactant. If the amount of this substance is inadequate, clinical symptoms are noticeable immediately after birth, including blueness **(cyanosis)** of the extremities, rapid breathing **(tachypnea),** flaring of the nostrils **(nares),** intercostal retraction, and a characteristic grunt audible during exhalation. Radiography shows a membrane that has a ground-glass appearance **(hyaline membrane).** Although severe cases of IRDS result in death, some forms of therapy are effective.

    Adult respiratory distress syndrome (ARDS) is caused by an impairment of surfactant production or by exposure to substances that remove surfactant from the lungs. Accidental inhalation of foreign substances, water, smoke, chemical fumes, and vomit is often the cause.

ONCOLOGY

Primary Pulmonary Cancer

Smoking is the leading cause of all types of lung cancers. The most common form of lung cancer in the United States is primary pulmonary cancer. The site most frequently involved is the epithelium of the bronchial passages; lung cancer located here is called bronchogenic carcinoma. In this type of cancer, the cells at the base of the epithelium **(basal cells)** divide repeatedly, until eventually the entire epithelium is involved. Within a short period of time the epithelium begins to invade the underlying tissues. Masses form and block air passages and alveoli, thereby reducing the surface area needed for gas exchange. Bronchogenic carcinoma spreads **(metastasizes)** rapidly to other areas of the body, frequently to lymph nodes, liver, bones, brain, or kidney. Surgery, radiation, and chemotherapy are common methods of treatment; however, lung cancer is difficult to control and survival rates are extremely low.

DIAGNOSTIC, SYMPTOMATIC, AND RELATED TERMS

Term	Meaning
anosmia ăn-ŎZ-mē-ăh	absence of the sense of smell
anoxia, hypoxia ăh-NŎK-sē-ăh, hī-PŎK-sē-ăh	absence or deficiency of O_2 in tissues
anoxemia, hypoxemia ăn-ŏk-SĒ-mē-ăh, hī-pŏk-SĒ-mē-ăh	absence or deficiency of O_2 in blood
asphyxia ăs-FĬK-sē-ăh	condition in which there is insufficient O_2; literally means "without pulse"
compliance kŏm-PLĪ-ăns	ease with which lung tissue can be stretched
coryza kŏ-RĪ-zăh	head cold; upper respiratory infection (URI)

DIAGNOSTIC, SYMPTOMATIC, AND RELATED TERMS
(Continued)

Term	Meaning
croup croop	condition resulting from an acute obstruction of the larynx caused by an allergen, foreign body, infection, or new growth; symptoms include resonant, barking cough; suffocative and difficult breathing; laryngeal spasm; and sometimes the formation of a membrane
Cheyne-Stokes respiration CHĀN-stōks	breathing characterized by fluctuation in the depth of respiration. The patient breathes deeply for a short time, then breathes very slightly, then not at all. This pattern occurs repeatedly. Cheyne-Stokes respiration is usually caused by diseases that affect the respiratory centers (e.g., heart failure or brain damage)
epistaxis ĕp-ĭ-STĂK-sĭs	nosebleed; nasal hemorrhage
eupnea ūp-NĒ-ăh	good, normal breathing
mucus MŪ-kŭs	viscous fluid secreted by mucuos membranes that communicate with the air
phlegm flĕm	abnormal amounts of mucus, especially expectorated from the mouth
pleurisy, pleuritis PLOOR-ĭ-sē, ploo-RĪ-tĭs	inflammation of the pleural membrane characterized by a stabbing pain that is intensified by coughing or deep breathing
pneumoconiosis, pneumoconioses (pl.) nū-mō-kō-nē-Ō-sĭs	respiratory disorder (usually occupational) caused by inhaling dust particles (e.g., anthracosis [coal dust], chalicosis [stone dust], siderosis [iron], asbestosis [asbestos])
postural drainage PŎS-tū-răl	positioning a patient so that gravity aids in the drainage of secretions from the bronchi and lobes of the lungs
pulmonary edema PŬL-mō-nĕ-rē ĕ-DĒ-mă	excessive fluid in the lungs that induces cough and dyspnea; common in left heart failure
pulmonary embolus PŬL-mō-nĕ-rē ĔM-bō-lŭs	a mass of undissolved matter (e.g., blood clot, tissue, air bubbles, bacteria) in the pulmonary arteries or its branches

DIAGNOSTIC, SYMPTOMATIC, AND RELATED TERMS (Continued)

Term	Meaning
rale, crackle răl, KRĂK-ĕl	abnormal respiratory sound heard on auscultation, caused by exudates, spasms, hyperplasia, or when air enters moisture-filled alveoli
rhonchus, rhonchi (pl.) RŎNG-kŭs, RŎNG-kĭ	rale or rattling in the throat, especially when it resembles snoring
sputum SPŪ-tŭm	pathological viscous fluid formed in the lower respiratory tract that often contains blood, pus, and bacteria
tracheostenosis trā-kē-ō-stĕn-Ō-sĭs	constricture or narrowing of the trachea
stridor STRĪ-dor	abnormal sound caused by a spasm or swelling of the larnyx

Special Procedures

DIAGNOSTIC IMAGING PROCEDURES

Term	Description
bronchography broŏng-KŎG-ră-fē	radiological evaluation of the trachea and bronchi following administration of a radiopaque contrast medium
chest radiographs RĀ-dē-ō-grăfs	series of x-ray images designed to evaluate the chest, heart, lungs, and rib cage
CT scan (thoracic) thō-RĂS-ĭk	provides a cross-sectional view of the chest, with or without an injected radiographic iodine contrast medium; used primarily to highlight blood vessels and tissue masses

CLINICAL PROCEDURES

Term	Description
bronchoscopy brŏng-KŎS-kō-pē	visual examination of the bronchi using a flexible bronchoscope inserted through the mouth and trachea into the bronchial tubes; used for suctioning, biopsy, removal of foreign bodies, and collection of fluid or sputum for examination and diagnosis

CLINICAL PROCEDURES (Continued)

Term	Description
laryngoscopy lăr-ĭn-GŎS-kō-pē	visual examination of the larynx with a laryngoscope; may be viewed directly or indirectly by transmitting image of the larynx via a laryngeal mirror; used for performing biopsies, collecting sputum samples, identifying tumors, and accounting for changes in the voice
mediastinoscopy mē-dē-ăs-tĭ-NŎS-kō-pē	allows direct visualization of the mediastinal structures, heart, trachea, esophagus, bronchus, thymus, and lymph nodes; especially important in early diagnosis of bronchogenic carcinoma
pulmonary function studies	series of tests to evaluate pulmonary volume and air-flow rate; sometimes calculated by computer attached to a sterile cylinder used by patient to perform various breathing exercises

SURGICAL PROCEDURES

Term	Description
bronchoplasty BRŎNG-kō-plăs-tē	surgical repair of the bronchus; surgical closure of a bronchial fistula
laryngectomy lăr-ĭn-JĔK-tō-mē	partial or total removal of the larynx, usually as cancer treatment
pleurectomy, decortication ploor-ĔK-tō-mē, dē-kŏr-tĭ-KĀ-shŭn	excision of part of the pleura
pneumonectomy nū-mō-NĔK-tō-mē	excision of a lung or lobe of the lung
thoracentesis, thoracocentesis thō-ră-sĕn-TĒ-sĭs, thō-răk-ō-sĕn-TĒ-sĭs	surgical puncture and drainage of pleural cavity

LABORATORY PROCEDURES

Test	Description
arterial blood gases (ABGs)	assessment of O_2 and CO_2 levels in arterial blood, important in treating disturbances of acid-base balance
sputum culture SPŪ-tŭm	bacteriological test performed using a sputum sample; identifies disease-causing organisms of lower respiratory tract, especially those that cause pneumonias
sweat test	measurement of the amount of salt (sodium chloride) in sweat; used almost exclusively in children to confirm cystic fibrosis
throat culture	bacteriological test used to identify throat pathogens, especially group A streptococci. It is important to treat streptococcal infections, as they may lead to serious secondary disorders

PHARMACOLOGY

Medication	Action
antihistamines	counteract the effects of histamines, which cause nasal passage swelling and inflammation; primary agents used to relieve allergic rhinitis (hay fever) symptoms
antitussives	suppress coughing
bronchodilators	cause dilation of the bronchi, thereby "opening up" the breathing passages
decongestants	reduce congestion or swelling, especially in the nasal passages, by constricting blood vessels and limiting blood flow to the area
expectorants	facilitate the removal of secretions from the lungs, bronchi, and trachea
mucolytics	liquify or break down tenacious, "sticky" mucus so that it can be coughed up more easily

ABBREVIATIONS

Diagnostic and Symptomatic	Meaning
ABGs	arterial blood gases
AP	anteroposterior
ARDS	adult respiratory distress syndrome
COPD	chronic obstructive pulmonary disease
CPR	cardiopulmonary resuscitation
CXR	chest x-ray film; chest radiograph
FEF	forced expiratory flow
FEV	forced expiratory volume
FVC	forced vital capacity
HMD	hyaline membrane disease
Hx	history
IPPB	intermittent positive-pressure breathing
IRDS	infant respiratory distress syndrome
PA	posteroanterior
PCP	*Pneumocystis carinii* pneumonia
PND	paroxysmal nocturnal dyspnea
RD	respiratory disease
RDS	respiratory distress syndrome
SOB	shortness of breath
TB	tuberculosis
TPR	temperature, pulse, and respiration
URI	upper respiratory infection
VC	vital capacity

Laboratory	Meaning
AFB	acid-fast bacillus (TB organism)
CO_2	carbon dioxide
O_2	oxygen

Case Study

Respiratory Evaluation

History of Present Illness. This 49-year-old man with known history of **COPD** is admitted because of **exacerbation** of **SOB** over the past few days. Patient was a heavy smoker and states that he quit smoking for a short while but now smokes three to four cigarettes a day. He has a **Hx** of difficult breathing, high blood pressure, COPD, and **peripheral vascular disease.** He underwent triple bypass surgery in 19XX. **PE** indicates scattered **bilateral** wheezes and **rhonchi** heard anteriorly and posteriorly.

Compared with a portable chest film from 4/17/XX, deterioration since the previous study is noted that most likely indicates **interstitial vascular congestion.** Some superimposed **inflammatory** change cannot be excluded. There may also be some **pleural** reactive change.

Dx. (a) Acute exacerbation of chronic obstructive pulmonary disease; (2) congestive heart failure; (3) hypertension; (4) peripheral vascular disease.

Worksheet 5 provides a dictionary and reading application and an analysis of this case study.

Worksheet 1

Use rhin/o (nose) to build a medical word meaning:

1. disease of the nose _____

2. inflammation of the (mucous membranes of the) nose _____

3. discharge from the nose _____

Use laryng/o (larynx or "voice box") to build a medical word meaning:

4. inflammation of the larynx _____

5. visual examination of the larynx _____

6. spasm of the larynx _____

7. stricture or narrowing of the larynx _____

8. pertaining to the larynx and the trachea _____

9. disease of the larynx _____

Use bronch/o or bronchi/o (bronchus) to build a medical word meaning:

10. instrument to view the bronchus _____

11. inflammation of the bronchus _____

12. dilation or expansion of the bronchus _____

13. spasm of the bronchus _____

14. disease of the bronchus _____

Use pneumon/o or pneum/o (air, lung) to build a medical word meaning:

15. inflammation of the lungs _____

16. x-ray of the lungs _____

Use thorac/o (chest) to build a medical word meaning:

17. pertaining to the chest _____

18. pain in the muscles of the chest _____

Use the suffix -pnea (breathing) to build a medical word meaning:

19. difficult or painful breathing _____

20. breathing in a straight (upright) position _____

21. not breathing (temporary) _____

22. good, normal breathing _____

23. slow breathing _____

Use the suffix -thorax (chest) to build a medical word meaning:

24. air in the chest _____

25. blood in the chest _____

Worksheet 2

Build a surgical term meaning:

1. forming an opening (mouth) in the larynx _____

2. puncture of the lung _____

3. excision of a lobe (of the lung) _____

4. surgical repair of the nose _____

5. puncture of the chest _____

6. suture of the larynx _____

7. fixation of the lung (to the thoracic wall) _____

8. surgical repair of the bronchus _____

9. forming an opening (mouth) in the trachea _____

10. excision of (part of) the pleura _____

Worksheet 3

Match the following medical terms with the definitions in the numbered list.

anosmia   epistaxis
anoxia   mucus
anoxemia   pulmonary edema
Cheyne-Stokes respiration   rales, crackles
compliance   sputum
coryza   stridor

1. _____ pathological fluid formed in the lungs or bronchi

2. _____ abnormal respiratory sounds heard in auscultation, indicating pathology

3. _____ ease with which lung tissue can be stretched

4. _____ viscous fluid secreted by mucous membranes

5. _____ excessive fluid in the lungs

6. _____ irregular breathing characterized by alteration in depth of respiration and apnea

7. _____ lack of sense of smell

8. _____ absence of or decrease in O_2 in the blood

9. _____ abnormal sound caused by a spasm or swelling of the larynx or a bronchus

10. _____ head cold; upper respiratory infection

Worksheet 4

SPECIAL PROCEDURES, PHARMACOLOGY, AND ABBREVIATIONS

Select a term that best describes the statements that follow.

antihistamines	FEV
antitussives	mucolytics
AP	pulmonary function studies
arterial blood gases	sputum culture
bronchography	sweat test
bronchoscopy	thoracentesis
COPD	throat culture
CXR	tomography
hemoptysis	

1. _____ tests designed to evaluate volume and air-flow rate of the lungs

2. _____ x-ray films of the bronchial tree following intratracheal injection of a contrast medium

3. _____ sequence of radiographs, each representing a "slice" of the lung at different depths

4. _____ bacteriological test to identify throat pathogens, especially group A streptococci

5. _____ anteroposterior

6. _____ chronic obstructive pulmonary disease

7. _____ prevent or relieve coughing

8. _____ primary agents used to relieve discomfort associated with allergic rhinitis by opposing the action of histamine

9. _____ liquify "sticky" mucus so that it can be coughed up more readily

10. _____ assesses the O_2 and CO_2 levels of arterial blood in order to evaluate and manage acid-base disturbances

11. _____ puncture of the chest to remove fluids

12. _____ measures the amount of salt for diagnosis of cystic fibrosis

13. _____ bacterial test used to identify lower respiratory tract pathogens

14. _____ chest x-ray examination; chest radiograph

15. _____ forced expiratory volume

Worksheet 5

RESPIRATORY EVALUATION DICTIONARY EXERCISE

Use a medical dictionary or other resource to define the terms and to determine their pronunciation; then practice reading the case study aloud (p. 135)

bilateral _____

COPD _____

Dx _____

exacerbation _____

Hx _____

inflammatory _____

interstitial vascular congestion _____

PE _____

peripheral vascular disease _____

pleural _____

rhonchi _____

SOB _____

ANALYSIS OF RESPIRATORY EVALUATION

1. What symptom caused the patient to seek medical help?

2. What was the patient's previous history?

3. What were the findings of the physical examination?

4. What changes were noted from the previous film?

5. What is the present Dx?

6. What new diagnosis was made that did not appear in the previous medical history?

7. What is the abbreviation for congestive heart failure?

Worksheet 6

Label the structures indicated on the following diagram. To check your answers, refer to Figure 8–1.

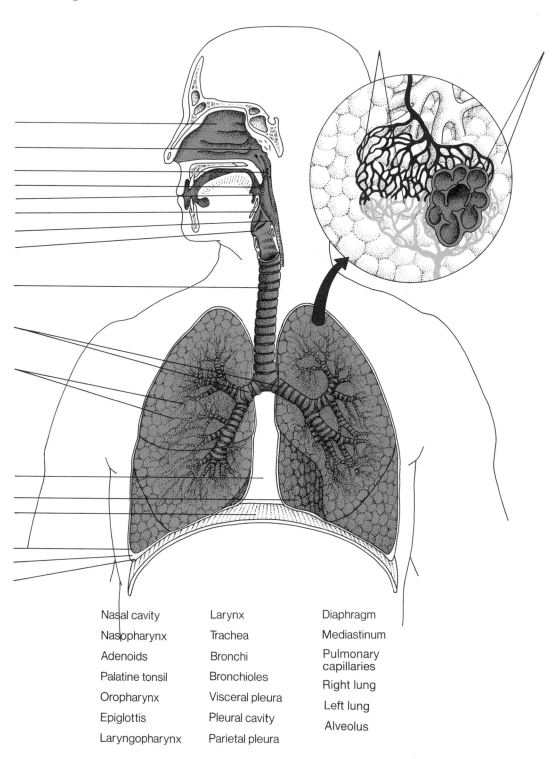

Nasal cavity

Nasopharynx

Adenoids

Palatine tonsil

Oropharynx

Epiglottis

Laryngopharynx

Larynx

Trachea

Bronchi

Bronchioles

Visceral pleura

Pleural cavity

Parietal pleura

Diaphragm

Mediastinum

Pulmonary capillaries

Right lung

Left lung

Alveolus

Chapter 9

Cardiovascular System

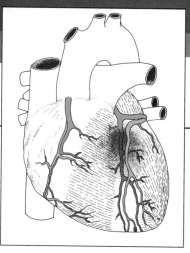

Chapter Outline

Student Objectives
Upon completion of this chapter, you will be able to do the following:

List and describe the structure and function of three types of blood vessels.

List and describe the major structures and functions of the heart.

Differentiate between systemic and pulmonary circulation.

Define systolic and diastolic blood pressures.

Discuss the function of the conduction system of the heart.

List the structures, in sequential order, through which electrical current passes during the cardiac cycle.

Student Objectives (Continued)

Identify the combining forms, suffixes, and prefixes related to the cardiovascular system.

Identify and discuss associated pathology related to the cardiovascular system.

Identify diagnostic imaging, clinical, surgical, and laboratory procedures and abbreviations related to the cardiovascular system.

Discuss pharmacology related to the treatment of disorders associated with the cardiovascular system.

Demonstrate your knowledge of the chapter by completing the worksheets.

Anatomy and Physiology

The cardiovascular system is composed of the heart and blood vessels. The heart is a hollow muscular organ lying in the mediastinum, the center of the thoracic cavity between the two lungs. It pumps blood through a vast network of blood vessels, which carry blood from the heart to body cells, and then return blood back to the heart.

The body is composed of trillions of cells, all requiring a constant supply of food and other vital products for survival. Cells also require a means of removing accumulated waste products. Because body cells are not always located near the source of the products they need and are not always near the organs necessary for elimination of waste, they require a transportation system. The cardiovascular system, in conjunction with the blood and lymphatic systems (discussed in Chapter 10), is responsible for transportation of products to and from body cells.

VASCULAR SYSTEM

Three types of vessels, **arteries, capillaries,** and **veins** (Figs. 9–1 and 9–2), carry blood throughout the body. Each type of vessel differs in structure, depending on its function.

Arteries

Arteries carry blood from the heart to body tissues and organs. Blood is propelled through arteries by the pumping action of the heart. Consequently, arterial walls are thick and muscular and capable of expanding to accommodate the surge of blood that results when the heart contracts. The surge of blood along the fibers of the arteries when blood is pumped from the heart is referred to as a **pulse.** Because of the pressure against arterial walls associated with the pumping action of the heart, a cut or severed artery may lead to profuse bleeding.

Arterial blood (except for that of the pulmonary artery) contains a high concentration of O_2. It appears bright red and is said to be **oxygenated.** Oxygenated blood is delivered to all capillary beds of the body, except those in the lungs.

Arteries branch to form smaller vessels called **arterioles** (little arteries). Arterioles further divide to form the smallest vessels of the circulatory system, the capillaries.

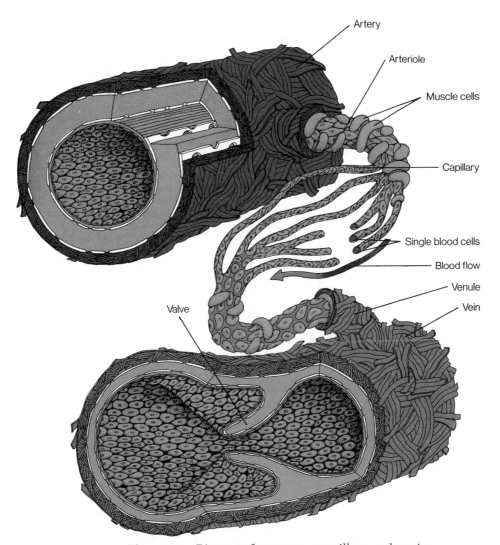

Artery

Arteriole

Muscle cells

Capillary

Single blood cells

Blood flow

Venule

Vein

Valve

Figure 9–1 Diagram of an artery, a capillary, and a vein.

Figure 9–2 Schematic representation of a capillary bed. The capillary system is the gateway for the return of blood to the heart. Blood flows from the heart through the arterial system to the capillaries. Transfer of products in and out of the blood vessels occurs at the capillary level.

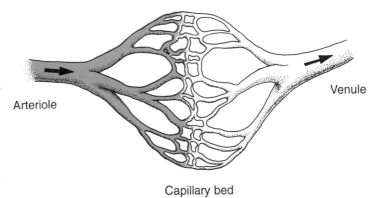

Arteriole

Venule

Capillary bed

Capillaries

Capillaries are microscopic vessels that join the arterial system with the venous system. Although seemingly the most insignificant of the three vessel types because of their microscopic size, capillaries are functionally the most important. Capillary walls are composed of a single layer of cells. The thinness of these walls makes it possible for substances to pass quite readily into and out of the vessels. Consequently, the primary function of the vascular system, that of providing cells with vital products and removal of waste products, occurs at the capillary level. The vast number of capillaries makes their combined diameter so great that blood flows through them very slowly, and the pulse that was present in the arteries can no longer be detected. The slow movement of blood through capillaries allows sufficient time for delivery of vital products and removal of waste. The pathway for this exchange is as follows:

$$\text{Blood} \underset{\text{Waste Products}}{\overset{\text{Vital Products}}{\rightleftarrows}} \text{Body Cells}$$

Veins

Veins return blood to the heart. They are formed from smaller vessels called **venules** (little veins), which develop from the union of capillaries. Because the extensive network of capillaries throughout the body absorbs the propelling pressure exerted by the heart, blood in veins use other methods to return to the heart, including:

- skeletal muscle contraction
- gravity
- respiratory activity
- valves

Valves are small structures within veins that prevent the backflow of blood. Valves are especially important for returning blood from the legs to the heart because blood must travel a long distance against the force of gravity to reach the heart.

Blood carried in the veins (except for the blood in the pulmonary veins) contains a low concentration of O_2 (deoxygenated) with a corresponding high concentration of CO_2. Deoxygenated blood takes on a characteristic purple color. It continuously circulates to the lungs, so that CO_2 can be expelled.

HEART

As you read the following material, refer to Figure 9–3 and identify the structures.

The heart is divided into four chambers: (1) **right atrium,** (2) **right ventricle,** (3) **left atrium,** and (4) **left ventricle.** The two upper chambers, the atria, collect blood; the two lower chambers, the ventricles, pump blood from the heart. The right side of the heart provides for the oxygenation of blood (pulmonary circulation) and the left side is responsible for the transportation of blood to body systems (systemic circulation). The muscular wall dividing the right side of the heart from the left is called the **septum.**

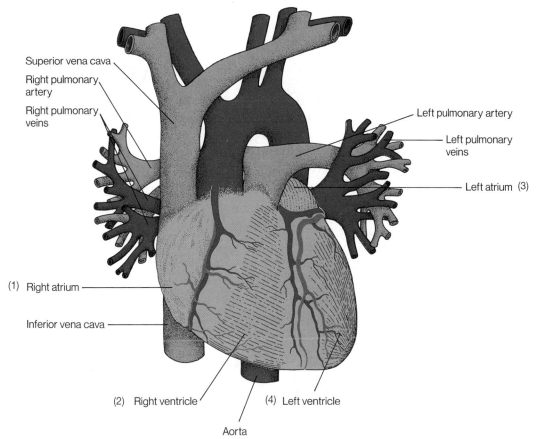

Figure 9–3 Diagram of the heart.

Refer to Figure 9–4 as you read the following paragraphs on blood flow through the heart and major blood vessels.

The heart has three distinct tissue layers:

- the (1) **endocardium,** a serous membrane that lines the four chambers of the heart and its valves, and is continuous with the arteries and veins
- the (2) **myocardium,** the muscular layer of the heart
- the (3) **epicardium,** the outermost layer of the heart

The heart is contained in a sac called the **pericardium.**

Deoxygenated blood returns to the heart by way of two large veins: the (4) **superior vena cava,** which collects and carries blood from the upper part of the body; and the (5) **inferior vena cava,** which collects and carries blood from the lower part of the body. The superior and inferior venae cavae (singular, vena cava) deposit deoxygenated blood into the upper right chamber of the heart, the (6) **right atrium.** From the right atrium, blood passes through the (7) **tricuspid valve** to the (8) **right ventricle.** During contraction of the ventricle, the tricuspid valve prevents a backflow of blood to the right atrium. When the heart contracts, blood leaves the right ventricle by way of the (9) **pulmonary artery** and

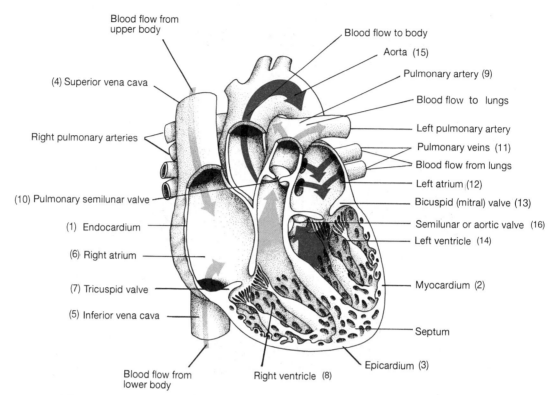

Figure 9–4 Diagram of the blood flow through the heart and major blood vessels.

travels to the lungs. The (10) **pulmonary semilunar valve** (or pulmonary valve) prevents a backflow of blood into the right ventricle. In the lungs, the pulmonary artery branches into millions of capillaries, each lying close to an alveolus. Here, CO_2 in the blood is replaced by O_2 that has been drawn into the lungs during inhalation.

Pulmonary capillaries unite to form four (11) **pulmonary veins,** the vessels that carry oxygenated blood back to the heart. Pulmonary veins deposit blood in the (12) **left atrium.** From here, blood passes through the (13) **bicuspid (mitral) valve** to the (14) **left ventricle.** Upon contraction of the heart, the oxygenated blood leaves the left ventricle through the largest artery of the body, the (15) **aorta.** Within the aorta is a valve called the (16) **semi-lunar valve** (or aortic valve), which permits blood to flow in only one direction—from the left ventricle to the aorta. The aorta branches into many smaller arteries that carry blood to all parts of the body. Some arteries derive their name from the organs or areas of the body that they vascularize. For example, the splenic artery vascularizes the spleen, the renal arteries vascularize the kidneys, and so forth.

It is important to recognize that O_2, present in the blood passing through the chambers of the heart, cannot be used by the myocardium. Instead, an arterial system composed of the coronary arteries branch from the aorta and provide the myocardium with its own blood supply. These arteries lie over the top of the heart much as a crown fits over a head; hence, the name **coronary** (pertaining to a crown). If blood flow in the coronary arteries is diminished, myocardial damage may result. When severe damage occurs, part of the heart muscle may die.

FETAL CIRCULATION

Because the lungs of the fetus are deflated and do not function in the breathing process, the circulatory system of the fetus is somewhat different from that just described. Oxygenation of fetal blood occurs in the placenta rather than in the lungs of the fetus. The umbilical cord, containing two arteries, carries deoxygenated blood from the fetus to the placenta. After oxygenation in the placenta, blood returns to the fetus via the umbilical vein. Most of the blood in the umbilical vein enters the inferior vena cava through the **ductus venosus,** where it is delivered to the right atrium. Some of this blood passes to the right ventricle, but most of it passes through a small opening in the atrial septum called the **foramen ovale** that closes shortly after birth.

An additional structure found in the fetal circulatory system is the **ductus arteriosus.** This structure shunts most blood out of the pulmonary arteries, causing it to flow into the aorta, thus bypassing the nonfunctional lungs of the fetus.

BLOOD PRESSURE

Blood pressure measures the force exerted by blood against the arterial walls during two phases of a heartbeat: the contraction phase, called **systole,** when the blood is forced out of the heart; and the relaxation phase, called **diastole,** when the ventricles are filling with blood. Systole is the maximum force exerted by blood against the arterial walls; diastole, the weakest. These measurements are recorded as two figures separated by a diagonal line; the systolic pressure is given first, followed by the diastolic pressure. For instance, blood pressure may be recorded as 120/80; in this example, 120 is the systolic pressure, 80 the diastolic pressure.

Several factors influence blood pressure:

- resistance of blood flow in blood vessels
- pumping action of the heart
- viscosity or thickness of blood
- elasticity of arteries
- quantity of blood in the vascular system

Elevated blood pressure is called **hypertension;** decreased blood pressure is called **hypotension.**

CONDUCTION SYSTEM OF THE HEART

Within the heart is specialized cardiac tissue known as **conductive tissue,** the sole function of which is to initiate and propagate contraction impulses. It consists of four masses of highly specialized cells (see Fig. 9–5 to identify the following structures):

- the (1) **sinoatrial (SA) node**
- the (2) **atrioventricular (AV) node**
- the (3) **bundle of His** (AV bundle)
- the (4) **Purkinje fibers**

The SA node, located in the upper portion of the right atrium, possesses its own intrinsic rhythm. Without being stimulated by external nerves, it has the ability to initiate

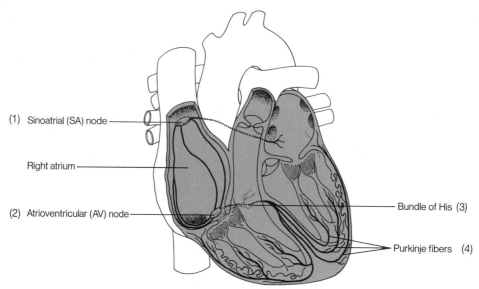

(1) Sinoatrial (SA) node

Right atrium

(2) Atrioventricular (AV) node

Bundle of His (3)

Purkinje fibers (4)

Figure 9–5 The conduction system of the heart.

and propagate each heartbeat, thereby setting the basic pace for the cardiac rate. For this reason, the SA node is commonly known as the pacemaker of the heart. Cardiac rate may be altered by impulses from the autonomic nervous system. Such an arrangement allows outside influences to accelerate or decelerate the rate of the heartbeat. For example, during physical exertion the heart beats faster, and during rest it beats slower.

Each electrical impulse discharged by the SA node is transmitted to the AV node, causing the atria to contract. The AV node is located at the base of the right atrium. From this point, a tract of conduction fibers called the bundle of His, composed of a right and left branch, relays the impulse to the Purkinje fibers. These fibers extend up the ventricle walls. The Purkinje fibers transmit the impulse to both the right and left ventricles, causing them to contract. Blood is now forced from the heart through the pulmonary artery and aorta.

In summary, the sequence of involvement of the four structures in the heart that are responsible for conduction of a contraction impulse is as follows:

SA node → AV node → bundle of His → Purkinje fibers

Impulse transmission through the conduction system generates weak electrical currents that can be detected on the surface of the body. These electrical impulses can be recorded on an instrument called an **electrocardiograph.** The needle deflection of the electrocardiograph produces waves or peaks designated by the letters P, Q, R, S, and T, each of which is associated with a specific electrical event. The P wave is the depolarization (contraction) of the atria, and the QRS complex is the depolarization (contraction) of the ventricles. The T wave, which appears a short time later, is the repolarization (recovery) of the ventricles (Fig. 9–6).

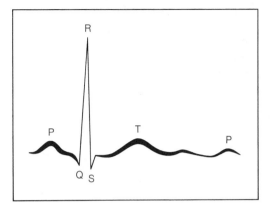

Figure 9–6 Normal ECG deflections. The ECG shows the spread of excitation to different parts of the heart. It is used in the diagnosis of abnormal cardiac rhythm and myocardial damage.

COMBINING FORMS

Combining Form	Meaning	Example	Pronunciation
angi/o	vessel	angi/o/rrhaphy suture	an-jē-ŎR-ăh-fē

vas/o		vas/o/spasm
		        involuntary contraction,
		        twitching
			VĂS-ō-spăzm

aort/o	aorta	aort/o/stenosis stricture, narrowing	ā-ŏr-tō-stĕ-NŌ-sĭs
arteriol/o	arteriole	arteriol/itis inflammation	ăr-tēr-ē-ō-LĪ-tĭs
arteri/o	artery	arteri/al pertaining to	ăr-TĔR-ĭ-ăl
ather/o	fatty plaque	ather/o/scler/ osis hardening abnormal condition	ăth-ĕr-ō-sklĕ-RŌ-sĭs
atri/o	atrium	atri/o/tome instrument to cut	Ā-trē-ō-tōm
cardi/o	heart	cardi/o/megaly enlargement	kăr-dē-ō-MĔG-ăh-lē
hemangi/o	blood vessel	hemangi/oma tumor	hē-MAN-jē-ō-mă
phleb/o	vein	phleb/o/tomy incision, cut into	flĕ-BŎT-ō-mē
ven/o		ven/ous pertaining to	VĒ-nŭs

COMBINING FORMS (Continued)

Combining Form	Meaning	Example		Pronunciation
thromb/o	blood clot	thromb/o/lysis	destruction, separation, loosening	thrŏm-BŎL-ĭ-sĭs
sphygm/o	pulse	sphygm/o/meter	instrument for measuring	sfĭg-MŎM-ĕt-ĕr

SUFFIXES

Suffix	Meaning	Example		Pronunciation
-gram	record, a writing	angi/o/gram	vessel	ĂN-jē-ō-grăm
-graph	instrument for recording	electr/o/ cardi/o/graph	electricity heart	ē-lĕk-trō-KĂR-dē-ō-grăf
-meter	instrument for measuring	therm/o/meter	heat	thĕr-MŎM-ĕ-tĕr

PREFIXES

Prefix	Meaning	Example		Pronunciation
endo-	within	endo/arter/itis	artery inflammation	ĕn-dō-ăr-tĕr-Ī-tĭs
extra-	outside	extra/atri/al	atrium pertaining to	ĔKS-tră-Ā-trē-ăl
peri-	around	peri/card/itis	heart inflammation	pĕr-ĭ-kăr-DĪ-tĭs
trans-	across, through	trans/sept/al	septum pertaining to	trăns-SĔP-tăl

Pathology

ATHEROSCLEROSIS

Atherosclerosis is a degenerative vascular disorder where fatty plaque **(atheromas)** accumulates in the innermost lining of the arteries **(tunica intima).** Plaque builds up over the years and hardens **(scleroses),** causing arteriosclerosis. One of the major risk factors for developing atherosclerosis is an elevated cholesterol level **(hypercholesterolemia).**

Other major risk factors include age, family history, smoking, hypertension, and diabetes. Cholesterol levels can sometimes be controlled by diet and exercise. With arteriosclerosis, vascular elasticity is lost and the vascular channel **(lumen)** narrows. As atheromas increase in size, they impede the flow of blood, leading to O_2 deficiency in surrounding tissues **(ischemia).** Ulcerations often occur on the surface of the plaque, leading to clot formation **(thrombosis)** and, ultimately, total blockage **(occlusion)** of the vessel. When a thrombus dislodges, it is called an embolus. Emboli that travel in venous circulation may cause death. Emboli that travel in arterial circulation frequently lodge in a capillary bed and cause a localized infarct. Sometimes plaque weakens the vessel wall to such an extent that it forms a bulge **(aneurysm)** that may rupture.

Atheromas may form in the abdominal aorta; in the coronary, cerebral, and renal arteries; and in the major arteries of the legs **(femoral arteries).** Removal of the innermost layer of the artery **(endarterectomy),** especially in the carotid or femoral arteries, is a common method of treatment.

CORONARY ARTERY DISEASE

Any disease that interferes with the ability of coronary arteries to deliver sufficient blood to the heart muscle is referred to as **coronary artery disease (CAD).** The usual cause of

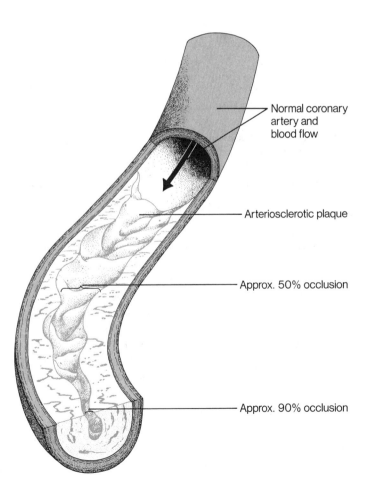

Normal coronary artery and blood flow

Arteriosclerotic plaque

Approx. 50% occlusion

Approx. 90% occlusion

Figure 9–7 Arteriosclerosis.

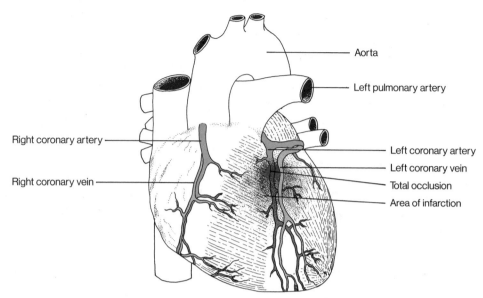

Figure 9–8 Myocardial infarction.

CAD, however, is arteriosclerosis (Fig. 9–7). About 20 percent of the total cardiac output is needed to supply the O_2 requirements of the heart muscle. When coronary arteries are unable to deliver this amount, localized areas of the heart experience ischemia. Myocardial ischemia causes a suffocating chest pain **(angina pectoris,** or **angina)** and difficulty in breathing **(dyspnea).** When pain cannot be controlled with medication, a small piece of vein, usually from the leg **(saphenous vein),** is used to bypass the obstruction. One end of the graft vessel is sutured to the aorta and the other end to the coronary artery below the blocked area **(anastomosis).** This re-establishes blood flow to the heart muscle. A less invasive treatment for an obstructed coronary artery is a technique in which a small deflated balloon is placed at the site of the occlusion and then inflated to compress the plaque against the arterial wall **(angioplasty; percutaneous transluminal coronary angioplasty [PTCA].** Some of the latest techniques involve using lasers and ultrasound to remove plaque.

Coronary artery disease may ultimately produce an acute myocardial infarction (MI). In this life-threatening condition, blood supply to part of the heart is totally suppressed, causing necrosis of the heart muscle **(myocardial infarction)** (Fig. 9–8). The clinical symptoms of an acute MI include intense angina, profuse sweating **(diaphoresis),** paleness **(pallor),** and dyspnea. An arrhythmic heartbeat, accompanied by either a rapid heart action **(tachycardia)** or a slow heart action **(bradycardia),** may also accompany MI.

As the heart muscle undergoes necrotic changes, several enzymes are released, including **glutamic oxaloacetic transaminase (GOT), creatine phosphokinase (CPK),** and **lactic dehydrogenase (LD).** The rapid elevation of these enzymes helps differentiate MI from pericarditis, aortic aneurysm, and acute pulmonary embolism.

INFECTIVE ENDOCARDITIS

Infection of the inner layer of the heart and, often, of the valves is called **infective endocarditis.** Either bacteria or, less commonly, fungi are the usual causes. The infecting organ-

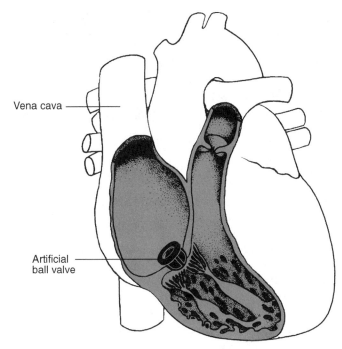

Vena cava

Artificial
ball valve

Figure 9–9 Replacement surgery may be performed to replace a damaged heart valve.

isms become imbedded in blood clots **(thrombi)** and form small masses **(vegetations)** that collect on the leaflets of the valves. Degeneration and scarring of the valves or the cords attached to the valves lead to a backflow of blood **(regurgitation).**

Birth **(congenital)** defects or some infections, especially those associated with scarlet fever or rheumatic fever, may produce valve scarring. When this occurs, there may be a narrowing of the valves **(stenosis)** or an inability of the valves to close properly **(insufficiency).** Although medications may prove helpful, heart surgery frequently is the only recourse. Whenever possible the original valve is repaired **(valvotomy** or **commissurotomy)**, but more often it is replaced with an artificial device (Fig. 9–9).

Patients who have had open heart surgery, rheumatic fever, scarlet fever, or valvular disease are susceptible to endocarditis. Thus, they are given antibiotic treatment before undergoing invasive procedures **(prophylactic treatment)** such as tooth removal, root canal procedures, and other minor surgeries.

VARICOSE VEINS

Varicose veins develop when the valves of the veins are damaged **(incompetent)** and fail to prevent the backflow of blood in the vein. Although found in almost any part of the body, they are most common in the esophagus **(varices,** anus **hemorrhoids)** and legs. Blood accumulates in flabby areas of the vein, and excess fluid eventually seeps from the vein, causing swelling in surrounding tissues **(edema).**

Varicose veins of the legs can result from a congenital weakness of the valves, pregnancy, occupations that require standing for long periods of time, injury **(trauma),** or inflammation of the vein wall **(phlebitis).** In phlebitis, there is usually pain and tenderness. A cordlike mass may develop under the skin but diminishes as the disease subsides. If infection occurs in a deep vein and involves the inner layer of vein tissue, clots may form

(thrombophlebitis). A more serious condition may develop when a thrombus breaks loose from a vein wall and begins to travel in the vascular system. Any masses, including blood clots that move within the vascular system are known as **emboli.** (singular, **embolus**). Death may result if an embolus lodges in a vital organ. Emboli may be removed directly by excision **(embolectomy)** or may be dissolved **(thrombolysis)** using medications.

Treatment of mild cases of varicose veins includes rest periods during which the legs are elevated and use of elastic stockings. In extreme cases, the affected vein is tied **(ligated)** and removed **(stripped).**

ONCOLOGY

The most common primary tumor of the heart is composed of mucous connective tissue **(myxoma);** however, these tend not to be malignant. Some myxomas originate in the endocardium of the heart chambers, but most arise in the left atrium. Occasionally they interfere with mitral valve function and cause a decrease in exercise tolerance, difficulty in breathing **(dyspnea),** fluid in the lungs **(pulmonary edema),** and systemic disturbances including joint pain **(arthralgia),** a feeling of discomfort and uneasiness **(malaise),** and anemia. These tumors are usually identified and located by two-dimensional echocardiography. The tumor should be removed **(excised)** surgically.

Most malignant tumors of the heart are the result of a malignancy **(primary tumor)** in another area of the body that has spread **(metastasized)** to the heart. The type usually found originates as a darkly pigmented mole or tumor **(malignant melanoma)** of the skin. Other primary sites of malignancy that metastasize to the heart are bone marrow and lymphatic tissue. Treatment of the metastatic tumor of the heart involves treating the primary tumor.

DIAGNOSTIC, SYMPTOMATIC, AND RELATED TERMS

Term	Meaning
Adams-Stokes syndrome	altered state of consciousness due to decreased blood flow to the brain
aneurysm ĂN-ū-rĭzm	localized abnormal dilation of a vessel, usually an artery
arrhythmia ăh-RĬTH-mē-ă	irregularity in heart action
ascites ă-SĪ-tēz	accumulation of serous fluid in the peritoneal cavity
bruit, murmur brwē or broot	soft blowing sound heard on auscultation; may result from vibrations associated with the movement of blood, valvular action, or both
cardiomyopathy kăr-dē-ō-mī-ŎP-ă-thē	any disease of heart muscle not caused by an impairment of coronary circulation and ischemia; may be caused by viral infections, metabolic disorders, or general systemic disease

DIAGNOSTIC, SYMPTOMATIC, AND RELATED TERMS
(Continued)

Term	Meaning
coarctation kō-ărk-TĀ-shŭn	narrowing of a vessel, especially the aorta
congestive heart failure (CHF)	failure of the heart to supply an adequate amount of blood to tissues and organs, most commonly caused by impaired coronary blood flow
edema ĕ-DĒ-mă	local or generalized condition in which body tissues contain an excess of tissue fluid
embolus, emboli (pl.) ĔM-bō-lŭs	mass of undissolved matter (foreign object, air, gas, tissue, thrombus) circulating in a blood or lymphatic channels until it becomes lodged in a vessel
extravascular ĕks-tră-VĂS-kū-lăr	outside a vessel
fibrillation fĭ-brĭl-Ā-shŭn	quivering or spontaneous muscle contractions, especially of the heart, causing ineffectual contractions; often may be corrected with a defibrillator
hemostasis hē-MŎS-tă-sĭs	arrest of bleeding or circulation
hyperlipidemia hī-pĕr-lĭp-ĭ-DĒ-mē-ă	excessive amounts of lipids (cholesterol, phospholipids, and triglycerides) in the blood
hypertension hī-pĕr-TĔN-shŭn	condition that is present when, on several separate occasions, blood pressure registers higher than normal
infarct ĭn-FĂRCT	area of tissue that undergoes necrosis following cessation of blood supply
ischemia ĭs-KĒ-mē-ă	local and temporary deficiency of blood supply owing to circulatory obstruction
mitral valve prolapse (MVP) MĪ-trăl, PRŌ-lăps	common and occasionally serious condition in which the leaflets of the mitral valve prolapse into the left atrium during systole; may cause nonanginal chest pain, palpitations, dyspnea, and fatigue
patent PĀ-tĕnt	open, unobstructed, or not closed (i.e., a patent artery)
patent ductus arteriosus PĀ-tĕnt DŬK-tŭs ăr-tē-rē-Ō-sŭs	failure of the ductus arteriosus to close after birth

DIAGNOSTIC, SYMPTOMATIC, AND RELATED TERMS (Continued)

Term	Meaning
tetralogy of Fallot tĕ-TRĂL-ō-jē, făl-Ō	congenital anomaly consisting of four elements (1) pulmonary artery stenosis; (2) interventricular septal defect; (3) transposition of the aorta, so that both ventricles empty into the aorta; (4) right ventricular hypertrophy caused by increased workload of the right ventricle
thrombus, thrombi (pl.) THRŎM-bŭs	blood clot that obstructs a vessel

Special Procedures

DIAGNOSTIC IMAGING PROCEDURES

Term	Description
aortography ā-or-TŎG-ră-fē	radiological examination of the aorta and its branches following the injection of a radiographic contrast medium via a catheter
cardiac catheterization KĂR-dē-ăk kăth-ĕ-tĕr-ĭ-ZĀ-shŭn	passage of a catheter into the heart through a vein or artery to evaluate valve function, septal defects, congenital anomalies, blood supply, or myocardial function
Doppler echocardiography DŎP-lĕr ĕk-ō-kăr-dē-ŎG-ră-fē	noninvasive adaptation of ultrasound technology, in which blood flow velocity is assessed in different areas of the heart. Sound waves strike moving red blood cells and are reflected back to a recording device that graphically records blood flow
echocardiography ĕk-ō-kăr-dē-ŎG-ră-fē	noninvasive diagnostic test using ultrasound to visualize internal cardiac structures and produce images of the heart. A transducer is placed on the chest to direct ultra-high–frequency sound waves toward cardiac structures. Reflected echoes are then converted to electrical impulses and displayed on a screen
phonocardiography fō-nō-kăr-dē-ŎG-ră-fē	provides a graphic display of heart sounds during the cardiac cycle. Transducer sends ultrasonic pulses through the chest wall, and the echoes are converted into images on a monitor to assess overall cardiac performance. An electrocardiograph is simultaneously displayed to provide a reference point for each of the sounds and their duration

DIAGNOSTIC IMAGING PROCEDURES (Continued)

Term	Description
ultrasonography ŭl-tră-sŏn-ŎG-ră-fē	used to produce an image or photograph of an organ or tissue; records ultrasonic echoes as they strike tissues of different densities
venography vē-NŎG-ră-fē	radiography of a vein after injection using a contrast medium; incomplete filling of a vein indicates obstruction

CLINICAL PROCEDURES

Term	Description
electrocardiogram (ECG, EKG) ē-lĕk-trō-KĂR-dē-ō-grăm	graphic record that shows the spread of electrical excitation to different parts of the heart; aids in diagnosing abnormal heart rhythms and myocardial damage
Holter monitor HŎL-tĕr	small portable ECG with a recording system capable of storing up to 24 hours of ECG recordings; particularly useful in obtaining a cardiac arrhythmia record that would be missed during an ECG of only a few minutes' duration
treadmill stress test	ECG taken under controlled exercise stress conditions; may show abnormal ECG tracings that do not appear during an ECG taken when the patient is resting

SURGICAL PROCEDURES

Term	Description
angioplasty ĂN-jē-ō-plăs-tē	reconstruction of a blood vessel
arterial anastomosis ăr-TĒ-rē-ăl ă-năs-tō-MŌ-sĭs	end-to-end union of two different arteries or two separate segments of the same artery
arterial biopsy ăr-TĒ-rē-ăl BI-ŏp-sē	removal and examination of a small segment of an arterial vessel wall; most frequently using temporal artery, but may use other arteries. Arterial biopsy most often confirms inflammation of the vessel wall, or arteritis, a type of vasculitis
atherectomy ăth-ĕr-ĔK-tō-mē	removal of material from an occluded vessel by using a specially designed radiological catheter

SURGICAL PROCEDURES (Continued)

Term	Description
intravascular thrombolysis ĭn-tră-VAS-kū-lăr thrŏm-BŎL-ĭ-sĭs	infusion of a thrombolytic agent to dissolve a vessel obstruction
ligation and stripping lī-GĀ-shŭn	tying a varicose vein followed by removal of the affected segment
percutaneous transluminal coronary angioplasty (PTCA) pĕr-kū-TĀ-nē-ŭs trăns-LŪ-mĭ-năl KOR-ō-nă-rē ĂN-jē-ō-plăs-tē	dilation of an occluded vessel by use of a balloon catheter under fluoroscopic guidance
pericardiocentesis pĕr-ĭ-kăr-dē-ō-sĕn-TĒ-sĭs	puncturing of the pericardium to remove fluid in order to test for protein, sugar, and enzymes or to determine the causative organism of pericarditis
phlebotomy, venipuncture flē-BŎT-ō-mē VĔN-ĭ-pŭnk-chŭr	incision of a vein to remove blood or introduce fluids or medications
valvotomy, mitral commissurotomy văl-VŎT-ō-mē, MI-trăl kŏm-ĭ-shŭr-ŎT-ō-mē	incision of a mitral valve to increase the size of the opening; used in treating mitral stenosis
vasoconstrictor infusion văs-ō-kŏn-STRĬK-tor ĭn-FŪ-zhŭn	infusion of a vasoconstrictor such as vasopressin via a radiological catheter to reduce blood flow to a lesion

LABORATORY PROCEDURES

Test	Description
cardiac enzyme studies KĂR-dē-ăk ĔN-zīm	blood test that assesses the concentration of three cardiac enzymes: glutamic oxaloacetic transaminase (GOT) (also called aspartate transaminase [AST]), CPK (also called creatine kinase [CK]), and LD, which are released by necrotic heart tissue. Each enzyme rises, peaks, and declines at predictable times after MI. These levels, along with a clinical evaluation and an ECG, help establish a diagnosis and extent of an MI
lipid profile LĬP-ĭd	panel of tests (glucose, total lipids, total cholesterol, triglycerides, phospholipids, and lipoprotein electrophoresis) used to assess risk factors of ischemic heart disease

PHARMACOLOGY

Medication	Action
antianginals	relieves angina pectoris by expanding the blood vessels of the heart; most common drug in this category is nitroglycerin
antihypertensives	agents used to lower blood pressure
beta-adrenergic blocking agents, beta blockers	agents used to relieve cardiac arrhythmias, angina pectoris, postmyocardial hypertension, and migraine headaches
calcium channel blockers	agents that selectively block the flow of calcium ions in the heart and are used to treat angina pectoris, some arrhythmias, and some forms of hypertension
diuretics	agents that reduce body fluid volume by stimulating urine flow; considered first step in management of hypertension
heparin	anticoagulant used in preventing and treating thrombosis and embolism
inotropics, cardiotonics	agents that alter the force of heart's contraction; used to treat cardiac arrhythmias and cardiac failure
vasodilators	drugs to expand blood vessels, used to treat angina pectoris and hypertension
peripheral vasodilators	agents used to expand blood vessels in the extremities and decrease blood pressure; also used to treat poor peripheral circulation and reduce pain caused by atherosclerosis

ABBREVIATIONS

Abbreviation	Meaning
ACG	angiocardiography
AS	aortic stenosis
ASD	atrial septal defect
ASHD	arteriosclerotic heart disease
BBB	bundle branch block
BP	blood pressure
CAD	coronary artery disease
CC	cardiac catheterization

ABBREVIATIONS (Continued)

Abbreviation	Meaning
CCU	coronary care unit
CHF	congestive heart failure
CPR	cardiopulmonary resuscitation
CV	cardiovascular
DVT	deep vein thrombosis
ECG, EKG	electrocardiogram
MI	myocardial infarction
MS	mitral stenosis
MVP	mitral valve prolapse
PAT	paroxysmal atrial tachycardia
PTCA	percutaneous transluminal coronary angioplasty
PVCs	premature ventricular contractions
SA	sinoatrial (node)
VSD	ventricular septal defect

Laboratory	Meaning
AST	aspartate transaminase
CK	creatine kinase
CPK	creatine phosphokinase
GOT	glutamic oxaloacetic transaminase
LD	lactic dehydrogenase
HDL	high-density lipoprotein
LDL	low-density lipoprotein
VLDL	very low–density lipoproteins

Case Study

Acute Myocardial Infarction

History of Present Illness. The patient is a 68-year-old woman hospitalized for **acute** anterior **myocardial infarction.** She had a history of sudden onset of chest pain. Approximately 2 hours before hospitalization she had severe **substernal pain** with radiation to the back. **ECG** showed evidence of abnormalities. She was given **streptokinase** and treated with **heparin** at 800 units per hour. She will be evaluated with a **partial thromboplastin time** and **cardiac enzymes** in the morning.

The patient had been seen in 19XX, with a history of an inferior MI in approximately 19XX or 19XX, but was stable and underwent a **treadmill test,** the results of which showed no **ischemia** and she had no chest pain. Her records confirmed an MI with **enzyme elevation** and evidence of a previous inferior MI.

At this time the patient is stable, is in the **CCU,** and will be given appropriate follow-up and supportive care.

Impression. **Acute lateral** anterior myocardial infarction and old healed inferior MI.

Worksheet 5 provides a dictionary and reading application and an analysis of this case study.

Worksheet 1

Use ather/o (fatty plaque) to build a medical word meaning:

1. a tumor of fatty plaque _____

2. condition of hardening of fatty plaque _____

Use phleb/o (vein) to build a medical word meaning:

3. inflammation of a vein _____

4. hardening of a vein (wall) _____

5. abnormal condition of a blood clot in a vein _____

Use ven/o (vein) to build a medical word meaning:

6. abnormal condition of hardening of a vein _____

7. spasm of a vein _____

8. pertaining to a vein _____

9. narrowing of a vein _____

Use cardi/o (heart) to build a medical word meaning:

10. enlargement of the heart _____

11. inflammation of the inner (lining) heart _____

12. inflammation of the epicardium _____

13. pertaining to the heart and lung _____

14. pertaining to heart (and blood) vessels _____

15. inflammation of the heart muscle _____

16. disease of the heart muscle _____

Use arteri/o (artery) to build a medical word meaning:

17. condition of hardening of the artery _____

18. spasm of the artery _____

19. rupture of an artery _____

20. pertaining to an artery _____

Worksheet 2

Build a surgical term meaning:

1. incision of the heart _____

2. puncture of the heart _____

3. fixation of a vein (in varicocele) _____

4. suture of an artery _____

5. (partial) excision of the pericardium _____

6. incision of a vein _____

7. surgical repair of an artery _____

8. surgical repair of a vessel _____

9. removal of an embolus _____

10. suture of a vein _____

Worksheet 3

Match the following words with the definitions in the numbered list.

Adams-Stokes syndrome   hypertension
aneurysm   hypotension
coarctation   infarction
extravascular   ischemia
fibrillations   patent
hyperlipidemia   thrombus

1. _____ narrowing of a vessel, especially the aorta

2. _____ outside a vessel

3. _____ high blood pressure

4. _____ altered state of consciousness owing to decreased blood flow to the brain

5. _____ open, unobstructed

6. _____ blood clot that obstructs a vessel

7. _____ local and temporary deficiency in blood supply

8. _____ quivering or spontaneous muscle contractions, especially in the heart

9. _____ excessive amounts of lipids in the blood

10. _____ local abnormal dilation of a vessel, usually an artery

Worksheet 4

SPECIAL PROCEDURES, PHARMACOLOGY, AND ABBREVIATIONS

Select the word(s) that best describes the following statements:

antianginals

arterial biopsy

arterial anastomosis

beta blockers

cardiac enzyme studies

diuretics

echocardiography

electrocardiography (ECG, EKG)

inotropics, cardiotonics

ligation and stripping

MI

MS

pericardiocentesis

phlebography, venography

phonocardiography

treadmill stress test
  vasodilators

1. _____ procedure that uses ultrasound to assess the structure of the heart

2. _____ procedure that graphically records the heart's electrical impulses on a paper strip

3. _____ puncturing the pericardium to remove fluid in order to test for protein, sugar, and LD or to determine the causative organism of pericarditis

4. _____ mitral stenosis

5. _____ medication to relieve chest pain

6. _____ drugs that affect the force of muscular contraction of the heart

7. _____ series of blood tests that establish a diagnosis and extent of MI

8. _____ radiographic study to identify and locate thrombi in the leg veins

9. _____ reduces heart workload by blocking the activity of epinephrine and norepinephrine

10. _____ measures the efficiency of the heart when subjected to a predetermined exercise

11. _____ specialized microphone records and graphically displays the sounds of the heart to assess abnormal acoustic events

12. _____ myocardial infarction

13. _____ tying off of a varicose vein, followed by removal of the affected segment

14. _____ end-to-end union of two different arteries or two separate segments of the same artery

15. _____ excision of a specimen of an arterial vessel wall for examination and testing

Worksheet 5

ACUTE MYOCARDIAL INFARCTION DICTIONARY EXERCISE

Use a medical dictionary or other resource to define the terms and to determine their pronunciation; then practice reading the case study aloud (p. 163).

acute _____

cardiac enzymes _____

CCU _____

ECG _____

enzyme elevation _____

heparin _____

infarction _____

ischemia _____

lateral _____

myocardial _____

partial thromboplastin time _____

streptokinase _____

substernal pain _____

treadmill _____

ANALYSIS OF CASE STUDY: ACUTE MYOCARDIAL INFARCTION

1. How long had the patient experienced chest pain before she was seen in the hospital?

2. Did she have a previous history of chest pain?   .

3. What are the cardiac enzymes that are tested to confirm the diagnosis of MI?

4. Initially, what medications were administered to stabilize the patient?

5. During the current admission, what part of the heart was damaged?

6. Was the location of damage to the heart for this admission the same as for the initial MI?

Worksheet 6

Label the structures indicated on the following diagram, and check your answers against Figure 9–3.

Aorta

Inferior vena cava

Right ventricle

Left pulmonary artery

Left atrium

Left pulmonary veins

Left ventricle

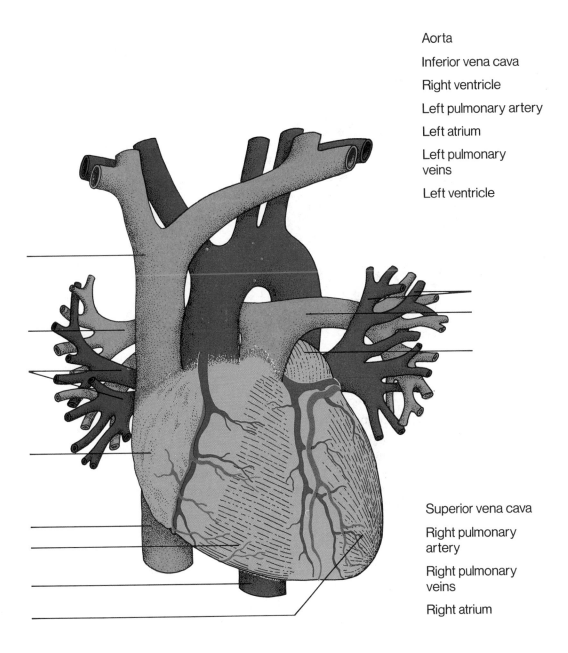

Superior vena cava

Right pulmonary artery

Right pulmonary veins

Right atrium

Worksheet 7

Label the structures indicated on the following diagram, and check your answers against Figure 9–4.

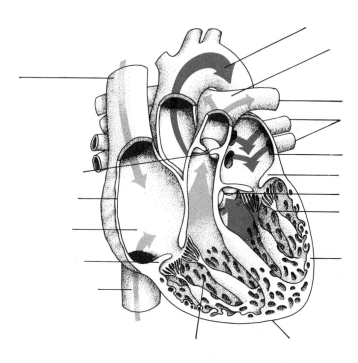

Aorta	Left pulmonary artery	Right atrium
Bicuspid valve	Left ventricle	Right ventricle
Endocardium	Myocardium	Semilunar or aortic valve
Epicardium	Pulmonary artery	Superior vena cava
Inferior vena cava	Pulmonary semilunar valve	Tricuspid valve
Left atrium	Pulmonary veins	

Chapter 10

Blood and Lymphatic System

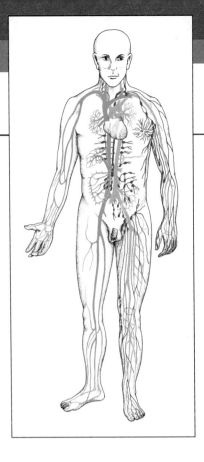

Chapter Outline

Student Objectives

Upon completion of this chapter, you will be able to do the following:

Describe the appearance and function of blood cells.

List the components of blood plasma, and briefly explain the function of plasma.

Describe the functions of the lymphatic system, and explain the relationship between plasma and lymph.

Briefly describe how protection is provided by each of the five types of white blood cells.

List the major blood groups, and explain their importance in clinical laboratory testing.

Identify combining forms, suffixes, and prefixes related to the blood and lymphatic system.

Identify and discuss pathology related to the blood and lymphatic system.

Identify diagnostic imaging, surgical and laboratory procedures, and abbreviations related to the blood and lymphatic system.

Discuss pharmacology related to the treatment of disorders of the blood and lymphatic system.

Demonstrate your knowledge of the chapter by completing the worksheets.

Anatomy and Physiology

Blood and lymph are specialized tissues of the body (Fig. 10–1). Both are composed of cells suspended in a liquid medium and both play a vital role in defending the body against infection. Because blood and lymph have the ability to move throughout the entire body, they provide a transportation system for body cells.

BLOOD

Blood is composed of a liquid medium called plasma and a solid portion that consists of three major types of blood cells: red blood cells **(erythrocytes),** white blood cells **(leukocytes),** and platelets **(thrombocytes).** Most blood cells in adults are formed in the bone marrow **(myelogenic)** tissue of the skull, ribs, sternum, vertebrae, and pelvis, as well as at the ends of the long bones of the arms and legs, but some white blood cells originate in lymphatic tissue.

Blood cells develop from an undifferentiated cell, the **hemocytoblast,** also called a stem cell (Fig. 10–2). The development and maturation of different blood cells is called **hematopoiesis.** Red blood cell development is called **erythropoiesis,** white blood cell development **leukopoiesis,** and platelet development **thrombopoiesis.** When blood cells mature, they enter the circulatory system. Figure 10–3 illustrates the composition of whole blood.

Erythrocytes

Erythrocytes are the most numerous of the circulating blood cells. During erythropoiesis, they develop a specialized iron-containing compound called **hemoglobin,** which gives

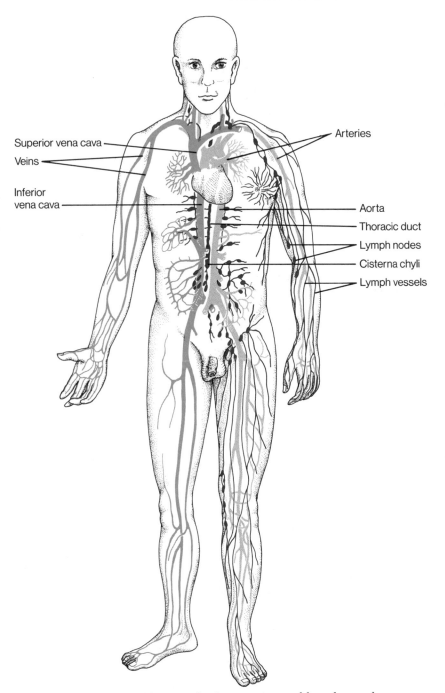

Figure 10–1   Diagram of veins, arteries, and lymph vessels.

them their red color. Hemoglobin carries oxygen (O_2) to body tissues, where it is exchanged for carbon dioxide (CO_2). The millions of hemoglobin molecules in each of the trillions of red blood cells attest to the magnitude of the job performed by erythrocytes. During erythropoiesis, the red blood cell decreases in size. Just before maturity, the nucleus passes from the cell. It leaves behind a small fragment of nuclear material that resembles a fine,

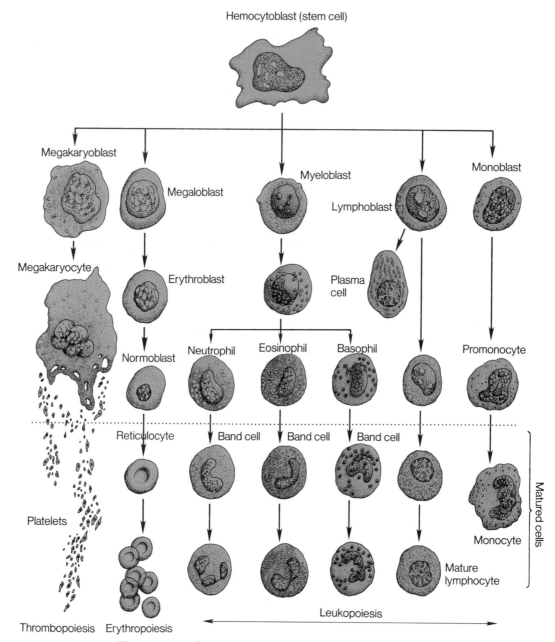

Hemocytoblast (stem cell)

Megakaryoblast

Megaloblast

Myeloblast

Lymphoblast

Monoblast

Megakaryocyte

Erythroblast

Plasma cell

Normoblast

Neutrophil   Eosinophil   Basophil

Promonocyte

Reticulocyte   Band cell   Band cell   Band cell

Monocyte

Platelets

Mature lymphocyte

Matured cells

Thrombopoiesis   Erythropoiesis

Leukopoiesis

Figure 10–2   The maturation of blood cells—hematopoiesis.

lacy net, which gives this cell its name, **reticulocyte.** Eventually, all of the nuclear material disappears and the mature erythrocyte enters the circulatory system.

Erythrocytes live about 120 days and then rupture, releasing hemoglobin and cell fragments. Hemoglobin breaks down into **hemosiderin,** a compound that contains iron, and several bile pigments. Most of the hemosiderin returns to the bone marrow and is used to manufacture new blood cells. The bile pigments are eventually excreted by the liver.

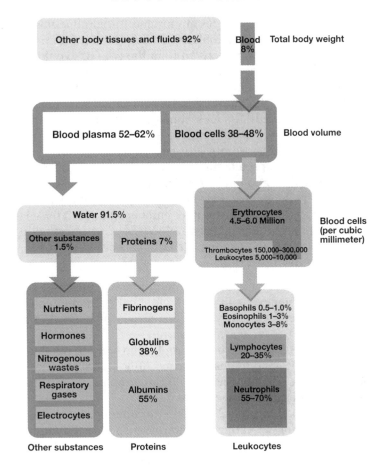

Figure 10–3 Components of blood and the relationship of blood to other body tissues. (Adapted from Scanlon, VC and Sanders, T: Essentials of Anatomy and Physiology, ed 2. FA Davis, Philadelphia, 1995, p 245, with permission.)

Leukocytes

The chief function of leukocytes is to protect the body against invasion of bacteria and foreign substances. Unlike erythrocytes, which remain exclusively in the vascular system, leukocytes are able to pass through capillary walls. They wander through tissue spaces to infection sites, where they destroy harmful substances and produce substances that aid in tissue repair.

Leukocytes are divided into two categories, depending on whether or not they have granules in their cytoplasm: **granulocytes** (those with granules) and **agranulocytes** (those without granules). Both of these categories are subdivided, as shown in Table 10–1.

Table 10–1   **Protection Provided by Leukocytes**

Granulocytes	Agranulocytes
neutrophils (phagocytic)	monocytes (phagocytic)
eosinophils (detoxification)	lymphocytes (immunologic)
basophils (release of substances that increase circulation)	B cells (humoral immunity)
	T cells (cellular immunity)

Granulocytes. Granulocytes are formed in red bone marrow from stem cells, which give rise to **myeloblasts.** Myeloblasts in turn develop into neutrophils, eosinophils, and basophils. These names are derived from the type of dye that stains the cytoplasmic granules when a blood smear is stained in the laboratory. In addition to the presence of granules, these cells are further characterized by a nucleus that is composed of several lobes in their mature form; hence, these cells are also called **polymorphonuclear** cells.

The neutrophil, the most numerous of the circulating white cells, is very motile and highly phagocytic, permitting it to ingest and devour bacteria and other particulate matter. Eosinophils and basophils, although capable of phagocytosis, rarely display this activity.

Eosinophils protect the body by releasing many substances that are capable of neutralizing toxic compounds, especially of a chemical nature. Eosinophils increase in number during allergic reactions and animal parasite infestations.

Basophils release **histamines** and **heparin** when tissue is damaged. Histamines initiate inflammation, which increases blood flow, to bring additional blood cells to damaged tissue for repair and healing. Heparin acts on blood vessels in the area of damaged tissue by preventing blood from clotting.

Agranulocytes. Agranulocytes include **monocytes** and **lymphocytes.** These cells have a single large nucleus and are therefore called **mononuclear cells.** In early development, monocytes and lymphocytes migrate from the bone marrow and enter the lymphatic system, where they change and mature.

Monocytes provide protection for the body in much the same manner as neutrophils; that is, by engaging in phagocytosis. After monocytes leave the vascular system and enter tissue spaces, they are then called **macrophages.** In this form, they can consume large numbers of bacteria and cellular debris.

Lymphocytes protect through immunologic activity. Two types of lymphocytes are responsible for activating an immune response: **T lymphocytes (T cells)** and **B lymphocytes (B cells).** B cells are believed to mature in bone marrow, and T cells mature in the thymus gland. T cells use one mode of attack called **cellular immunity;** B cells use another called **humoral immunity.** T cells determine a specific weakness of the invading foreign substance or **antigen** and use this weakness as a point of attack to destroy the antigen. B cells produce a clone of cells called **plasma cells** that produce proteins called **antibodies.** Antibodies enter the circulatory system and travel throughout the body. When antibodies encounter an antigen, they destroy it, neutralize it, or render it harmless.

A memory component in the immune system allows an immediate disposal of the same antigen if it is encountered again. Memory cells are produced by B and T cells during the initial exposure to an antigen. These memory cells migrate to and remain in lymphoid tissue. In the event of future exposures to the same antigen, memory cells "recall" how they previously disposed of the antigen and repeat the process. Disposing of the antigen during the second and all subsequent exposures is extremely rapid and much more effective than it was during the first exposure.

Thrombocytes

The smallest formed elements within the blood are thrombocytes, or platelets (so named for their small platelike appearance). The purpose of thrombocytes is to initiate blood clotting when injury occurs.

Blood clotting is not a single reaction, but rather a chain of interlinked reactions. At least 13 separate steps are involved, but these steps can be combined into three major reactions, as shown here.

Platelet factors Calcium ions Other clotting factors	Thromboplastin →	Prothrombin activator
Prothrombin Calcium ions	Prothrombin activator →	Thrombin
Fibrinogen (soluble)	Thrombin →	Fibrin (insoluble)

Stage 1. Thromboplastin may be either released by traumatized tissue at the injury site or formed when platelets rupture. Thromboplastin and other blood clotting factors combine with calcium ions to form prothrombin activator.

Stage 2. Prothrombin activator reacts with prothrombin and calcium ions to form thrombin.

Stage 3. Thrombin converts the soluble blood protein fibrinogen to fibrin. Fibrin, a thread-like insoluble protein, forms a meshwork entangling blood cells and platelets. This jelly-like mass of protein, blood cells, and platelets is known as a blood clot.

Plasma

Plasma is the liquid portion of the blood in which blood cells are suspended. It is composed of about 92 percent water and contains the plasma proteins (albumins, globulins, and fibrinogen), gases, nutrients, salts, hormones, and excretory products. Plasma makes possible the chemical communication between all body cells by carrying these products to different parts of the body. When free of blood cells, plasma is a thin, almost colorless fluid.

Blood serum is a product of blood plasma. It differs from plasma only in that it does not contain fibrinogen, which can be represented as follows:

Plasma − Fibrinogen = Serum

When a blood sample is placed in a test tube and permitted to clot, the resulting clear fluid that remains after the removal of the clot from the test tube is serum. The formation of the clot has removed fibrinogen from the plasma.

Blood Groups

Human blood is divided into four groups based on the presence or absence of blood antigens **(agglutinogens)** on the surface of red blood cells. These four groups are A, B, AB, and O. Type A blood has A antigen; type B blood, B antigen; type AB blood, both A and B antigens; and type O has neither A nor B antigens. In each of these four blood groups, the plasma does not contain the antibody **(agglutinin)** against the antigen that is present on

Table 10–2 **Agglutinogens and Agglutinins of the ABO System**

Blood Type	Agglutinogen (RBC Antigen)	Agglutinin (Plasma Antibody)
type A	A	anti-B
type B	B	anti-A
type AB	A and B	none
type O	None	anti-A and anti-B

the red blood cells. Rather, the plasma contains the opposite antibodies. These antibodies occur naturally; that is, they are present even though there has been no exposure to the antigen (Table 10–2).

In addition to the blood groups just listed, there are numerous other antigens that may be present on red blood cells. One such factor includes the Rh blood group. This particular factor may cause hemolytic disease of the newborn (HDN) because of an incompatibility between maternal and fetal blood.

Although more than 300 different blood antigens have been identified by hematologists, most of these are not highly antigenic and do not cause concern in pregnancy or transfusions.

LYMPHATIC SYSTEM

The lymphatic system consists of a fluid called lymph and a network of transporting structures called lymph vessels, lymph nodes, the spleen, thymus, and tonsils. The primary function of the lymphatic system is to drain fluid from tissue spaces and return it to the blood. Other functions provided by the lymphatic system include transporting materials (nutrients, hormones, and oxygen) to body cells and carrying waste products from body tissues back to the bloodstream. The lymphatic system also transports lipids away from the digestive organs. Finally, it aids in the control of infection by providing lymphocytes and monocytes, which defend against infections caused by microorganisms.

Lymph originates from blood plasma. As whole blood circulates through the capillaries, some of the plasma seeps out of these thin-walled vessels. This fluid, now called interstitial fluid, or tissue fluid, resembles plasma, except that it contains less protein. Interstitial fluid nourishes and cleanses the body tissues through which it circulates. It also collects cellular debris, bacteria, and particulate matter. Eventually, interstitial fluid either returns to blood capillaries or enters into blind-ended vessels called lymph capillaries (Fig. 10–4). Once it enters a lymph capillary it is called lymph. Lymph passes from capillaries to larger vessels and to lymph nodes, which serve as depositories for cellular debris. As lymph passes through the nodes it is filtered and replenished with lymphocytes and antibodies. Bacteria and debris are phagocytized by macrophages that line the nodes. When a local infection exists, the number of bacteria entering a node is so great that the node frequently enlarges and becomes tender.

Lymph vessels from the right chest and arm join the right lymphatic duct. This duct drains into the right subclavian vein, a major vessel in the cardiovascular system. Lymph from all other parts of the body enters the thoracic duct and drains into the left subclavian

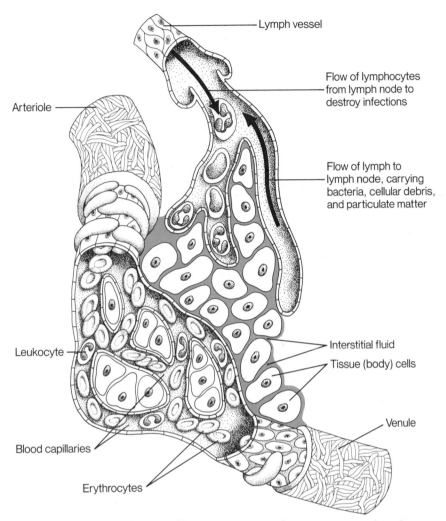

Lymph vessel

Flow of lymphocytes from lymph node to destroy infections

Flow of lymph to lymph node, carrying bacteria, cellular debris, and particulate matter

Arteriole

Interstitial fluid

Tissue (body) cells

Leukocyte

Venule

Blood capillaries

Erythrocytes

Figure 10–4 As plasma seeps from capillaries into surrounding tissue, it is referred to as *interstitial fluid,* or *tissue fluid.* When it finally enters into the blind-ended lymph vessels, it is called *lymph.*

vein. Lymph is redeposited into the circulating blood and becomes plasma. This cycle repeats itself over and over (Fig. 10–5).

The three organs associated with the lymphatic system are the spleen, thymus gland, and tonsils. Like lymph nodes, the spleen acts as a filter for lymph. Phagocytic cells within the spleen lining remove cellular debris, bacteria, parasites, and other infectious agents, thereby cleansing the lymph. The spleen also destroys old red blood cells and serves as a repository for healthy blood cells that are placed into circulation when needed.

The thymus gland is located in the mediastinum, the upper part of the chest. It partially controls the immune system. The thymus changes lymphocytes to T cells, which provide cellular immunity, as described previously.

Tonsils are masses of lymphatic tissue that act as a filter to protect the body from invasion by pathogens. They also aid in the development of leukocytes.

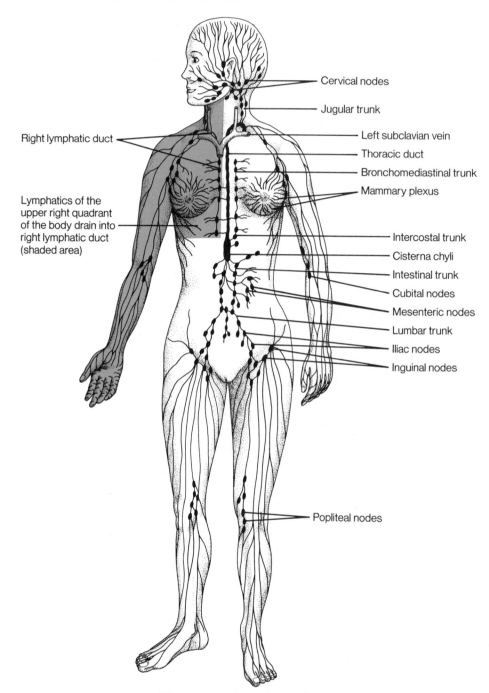

Figure 10–5 Lymphatic system.

COMBINING FORMS

Combining Form	Meaning	Example	Pronunciation
aden/o	gland	aden/o/pathy — disease	ăd-ĕ-NŎP-ăh-thē
blast/o	embryonic cell	erythr/o/blast/osis — red — abnormal condition	ĕ-rĭth-rō-blăs-TŌ-sĭs
chrom/o	color	hypo/chrom/ic — decrease — pertaining to	hī-pō-KRŌM-ĭk
eosin/o	dawn (rose colored)	eosin/o/phil — attraction to	ē-ō-SĬN-ō-fĭl
erythr/o	red	erythr/o/cyte — cell	ĕ-RĬTH-rō-sīt
granul/o	granule	granul/o/cyte — cell	GRĂN-ū-lō-sīt
hem/o ⎫ hemat/o ⎭	blood	hem/o/lysis — destruction hemat/oma — tumor	hē-MŎL-ĭ-sĭs hē-mă-TŌ-mă
immun/o	safe	immun/o/logist — specialist in the study	ĭm-ŭ-NŎL-ō-jĭst
kary/o ⎫ nucle/o ⎭	nucleus	kary/o/lysis — destruction nucle/ar — pertaining to	kăr-ē-ŌL-ĭ-sĭs NU-klē-ăr
leuk/o	white	leuk/o/cyte — cell	LOO-kō-sīt
lymph/o	lymph	lymph/oma — tumor	lĭm-FŌ-măh
morph/o	shape	morph/o/logy — study of	mŏr-FŎL-ō-jē
myel/o	bone marrow, spinal cord	myel/oid — resembling	MĪ-ĕ-loid

COMBINING FORMS (Continued)

Combining Form	Meaning	Example	Pronunciation
phag/o	swallowing, eating	phag/o/cyte cell	FĂG-ō-sīt
poikil/o	varied, irregular	poikil/o/cyte cell	POY-kĭl-ō-sīt
reticul/o	net, mesh	reticul/o/cyte cell	rĕ-TĬK-ū-lō-sīt
sider/o	iron	hem/o/sider/osis blood abnormal condition	hē-mō-sĭd-ĕr-Ō-sĭs
splen/o	spleen	splen/o/megaly enlargement	splē-nō-MĔG-ăh-lē
thromb/o	blood clot	thromb/o/lysis destruction	thrŏm-BŎL-ĭ-sĭs
thym/o	thymus	thym/ectomy excision	thī-MĔK-tō-mē

SUFFIXES

Suffix	Meaning	Example	Pronunciation
-blast	embryonic cell	myel/o/blast bone marrow	MĪ-ĕl-ō-blăst
-globin	protein	hem/o/globin blood	hē-mō-GLŌ-bĭn
-emia	blood condition	an/ emia without	ă-NĒ-mē-ăh
-osis	abnormal condition, abnormal increase (when used with blood cells)	erythr/o/cyt/osis red cell	ĕ-rĭth-rō-sī-TŌ-sĭs
-penia	decrease, deficiency	leuk/o/cyt/o/penia white cell	loo-kō-sī-tō-PĒ-nē-ăh
-phil	attraction to	eosin/o/phil eosin (dye)	ē-ŏ-SĬN-ō-fĭl
-phoresis	borne, carried	electr/o/phoresis electricity	ē-lĕk-trō-fō-RĒ-sĭs

SUFFIXES (Continued)

Suffix	Meaning	Example	Pronunciation
-poiesis	formation, production	hem/o/poiesis blood	hē-mō-poy-Ē-sĭs
-stasis	standing still	hem/o/stasis blood	hē-mō-STĀ-sĭs

PREFIXES

Prefix	Meaning	Example	Pronunciation
a-	without, not	a/granul/o/cyte granule cell	ă-GRĂN-ŭ-lō-sīt
aniso-	unequal, dissimilar	aniso/cyt/osis cell abnormal condition	ăn-ī-sō-sī-TŌ-sĭs
hetero-	different	hetero/phil attraction to	HĔT-ĕr-ō-fĭl
homo-	same	homo/graft transplant	HŌ-mō-grăft
iso-	same	iso/chrom/ic color pertaining to	ī-sō-KRŌ-mĭk
macro-	large	macr/o/cyt/ic cell pertaining to	măk-rō-SĬ-tĭk
micro-	small	micr/o/cyt/osis cell abnormal increase	mī-krō-sī-TŌ-sĭs
mono-	one	mono/cyte cell	MŎN-ō-sīt
poly-	many, much	poly/morph/o/nucle/ar shape nucleus pertaining to	pŏl-ē-mor-fō-NŪ-klē-ăr

Pathology

ANEMIAS

Anemia is any condition in which the oxygen-carrying capacity of blood is reduced. It is not a disease but rather a symptom of various diseases. It is caused when there is a decrease in the number of circulating red blood cells **(erythropenia),** a decrease in the amount of hemoglobin within them, or a decrease in the volume of packed erythrocytes **(hematocrit).**

Anemias are identified according to their etiology or by the appearance of the erythrocytes. In healthy individuals, red blood cells **(RBCs)** fall within a normal reference range as to size **(normocytic)** and amount of hemoglobin **(normochromic).** Variations from these normal values include RBCs that are excessively large **(macrocytic)** or excessively small

Table 10–3   **Morphology and Etiology of Common Anemias**

Causes of Various Common Anemias	Appearance of RBCs
excessive blood loss (acute or chronic hemorrhage)	normochromic, normocytic
bone marrow failure (hypoplastic, aplastic)	
hemolytic anemias (RBC defects)	
extra erythrocytic factors (infections, systemic diseases, autoimmune reactions)	
iron deficiency, thalassemia	microcytic, hypochromic
vitamin B_{12} deficiency, folic acid deficiency	microcytic, normochromic
gastric resection, intestinal anastomosis, parasites	macrocytic, hypochromic

(microcytic) or have decreased amounts of hemoglobin **(hypochromic).** Some of the causes of anemias include excessive blood loss, excessive blood cell destruction, decrease blood formation, and faulty hemoglobin production. Table 10–3 summarizes some of the types of anemias according to morphology and etiology.

The signs and symptoms associated with most anemias include difficulty in breathing **(dyspnea),** weakness, rapid heart beat **(tachycardia),** paleness **(pallor),** low blood pressure **(hypotension),** and often a slight fever.

ACQUIRED IMMUNODEFICIENCY SYNDROME

Acquired immunodeficiency syndrome (AIDS) is a transmissible infectious disease caused by the human immunodeficiency virus (HIV), which slowly destroys the immune system. Eventually the immune system becomes so weak **(compromised)** that in the final stage of the disease, the patient falls victim to disorders that usually do not affect healthy individuals.

The disease was first identified in 1981 in homosexual men. Since that time, it has been found throughout the world and in all populations. In the United States, homosexuals, bisexuals, and intravenous drug users constitute the highest risk group. However, the number of cases in heterosexual women, adolescents, and babies is rising. Statistics released in 1992 by the Centers for Disease Control (CDC) indicate that one in every 100 adult men and one in every 600 adult women is infected with HIV.

Transmission of HIV occurs primarily through the exchange of body fluids—mostly blood, semen, and vaginal secretions. The virus attacks the most important cell in the immune system, the helper T cell. Once infected by HIV, the helper T cell becomes a "mini-factory" for the replication of the virus. The incubation time from exposure to manifesting the signs and symptoms of AIDS may be quite long, usually about 7 to 10 years. Antibodies to the disease begin to appear in the blood **(seroconversion)** about 3 months after exposure. Although these antibodies are ineffective in destroying HIV, they are useful in serological tests used to diagnose the infection.

Eventually the entire immune system is affected and no longer functions. Gradually the patient begins to display the symptoms of AIDS: swollen lymph glands **(lymphadenopathy),** malaise, fever, night sweats, and weight loss. Infections caused by organisms that are normally considered harmless **(opportunistic infections)** become established in the patient. Kaposi's sarcoma, a neoplastic disorder, and *Pneumocystis carinii* pneumonia

(PCP) are two very important diseases associated with AIDS. The immune system ultimately fails, and the patient dies. There is no effective treatment, nor are vaccines available. Controlling the spread of the disease depends on avoiding behaviors that cause its spread.

AUTOIMMUNE DISEASES

Failure of the body to distinguish accurately between what is self and what is nonself leads to a phenomenon called **autoimmunity.** In this abnormal immunologic response, the body produces antibodies against antigens found on its own cells. The antibodies attack the antigens to such an extent that it causes tissue injury. Types of autoimmune disorders range from those that affect only a single organ to those that affect many organs and tissues **(multisystemic).**

Myasthenia gravis is an autoimmune disorder that affects the neuromuscular junction. Muscles of the limbs and eyes and those affecting speech and swallowing are usually involved. Other autoimmune diseases include **rheumatoid arthritis, idiopathic thrombocytopenic purpura (ITP), vasculitis,** and **systemic lupus erythematosus (SLE).** Treatment consists of attempting to reach a balance between suppressing the immune response in order to avoid tissue damage while still maintaining the immune mechanism sufficiently to protect against disease. Administration of steroids is often the chosen treatment. Most autoimmune diseases have periods of flare-ups **(exacerbations)** and remissions **(latent periods).**

EDEMA

Edema is an abnormal accumulation of fluids in the intercellular spaces of the body. One of the major conditions that cause edema is a decrease in the blood protein level **(hypoproteinemia).** This lowers osmotic pressure within the blood. Consequently, large amounts of plasma pass out of blood vessels and into the surrounding tissues. Other causes of edema include poor lymph drainage, increased capillary permeability, and congestive heart failure.

Edema limited to a specific area **(localized edema)** may be relieved by elevation of that body part and application of cold packs. Systemic edema may be treated with medications that promote urination **(diuretics).**

Closely associated with edema is a condition called **ascites,** in which fluid collects within the peritoneal cavity. The chief causes of ascites are interference in venous return during cardiac disease, obstruction of lymphatic flow, disturbances in electrolyte balance, and liver disease.

HEMOPHILIA

Hemophilia is a hereditary disorder in which the blood clotting mechanism is impaired. It results from the failure of prothrombin to form thrombin. The disease is sex-linked and found most often in men. Women are the carriers of the trait but generally do not have symptoms of the disease.

Patients with hemophilia lack factor VIII **(antihemophilic factor [AHF]),** an essential blood clotting factor. The amount and site of bleeding depends on the degree of deficiency.

Mild symptoms include nosebleeds, easy bruising, and bleeding from the gums. Severe symptoms produce **hematomas** deep within muscles. If blood enters joints, it is associated with pain and possible permanent deformity. Uncontrolled bleeding any place in the body may lead to shock and death.

INFECTIOUS MONONUCLEOSIS

One of the acute infections caused by the Epstein-Barr virus (EBV) is **infectious mononucleosis.** It is found mostly in young adults and appears in greater frequency in early spring and early fall. This disease is characterized by a sore throat, fever, and enlarged cervical lymph nodes. Other signs and symptoms include gum infection **(gingivitis),** headache, tiredness, loss of appetite **(anorexia),** and general malaise. Occasionally, the liver and spleen enlarge **(hepatomegaly** and **splenomegaly).** Less common clinical findings include hemolytic anemia with jaundice, thrombocytopenia, and occasionally a ruptured spleen **(splenorrhexis).** Recovery usually ensures a lasting immunity.

ONCOLOGY

Leukemias

The major oncological disorder of the blood-forming organs is leukemia. With this condition, healthy bone marrow cells are replaced by malignant cells. The disease may be generally categorized as to the type of leukocyte population affected, that is, granulocytic (myelogenous) or **lymphocytic.** The overgrowth **(proliferation)** of malignant cells may be either chronic or acute. In acute leukemias, the cells are highly embryonic **(blastic)** and the disease is more severe. In chronic leukemias, the cells are more mature and the disease is less severe. All forms of leukemias, if left untreated, are usually fatal.

The most common type of leukemia in adults is **acute myelogenous leukemia (AML).** The survival rate with this type of leukemia, even with very aggressive treatment, is poor, and most individuals die within 1 year after diagnosis.

Acute lymphocytic leukemia (ALL) is primarily a disease of children. Some predisposing factors associated with acute forms of leukemia are ionizing radiation, viruses, genetic predisposition, and chemicals.

Chronic myelogenous leukemia (CML) is associated with a unique chromosome called the Philadelphia (Ph') chromosome. The onset of CML is usually between 40 and 50 years old.

Chronic lymphocytic leukemia (CLL) is found primarily in patients older than 50 years of age.

Hodgkin's Disease

Hodgkin's disease is a malignant disease that primarily affects the lymph nodes **(lymphadenopathy).** However, the spleen, gastrointestinal tract, liver, or bone marrow may also be involved.

Hodgkin's disease usually begins with a painless enlargement of lymph nodes, usually on one side of the neck. Other symptoms include itching **(pruritus),** weight loss, progressive anemia, and fever. If nodes in the neck become excessively large, they may press on the trachea, causing difficulty in breathing **(dyspnea),** or on the esophagus, causing difficulty in swallowing **(dysphagia).**

Radiation and chemotherapy are important methods of controlling the disease. Newer methods of treatment include bone marrow transplants.

DIAGNOSTIC, SYMPTOMATIC, AND RELATED TERMS

Term	Meaning
anisocytosis ăn-ī-sō-sī-TŌ-sĭs	condition of marked variation in size of erythrocytes
antibody ĂN-tĭ-bŏd-ē	immunoglobulin produced by B lymphocytes in response to the presence of an antigen
antigen ĂN-tĭ-jĕn	usually a protein marker on the surface of cells that identifies the cell as self or nonself and can cause the formation of antibodies
ascites ă-SĪ-tēz	collection of serous fluid in the peritoneal cavity
coagulopathy kō-ăg-ū-LŎP-ă-thē	disease affecting the clotting mechanism of the blood
dyscrasia dĭs-KRĀ-zē-ăh	any blood abnormality
edema e-DĒ-mă	localized or general condition in which body tissues contain an excessive amount of tissue fluid
graft versus host reaction (GVHR) grăft	pathological reaction between the host and grafted tissue, resulting in rejection of a transplanted tissue
hemolysis hē-MŎL-ĭ-sĭs	destruction of erythrocytes with a release of hemoglobin that diffuses into the surrounding fluid
hemostasis hē-MŎS-tă-sĭs	arrest of bleeding or circulation
lymphadenopathy lĭm-făd-ĕ-NŎP-ă-thē	disease of the lymph nodes
lymphosarcoma lĭm-fō-săr-KŌ-măh	malignant neoplastic disorder of lymphatic tissue, not related to Hodgkin's disease
seroconversion SĔR-ō-kon-VER-zhŭn	development of detectable antibodies in serum as a result of infection or immunization
serology sē-RŎL-ō-jē	study of blood serum, especially antigen-antibody reactions

Special Procedures

DIAGNOSTIC IMAGING PROCEDURES

Term	Description
lymphadenography lĭm-făd-ĕ-NŎG-ră-fē	x-ray examination of lymph glands after injection of radiopaque material
lymphangiogram lĭm-FĂN-jē-ō-grăm	x-ray examination of a lymph vessel
splenography splē-NŎG-ră-fē	radiographic image of the spleen

CLINICAL PROCEDURES

Term	Description
autologous transfusion aw-TŎL-ō-gŭs	transfusion prepared from the recipient's own blood
bleeding time	test to determine time required for a small stab wound made in the earlobe or forearm to stop bleeding; test evaluates the vascular and platelet factors associated with hemostasis
bone marrow aspiration ăs-pĭ-RĀ-shŭn	removal of a bone marrow specimen for examination and diagnosis, using a surgical aspirating needle
bone marrow transplantation	transplantation of bone marrow from one individual to another; used for treating aplastic anemia and immunodeficiency disorders
bone marrow transplantation (autologous)	harvesting, freezing (cryopreserving), and reinfusing of the patient's own bone marrow; used to treat bone marrow hypoplasia following cancer therapy
homologous transfusion	transfusion prepared from another individual whose blood is compatible with that of the recipient

SURGICAL PROCEDURES

Term	Description
lymphangiectomy lĭm-făn-jē-ĔK-tō-mē	removal of a lymph vessel
splenolaparotomy splē-nō-lăp-ă-RŎT-ō-mē	incision through the abdominal wall into the spleen
splenolysis splē-NŎL-ĭ-sĭs	destruction of splenic tissue
splenopexy SPLĒ-nō-pĕk-sē	fixation of a movable spleen

LABORATORY PROCEDURES

Test	Description
activated partial thromboplastin time (APTT) thrŏm-bō-PLĂS-tĭn	evaluation of many of clotting factors necessary for hemostasis; valuable for preoperative screening for bleeding tendencies
coagulation time	time required for blood to clot in a test tube
complete blood count (CBC)	series of tests that include hemoglobin, hematocrit, red and white blood cell counts, differential white blood cell (WBC) count, RBC indices, and RBC and WBC morphology
differential WBC count	enumerates the distribution of leukocytes in a stained blood smear. The different kinds of WBCs are counted and reported as a percentage of the total examined. Because the differential values change considerably in pathology, this test is often used as a first step to diagnose a disease
erythrocyte sedimentation rate (ESR; sed rate)	assessment of the rate at which RBCs settle to the bottom of a narrow tube (rate increases in inflammatory diseases, cancer, and pregnancy, and decreases in liver disease)
hemoglobin (Hgb, Hb)	measurement of the amount of hemoglobin found in whole blood (decreases in anemia; increases in dehydration, polycythemia vera, and thrombocytopenia purpura)
hematocrit (Hct, crit)	measurement of the percentage of packed RBCs in a whole blood sample

LABORATORY PROCEDURES (Continued)

Test	Description
Monospot	serological test performed on a blood sample to detect the presence of a nonspecific antibody called the heterophile antibody that is present in the serum of patients with infectious mononucleosis
prothrombin time (pro-time, PT)	test that determines the time required for a clot to form in a test tube containing plasma, after the addition of calcium; commonly used to manage patients undergoing anticoagulant therapy
partial thromboplastin time (PTT)	test similar to APTT but less sensitive
RBC indices	evaluation of RBCs by providing the approximate size, volume, and concentration of hemoglobin in an average RBC
Schilling test	definitive test for pernicious anemia; assesses the absorption of radioactive vitamin B_{12} by the gastrointestinal system (in pernicious anemia, B_{12} is not absorbed and passes in the stool)

PHARMACOLOGY

Medication	Action
anticoagulants	agents that inhibit or delay the clotting process; used to prevent clots from forming in blood vessels in patients predisposed to this condition, and to preserve stored whole blood and blood products
fibrinolytics	agents that trigger the body to produce plasmin, an enzyme that dissolves clots; used to treat acute pulmonary embolism and, occasionally, deep vein thromboses
hemostatics	drugs, medicines, or blood components that serve to stop bleeding

ABBREVIATIONS

Diagnostic and Symptomatic	Meaning
AHF	antihemophilic factor VIII
AHG	antihemophilic globulin factor VIII

ABBREVIATIONS (Continued)

Diagnostic and Symptomatic	Meaning
AIDS	acquired immunodeficiency syndrome
ALL	acute lymphocytic leukemia
AML	acute myelogenous leukemia
CDC	Centers for Disease Control
CLL	chronic lymphocytic leukemia
CML	chronic myelogenous leukemia
EBV	Epstein-Barr virus
HDN	hemolytic disease of the newborn
HIV	human immunodeficiency virus
Ig	immunoglobulin
ITP	idiopathic thrombocytopenia purpura
PA	pernicious anemia
PCP	*Pneumocystis carinii* pneumonia
SLE	systemic lupus erythematosus

Laboratory	Meaning
AC	anticoagulant
APTT	activated partial thromboplastin time
baso	basophil
CBC	complete blood count
CO_2	carbon dioxide
diff	(white cell) differential blood count
eos	eosinophil
ESR, SR	erythrocyte sedimentation rate; sedimentation rate
HCT, Hct	hematocrit
HGB, Hgb, Hb	hemoglobin
lymphs	lymphocytes
MCH	mean corpuscular hemoglobin
MCHC	mean corpuscular hemoglobin concentration
MCV	mean corpuscular volume
mono	monocyte

ABBREVIATIONS (Continued)

Laboratory	Meaning
mL, ml	milliliter; 0.001 liter
O_2	oxygen
PCV	packed cell volume (hematocrit)
PMN, seg, poly	polymorphonuclear neutrophil
PTT	partial thromboplastin time
PT	prothrombin time
RBC	red blood cell
WBC	white blood cell

Case Study

Therapeutic Plasmapheresis

Procedure. Therapeutic plasmapheresis

Diagnosis. Thrombotic thrombocytopenic purpura/hemolytic uremic syndrome

Technique. Plasmapheresis was carried out in the patient's room on 4 West. A Cobe Spectra machine was used. The patient tolerated the procedure well and her **vital signs** remained stable. **Hemodialysis** nurse Angie Greco, RN, attended the patient. The following figures represent the amount of **plasma** removed and the **infusion** of plasma and other fluids. The procedure was begun at 1350 hours and ended at 1540 hours. **Hgb:** 12.5; **Hct:** 42.6; **WBC** count: 9.1; **platelets:** 133; estimated total blood volume: 3648 **mL;** estimated plasma volume: 2116 mL; plasma removed: 3106 mL; AC infused: 712 mL; **saline** rinse back: 195 mL.

Fresh frozen plasma infused: 1946 mL
Total volume infused: 2853 mL
Net volume lost: minus 253 mL

Comment. The patient's blood pressure dropped slightly to 90 **systolic,** but returned to normal when the procedure was slowed. She tolerated the procedure extremely well. She seemed a bit more alert and less confused today.

Plans. The plans are to perform the next therapeutic plasmapheresis on Saturday, 9/25/XX and again next week on Tuesday and Friday.

Worksheet 5 provides a dictionary and reading application and an analysis of this case study.

Worksheet 1

Use the suffix -osis (abnormal increase) to build a medical word meaning:

1. abnormal increase in RBCs _____

2. abnormal increase in WBCs _____

3. abnormal increase in granulocytes _____

4. abnormal increase in thrombocytes _____

5. abnormal increase in lymphocytes _____

6. abnormal increase in reticulocytes _____

Use the suffix -penia (deficiency, decrease) to build a medical word meaning:

7. decrease in RBCs _____

8. decrease in WBCs _____

9. decrease in platelets _____

10. decrease in granulocytes _____

11. decrease in lymphocytes _____

Use the suffix -poiesis (production or formation) to build a medical word meaning:

12. production of blood _____

13. production of red cells _____

14. production of white cells _____

15. production of lymphocytes _____

Use immun/o (protection, safety, immunity) to build a medical word meaning:

16. specialist in the study of immunity _____

17. study of immunity _____

Use splen/o (spleen) to build a medical word meaning:

18. herniation of the spleen _____

19. inflammation of the spleen _____

Worksheet 2

Build surgical terms meaning:

1. excision of the spleen _____

2. incision of the spleen _____

3. removal of the thymus _____

4. destruction of the thymus _____

5. incision of the spleen through the abdominal wall _____

6. fixation of (a displaced) spleen _____

Worksheet 3

Match the words below with the definitions in the numbered list.

anisocytosis	hemolysis
antibody	hemostasis
antigen	lymphosarcoma
coagulopathy	microcytosis
dyscrasia	reticulocytosis
edema	serology

1. _____ study of antigen-antibody reactions

2. _____ usually a protein marker on the surface of cells that identify the cell as self or nonself

3. _____ destruction of erythrocytes with the release of hemoglobin

4. _____ arrest of bleeding or circulation

5. _____ condition of marked variations in the size of erythrocytes

6. _____ immunoglobulin produced by B cell lymphocytes in response to the presence of an antigen

7. _____ malignant neoplastic disorder of lymphatic tissue, unrelated to Hodgkin's disease

8. _____ any blood abnormality

9. _____ defect in the clotting mechanism

10. _____ localized or general condition in which body tissues contain excessive amounts of tissue fluid

Worksheet 4

SPECIAL PROCEDURES, PHARMACOLOGY, AND ABBREVIATIONS

Match the following words to the statements in the numbered list:

anticoagulants   hemoglobin
bleeding time   hemostatics
coagulation time   Ig
complete blood count (CBC)   Monospot
diff   monocyte
EBV   PMN
erythrocyte sedimentation rate   prothrombin time
fibrinolytics   splenography
hematocrit

1. _____ substances that control blood flow

2. _____ test that assesses the amount of iron-containing pigment in RBCs

3. _____ measurement of the speed at which RBCs settle when placed in a narrow tube

4. _____ volume of packed RBCs expressed as a percentage of whole blood

5. _____ immunoglobulin

6. _____ polymorphonuclear neutrophil

7. _____ time required for a clot to form in a test tube

8. _____ nonspecific test for the presence of the heterophile antibody, present in patients with infectious mononucleosis

9. _____ time required for a small puncture wound to stop bleeding

10. _____ series of blood tests that includes WBC, RBC, diff, Hgb, Hct, RBC indices, and RBC and WBC morphology

11. _____ trigger the body to produce plasmin, an enzyme that dissolves clots

12. _____ agents that delay or inhibit clotting

13. _____ time required for blood to clot in a tube after the addition of calcium

14. _____ Epstein-Barr virus

15. _____ x-ray examination of the spleen

Worksheet 5

THERAPEUTIC PLASMAPHERESIS DICTIONARY EXERCISE

Use a medical dictionary or other resource to define the terms and to determine their pronunciation; then practice reading the case aloud (p. 194).

hemodialysis _____

hemolytic uremic syndrome _____

Hgb _____

Hct _____

infusion _____

mL _____

plasma _____

plasmapheresis _____

platelets _____

purpura _____

saline _____

systolic _____

therapeutic _____

thrombocytopenic _____

vital signs _____

WBC _____

ANALYSIS OF THERAPEUTIC PLASMAPHERESIS

1. What is the name of the dialysis machine used to perform the plasmapheresis?

2. What vital sign showed a slight abnormality but returned to normal when the procedure was slowed down?

3. If 250 mL is the equivalent of 1 cup, approximately how many cups of plasma were removed?

4. What was the net volume loss?

5. Were the Hgb, Hct, WBC count, and platelets within the reference range?

6. How long did the procedure take?

Chapter 11

Musculoskeletal System

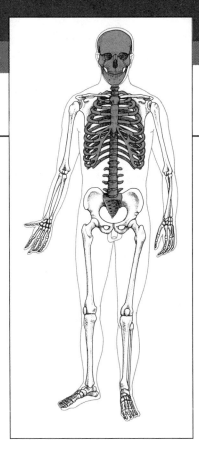

Chapter Outline

Student Objectives
Upon completion of this chapter, you will be able to do the following:

Describe the functions of the skeletal system.

Locate and identify the major bones of the body.

Identify two main divisions of the skeletal system.

List four types of bones.

Explain the function of the vertebral column.

Identify the bones of the five regions of the vertebral column.

Describe the function of the thorax, and list five parts that compose its skeletal framework.

List three classifications of joints, and describe their function.

Explain the purpose of bone markings.

Describe three types of bone projections and depressions.

Identify five common types of fractures.

List three functions of muscles.

Identify combining forms, suffixes, and prefixes related to the musculoskeletal system.

Identify and discuss associated pathology related to the musculoskeletal system.

Identify diagnostic imaging, surgical procedures, and abbreviations related to the musculoskeletal system.

Explain pharmacology related to the treatment of musculoskeletal disorders.

Demonstrate your knowledge of the chapter by completing the worksheets.

Anatomy and Physiology

The musculoskeletal system consists of bones, joints, and muscles. Bones perform mechanical functions of support, protection, body movement, and metabolic functions of **hematopoiesis** (production of blood cells) and mineral storage. Muscle tissue is composed of contractile cells or fibers that affect movement of an organ or part of the body.

SKELETAL SYSTEM

Functions

Bones protect many vital organs. For example, the bones of the skull and the bones of the thorax are hard shields that protect the brain, heart, and lungs, respectively. Besides **support** and **protection,** the skeletal system provides a number of other important functions. **Movement** is possible because bones provide points of attachment for muscles, tendons, and ligaments. Bone marrow, found within the larger bones, is responsible for hematopoiesis, continuously producing millions of blood cells to replace those that have been destroyed. Bones serve as a **storehouse for minerals,** particularly phosphorus and calcium. When the body experiences a need for a certain mineral, such as calcium during pregnancy, it is withdrawn from the bones.

Structure and Types of Bones

The four principal types of bones are: long bones, short bones, flat bones, and irregular bones.

    Long bones are found in the extremities of the body (e.g., legs, arms, and fingers). Figure 11–1 shows the parts of a long bone.

- The (1) **diaphysis** is the shaft or long, main portion of a bone. It consists mainly of **compact bone.**
- On each end of the diaphysis is (2) an **epiphysis,** whose somewhat bulbous shape provides space for muscle and ligament attachments.
- The (3) **articular cartilage** is a thin layer of resilient hyaline cartilage. The elasticity of hyaline cartilage provides joints with a cushion against jars and blows.
- The (4) **periosteum,** a dense white fibrous membrane, covers the remaining surface of the bone. It contains numerous blood and lymph vessels and nerves. In growing

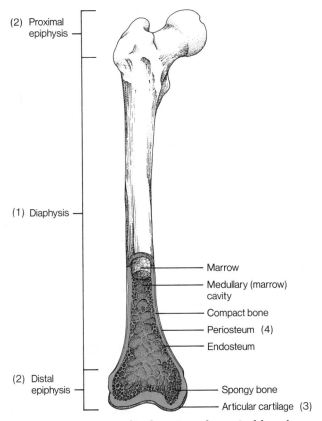

Figure 11–1 Longitudinal section of a typical long bone.

bones, the inner layer contains the bone-forming cells, called **osteoblasts.** Because blood vessels and osteoblasts are located here, the periosteum provides a means for bone repair and general bone nutrition. It also serves as a point of attachment for muscles, ligaments, and tendons.

Short bones are somewhat cubed-shaped. They consist of a core of **cancellous** (spongy) bone that is enclosed in a thin layer of compact tissue (e.g., bones of the ankles, wrists, and toes).

Irregular bones include the bones that cannot be grouped under the previous headings because of their complex shapes (e.g., bones of the middle ear, vertebrae). **Flat bones** are exactly what their name suggests. They provide broad surfaces for muscular attachment or protection for internal organs (e.g., bones of the skull, shoulder blades, and sternum).

Divisions of the Skeletal System: Axial and Appendicular Skeleton

The axial and appendicular portions of the human skeleton is composed of 206 bones. Only the major bones are identified in Figure 11–2.

The **axial skeleton** consists of the bones of the skull, thorax, and vertebral column. These bones contribute to the formation of body cavities and provide protection for internal organs.

The **appendicular skeleton** consists of the bones of the shoulder, the upper extremities, the hips, and the lower extremities. They attach to the axial skeleton as appendages.

Vertebral Column. The vertebral column of the adult is composed of 26 bones called vertebrae (singular, vertebra). The vertebral column supports the body and provides a protective bony canal for the spinal cord. As you read the following material, refer to Figure 11–3.

Five regions of bones comprise the vertebral column. Each region derives its name from its location within the spinal column. The seven (1) **cervical vertebrae** form the skeletal framework of the neck. The first cervical vertebra, the (2) **atlas,** supports the skull. The second cervical vertebra, the (3) **axis,** makes it possible to rotate the skull on the neck. Under these are twelve (4) **thoracic or dorsal vertebrae,** which support the chest and serve as a point of articulation for the ribs. The next five vertebrae, the (5) **lumbar vertebrae,** are situated in the lower back area and carry most of the weight of the torso. Below this area, the five sacral vertebrae are fused into a single bone in the adult and are referred to as the (6) **sacrum.** The tail of the vertebral column consists of four or five fragmented vertebrae fused together, referred to as the (7) **coccyx.**

Vertebrae are separated by flat, round structures, the (8) **intervertebral disks,** which are composed of a fibrocartilaginous substance with a gelatinous mass in the center (nucleus pulposus). When disk material protrudes into the neural canal, pressure on the adjacent nerve root causes pain. This condition is referred to as herniation of an intervertebral disk, herniated nucleus pulposus (HNP), ruptured disk, or slipped disk.

Thorax. Two important internal organs of the thorax (chest) are the heart and lungs. Together with other soft tissue, the internal organs are enclosed and protected by the thorax. As you read the following paragraph, refer to Figure 11–4.

The ribs, the (1) **sternum** (chest plate), and the thoracic vertebrae form the skeletal framework of the rib cage. There are 12 pairs of ribs, each pair is attached posteriorly to a thoracic vertebra. The (2) **true ribs** are the first seven pairs of ribs. These are attached

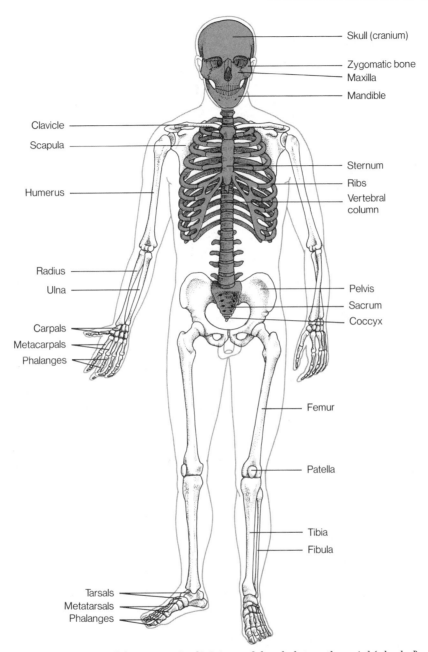

Figure 11–2 Anterior view of the two main divisions of the skeleton: the axial (*shaded*) and appendicular portions.

directly to the sternum by a strip of (3) **costal cartilage.** The costal cartilage of the next five pairs of ribs is not fastened directly to the sternum. These are known as (4) **false ribs.** The last two pairs of false ribs are not joined, even indirectly, to the sternum but attach posteriorly to the thoracic vertebrae and are known as (5) **floating ribs.**

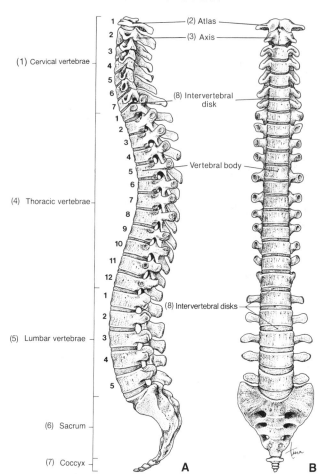

(1) Cervical vertebrae
1
2 — (2) Atlas
3 — (3) Axis
4
5
6
7
(8) Intervertebral disk

(4) Thoracic vertebrae
1
2
3
4
5 — Vertebral body
6
7
8
9
10
11
12

(5) Lumbar vertebrae
1
2
3 — (8) Intervertebral disks
4
5

(6) Sacrum

(7) Coccyx

A   B

Figure 11–3 Vertebral column. *A,* Lateral view of left side. *B,* Anterior view. (Adapted from Scanlon, VC and Sanders, T: Essentials of Anatomy and Physiology, ed 2. FA Davis, Philadelphia, 1995, p 117, with permission.)

Pelvic Girdle (Pelvis). The pelvis is a basin-shaped structure that supports the sigmoid colon, the rectum, the urinary bladder, and other soft organs of the abdominopelvic cavity. It also provides a point of attachment for the legs, as shown in Figure 11–2.

Male and female pelves differ considerably in size and shape. Some of the differences are attributable to the function of the female pelvis during the stages of childbearing. The female pelvis is more shallow than the male pelvis but wider in every direction. The female pelvis not only supports the enlarged uterus as the fetus matures, but also provides a large enough opening to allow the infant to pass through during birth.

Refer to Figure 11–5 as you read the following material.

Both the female and male pelves are divided into the (1) **ilium,** (2) **ischium,** and (3) **pubis.** These are fused together in the adult to form a single bone called the innominate bone. Nevertheless, the individual names are retained in order to identify the respective areas of the hip bone. The bladder is located behind the (4) **symphysis pubis;** the rectum is in the curve of the (5) **sacrum** and (6) **coccyx.** In the female, the uterus, fallopian tubes, ovaries, and vagina are located between the bladder and the rectum.

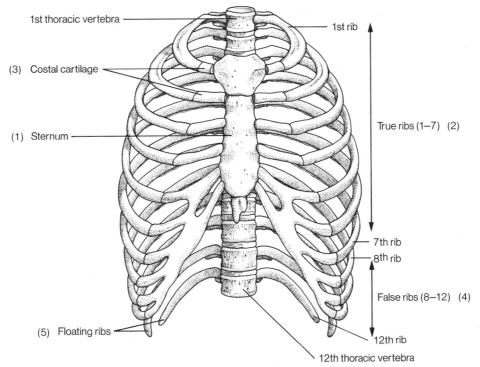

1st thoracic vertebra

(3) Costal cartilage

(1) Sternum

1st rib

True ribs (1–7) (2)

7th rib

8th rib

False ribs (8–12) (4)

12th rib

12th thoracic vertebra

(5) Floating ribs

Figure 11–4 The thorax.

Projections and Depressions in Bones

Surfaces of bones have both projections and depressions to provide attachments for muscles, to join one bone to another, or to furnish cavities and pathways for nerve and blood supplies. The portion of the bone that projects is called a **process.** Various types of projections, or processes, are evident in bones. They may be rounded, sharp, narrow, or have a large ridge, called a **crest. Depressions** are cavities or openings in a bone. There are several distinct types. The anatomical terms for the most common types of projections and depressions are summarized in Table 11–1.

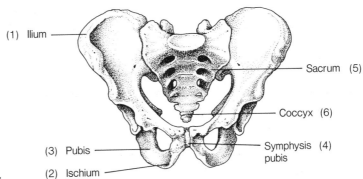

(1) Ilium

Sacrum (5)

Coccyx (6)

(3) Pubis

Symphysis (4)
pubis

(2) Ischium

Figure 11–5 The male pelvis.

Table 11–1 **Projections and Depressions**

	Description	Example
Projection		
Condyle	Rounded articulating knob	Condyle of the humerus
Trochanter	Massive process found only on the femur	Greater trochanter of the femur
Tubercle	Small, rounded process	Tubercle of the femur
Tuberosity	Large, rounded process	Tuberosity of the humerus
Depression		
Foramen	Rounded opening through a bone to accommodate blood vessels and nerves	Foramen of the skull through which cranial nerves pass
Fossa	Flattened or shallow basin	Axillary (armpit)
Sulcus	Groove, slight depression, or fissure	Deep furrows in the brain
Sinus	Cavity or hollow space in a bone	Frontal sinus

Joints or Articulations

To allow for body movements, bones must have surfaces that join together **(articulate).** These surfaces form joints, or articulations, with various degrees of mobility. Some are freely movable **(diarthroses);** others are only slightly movable **(amphiarthroses);** and the remaining are totally immovable **(synarthroses).** All three types are necessary for smooth, coordinated body movements.

Joints are covered with connective tissue and cartilage, which permit bones to be connected to each other. Muscles attached to freely movable joints permit a great deal of body movement. The synovial membrane lining the joint cavity secretes synovial fluid, which acts as a joint lubricant. The bones in a synovial joint are separated by a joint capsule. The joint capsule is strengthened by ligaments (fibrous bands, or sheets, of connective tissues) that often anchor bones to each other. All of the foregoing structures, working together in a complementary manner, make various body movements possible.

MUSCLES

All muscles, through contraction, provide the body with motion or body posture. The less apparent motions provided by muscles are the passage and elimination of food through the digestive system, propulsion of blood through the arteries, and contraction of the bladder to eliminate urine.

There are three types of muscle tissue in the body: skeletal, cardiac, and smooth. **Skeletal muscles,** also called **voluntary** or **striated muscles,** are muscles whose action is controlled by will. Some examples of voluntary muscles are the muscles that move the eyeballs, tongue, and bones. Except for cardiac muscle, all striated muscles are voluntary.

Cardiac muscle makes up most of the wall of the heart. Like skeletal muscle, cardiac muscle is striated; but unlike skeletal muscle, it experiences rhythmical involuntary contractions.

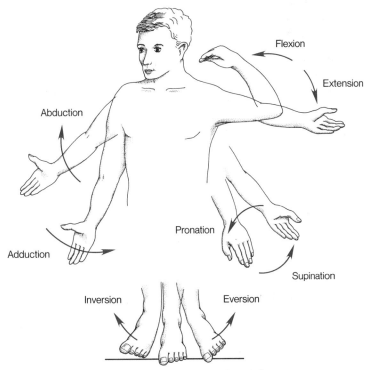

Figure 11–6   Actions of muscles.

Smooth muscles (involuntary or **visceral muscles)** are muscles whose action is not controlled by will. They are found principally in the visceral organs, the walls of arteries, the walls of respiratory passages, and in the urinary and reproductive ducts. The contraction of smooth muscle is under autonomic (involuntary) nervous control.

Figure 11–6 and Table 11–2 show the actions provided by muscles.

Table 11–2   **Actions of Muscles**

Motion	Action
Flexion	Decreases the angle of a joint
Extension	Increases the angle of a joint
Adduction	Moves closer to the midline
Abduction	Moves away from the midline
Pronation	Turns the palm down
Supination	Turns the palm up
Dorsiflexion	Elevates the foot
Plantar flexion	Lowers the foot (points the toes)
Rotation	Moves a bone around its longitudinal axis

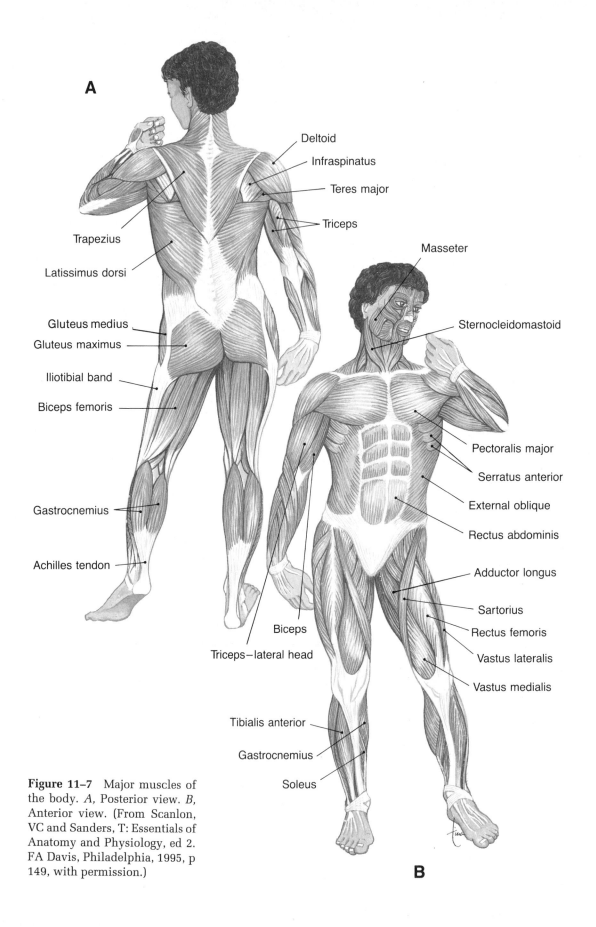

Figure 11-7 Major muscles of the body. *A,* Posterior view. *B,* Anterior view. (From Scanlon, VC and Sanders, T: Essentials of Anatomy and Physiology, ed 2. FA Davis, Philadelphia, 1995, p 149, with permission.)

A

Deltoid
Infraspinatus
Teres major
Triceps

Trapezius

Latissimus dorsi

Gluteus medius
Gluteus maximus

Iliotibial band

Biceps femoris

Gastrocnemius

Achilles tendon

Masseter

Sternocleidomastoid

Pectoralis major

Serratus anterior

External oblique

Rectus abdominis

Adductor longus

Sartorius
Rectus femoris
Vastus lateralis
Vastus medialis

Biceps

Triceps–lateral head

Tibialis anterior
Gastrocnemius
Soleus

B

ATTACHMENTS

Muscles attach to bones either by fleshy or fibrous attachments. In **fleshy attachments,** muscle fibers arise directly from bone. These fibers distribute force over wide areas, but a fleshy attachment is weaker than a fibrous attachment. In **fibrous attachments,** the connective tissue of the **epimysium, perimysium,** and **endomysium** converges at the end of the muscle to become continuous and indistinguishable from the periosteum. In some instances, this connective tissue penetrates the bone itself. When connective tissue fibers form a cord or strap, it is referred to as a **tendon.** This localizes a great deal of force in a small area of bone. Ligaments are composed of connective tissue and attach one bone to another. When the fibrous attchment spans a large area of a particular bone, the attachment is called an **aponeurosis.** Such attachments are found in the lumbar region of the back.

To become familiar with the names of major muscles, review Figure 11–7.

Combining Forms

SKELETAL SYSTEM

Combining Form	Meaning	Example	Pronunciation
Bones of Upper Extremities			
brachi/o	arm	brachi/o/cephal/ic head pertaining to	brăk-ē-ō-sě-FĂL-ĭk
carp/o	carpus (wrist bones)	carp/o/ptosis downward displacement, prolapse	kăr-pŏp-TŌ-sĭs
cephal/o	head	cephal/ad toward	SĚF-ă-lăd
cervic/o	neck	cervic/o/facial face	sěr-vĭ-kō-FĀ-shē-ăl
cost/o	ribs	cost/o/chondr/ itis cartilage inflammation	kŏs-tō-kŏn-DRĪ-tĭs
crani/o	cranium (skull)	crani/o/tomy incision	krā-nē-ŎT-ō-mē
dactyl/o	digit (a finger or toe)	syn/ dactyl/ism joined condition together	sĭn-DĂK-tĭl-ĭzm
humer/o	humerus	humer/al pertaining to	HŪ-měr-ăl
metacarp/o	metacarpus (bones of the hand)	metacarp/ectomy excision	mět-ă-kăr-PĔK-tō-mē

SKELETAL SYSTEM (Continued)

Combining Form	Meaning	Example	Pronunciation
phalang/o	phalanges (bones of fingers and toes)	phalang/eal — pertaining to	fă-LĂN-jē-ăl
rachi/o	spine	rachi/o/plegia — paralysis	rā-kē-ō-PLĒ-jē-ă
spondyl/o (used to make words about conditions of the structure)		spondyl/itis — inflammation	spŏn-dĭl-Ī-tĭs
vertebr/o (used to make words that describe the structure)	vertebrae (backbone)	cost/o/vertebr/al ribs — pertaining to	kŏs-tō-VĔR-tĕ-brăl
stern/o	sternum (breastbone)	stern/al — pertaining to	STĔR-năl
thorac/o	chest	thorac/o/dynia — pain	thō-răk-ō-DĬN-ē-ă

Bones of Lower Extremities

Combining Form	Meaning	Example	Pronunciation
calcane/o	calcaneum (heel bone)	calcane/o/dynia — pain	kăl-kā-nē-ō-DĬN-ē-ă
femor/o	femur (thigh bone)	femor/al — pertaining to	FĔM-or-ăl
fibul/o	fibula (smaller, outer bone of lower leg)	fibul/ar — pertaining to	FĬB-ū-lăr
ili/o	ilium (lateral flaring portion of hip bone)	ili/ac — pertaining to	ĬL-ē-ăk
ischi/o	ischium (lower portion of hip bone)	ischi/al — pertaining to	ĬS-kē-ăl
lumb/o	loins	lumb/o/dynia — pain	lŭm-bō-DĬN-ē-ăh

SKELETAL SYSTEM (Continued)

Combining Form	Meaning	Example	Pronunciation
patell/o	patella (kneecap)	patell/a/pexy fixation	păh-TĔL-ăh-pĕk-sē
ped/i	foot	ped/i/cure care	PĔD-ĭ-kūr
pod/o		pod/iatry treatment	pō-DĪ-ă-trē
pelv/i	pelvis	pelv/i/metry measuring	pĕl-VĬM-ĕt-rē
pub/o	pelvic bone (anterior)	pub/is noun ending	PŪ-bĭs
tibi/o	tibia (larger, inner bone of lower leg)	tibi/o/femor/al femur pertaining to	tĭb-ē-ō-FĔM-ŏr-ăl

Other Combining Forms

Combining Form	Meaning	Example	Pronunciation
arthr/o	joint	arthr/o/desis fixation (of a bone or joint)	ăr-thrō-DĒ-sĭs
acromi/o	acromion (projection of scapula)	acromi/o/clavic/ular collar pertaining to bone	ă-krō-mē-ŏ-klă-VĬK-ū-lăr
ankyl/o	stiffness, bent, crooked	ankyl/osis abnormal condition	ăng-kĭ-LŌ-sĭs
condyl/o	condyle (rounded protuberance at end of bone forming an articulation)	condyl/ectomy excision	kŏn-dĭl-ĔK-tō-mē
lamin/o	lamina (part of the vertebral arch)	lamin/ectomy excision	lăm-ĭ-NĔK-tō-mē
myel/o	bone marrow, spinal cord	myel/o/cele herniation	MĪ-ĕl-lō-sēl

SKELETAL SYSTEM (Continued)

Combining Form	Meaning	Example	Pronunciation
orth/o	straight	orth/o/ped/ ic child pertaining to	ŏr-thō-PĒ-dĭk
oste/o	bone	oste/oma tumor	ŏs-tē-Ō-mă

MUSCULAR SYSTEM

Combining Form	Meaning	Example	Pronunciation
chondr/o	cartilage	chondr/itis inflammation	kŏn-DRĪ-tĭs
leiomy/o	smooth muscle (visceral)	leiomy/oma tumor	lī-ō-mī-Ō-mă
my/o	muscle	my/oma muscle	mī-Ō-mă
rhabd/o	rod-shaped (striated)	rhabd/oid resembling	RĂB-doyd
rhabdomy/o	rod-shaped muscle (striated)	rhabdomy/oma tumor	răb-dō-mī-Ō-mă
ten/o tend/o tendin/o	tendon	ten/o/tomy incision tend/o/tome instrument to cut tendin/itis inflammation	tĕn-ŎT-ō-mē TĔN-dō-tōm tĕn-dĭn-Ī-tĭs

SUFFIXES

Suffix	Meaning	Example	Pronunciation
-blast	embryonic cell	oste/o/blast bone	ŎS-tē-ō-blăst
-clasis	break, refracture	oste/o/clasis bone	os-tē-ō-KLĂ-sĭs
-desis	binding, fixation (of a bone or joint)	arthr/o/desis joint)	ăr-thrō-DĒ-sĭs
-malacia	softening	oste/o/malacia bone	ŏs-tē-ō-măh-LĀ-shē-ăh

SUFFIXES (Continued)

Suffix	Meaning	Example	Pronunciation
-physis	to grow	dia/physis through	dī-ĂF-ĭ-sĭs
-plasty	surgical repair	arthr/o/plasty joint	ĂR-thrō-plăs-tē
-porosis	porous	oste/o/porosis bone	ŏs-tē-ō-pŏ-RŌ-sĭs
-schisis	a splitting	rachi/schisis spine	ră-KĬS-kĭ-sĭs
-scopy	visual examination	arthr/o/scopy joint	ăr-THRŎS-kō-pĕ

PREFIXES

Prefix	Meaning	Example	Pronunciation
epi-	above, upon	epi/physis to grow	ĕ-PĬF-ĭ-sĭs
sub-	under, below	sub/stern/ al sternum pertaining to	sŭb-STĔR-năl

Pathology

BONES

Osteomyelitis, an infection of bone and bone marrow, is commonly caused by pus-forming **(pyogenic)** bacteria. The disease usually begins with local trauma to the bone causing a blood clot **(hematoma).** Bacteria from an acute infection in another area of the body find their way to the injured bone and are frequently responsible for bone infection.

Most bone infections are more difficult to cure than soft-tissue infections. Eventually they may result in bone destruction **(necrosis)** and stiffening, or freezing, of the joints **(ankylosis).** Osteomyelitis may be acute or chronic. With early treatment, prognosis for acute osteomyelitis is good; prognosis for the chronic form of the disease is poor.

Paget's disease, also known as **osteitis deformans,** is a chronic inflammation of bones, resulting in thickening and softening of bones. It can occur in any bone but most often affects the long bones of the legs, the lower spine, the pelvis, and the skull. This disease is found in the population over age 40. Although a variety of causes have been proposed, a slow virus (not yet isolated) is currently thought to be the most likely cause.

Fractures

A fracture means that a bone has been broken. The different types of fractures are classified as to extent of damage (Fig. 11–8).

A (1) **closed** or **simple fracture** is one in which the bone is broken but no external wound exists. An (2) **open** or **compound fracture** involves a broken bone and an external wound that leads to the site of fracture. Fragments of bone often protrude through the skin. A (3) **complicated fracture** occurs when a broken bone has injured some internal organ, such as when a broken rib pierces a lung. In a (4) **comminuted fracture,** the bone has broken or splintered into pieces. An (5) **impacted fracture** occurs when the bone is broken and one end is wedged into the interior of the other. An (6) **incomplete fracture** is when the line of fracture does not include the whole bone. (7) A **greenstick fracture** occurs when the bone is partially bent and partially broken, as when a green stick breaks. It occurs in children because their bones contain more collagen than do adult bones and tend to splinter rather than break completely. A **hairline fracture** is a minor fracture in which all portions of the bone are in perfect alignment. The fracture is seen on x-ray examination as a very thin hairline between the two segments but not extending entirely through the bone. **Pathological** (spontaneous) **fractures** are those which are usually caused by a disease process such as neoplasm or osteoporosis.

Unlike other repairs of the body, bones sometimes require months to heal. Several factors influence the rate at which fractures heal. Broken bones that lie close together heal

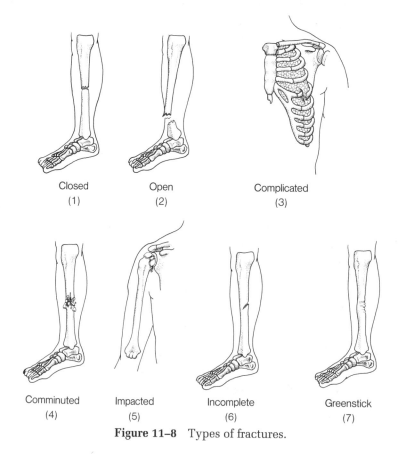

Closed
(1)

Open
(2)

Complicated
(3)

Comminuted
(4)

Impacted
(5)

Incomplete
(6)

Greenstick
(7)

Figure 11–8 Types of fractures.

faster than those that do not. Because of this, fractured bones are set in a cast **(immobilized).** Some bones have a natural tendency to heal more rapidly than others. For instance, the long bones of the arms have an inclination to mend twice as fast as those of the legs. Age also plays an important role in bone fracture healing rate. Older patients require more time for healing. Also, an adequate blood supply to the injured area and the nutritive state of the individual are crucial to the healing process.

Osteoporosis

Porous bone **(osteoporosis)** is a common bone disorder in older persons, especially women older than 60 years of age. A decrease of bone density occurs when the rate of bone resorption (loss of substance) exceeds that of bone formation. Among the many causes of osteoporosis are disturbances of protein metabolism, protein deficiency, disuse of bones because of prolonged periods of immobilization, estrogen deficiencies associated with menopause, a diet lacking vitamins or calcium, and long-term administration of high doses of corticosteroids.

Patients with osteoporosis frequently complain of bone pain, most commonly in the back, which may be caused by repeated microscopic fractures. Thin areas of porous bone are also evident. Deformity associated with osteoporosis is usually the result of pathological fractures.

Spinal Disorders

Because of various conditions, the normal curvature of the spine may become abnormally bent, causing **curvature** of the spine. A lateral curvature deviation of the spine to the right or left is called **scoliosis.** Scoliosis or C-shaped curvature of the spine may be congenital, caused by chronic poor posture during childhood while the vertebrae are still growing, or the result of one leg being longer than the other. Surgery, braces, casts, and corrective exercise may alleviate abnormal spine curvatures. Untreated scoliosis may result in pulmonary insufficiency (curvature may decrease lung capacity), back pain, sciatica, disk disease, or even degenerative arthritis.

Hunchback or humpback **(kyphosis)** is an exaggeration or angulation of the thoracic curve of the vertebral column. This condition may be caused by rheumatoid arthritis, rickets, poor posture, or chronic respiratory diseases. Treatment for kyphosis caused by poor posture may consist of bed rest, therapeutic exercise, and a brace to straighten the kyphotic curve until growth is completed. Treatment for both adolescent and adult kyphosis includes appropriate measures for the underlying cause and, possibly, spinal arthrodesis for relief of symptoms. Surgery may be necessary when kyphosis causes neurological damage or intractable and disabling pain, but it is rarely necessary.

Swayback **(lordosis),** a forward curvature of the lumbar spine, may be caused by increased weight of the abdominal contents, resulting from obesity or excessive weight gain during pregnancy.

Spina bifida is a congenital defect characterized by defective closure of the spinal canal through which the spinal cord and meninges may or may not protrude. It usually occurs in the lumbosacral area and has several forms. **Spina bifida occulta** is the most common and least severe form. There is no protrusion of the spinal cord or meninges. **Spina bifida cystica** is a more severe type involving protrusion of the meninges **(meningocele),** spinal cord **(myelocele),** or both **(meningomyelocele).**

An inflammation of the vertebrae **(spondylitis)** is a serious chronic disorder. When it is associated with tuberculosis of the bones, it is called **Pott's disease.** Vertebrae become eroded and collapse, causing kyphosis. Spondylitis may also be associated with other infectious diseases. The intervertebral disks and the vertebrae are affected and sometimes destroyed, with resultant permanent stiffening or ankylosis of the back.

JOINTS

Because of their location and constant use, joints are prone to stress injuries and inflammation. The main diseases affecting the joints are rheumatoid arthritis, osteoarthritis, and gout.

Rheumatoid arthritis, a systemic disease characterized by inflammatory changes in joints and their related structures, results in crippling deformities. This form of arthritis is believed to be caused by an autoimmune reaction of joint tissue. It begins most often in women between the ages of 23 and 35 years but can affect people of any age group. Intensified aggravations **(exacerbations)** of this disease are frequently associated with periods of increased physical or emotional stress. In addition to joint changes, muscles, bones, and skin adjacent to the affected joint atrophy. There is no specific cure, but nonsteroidal anti-inflammatory drugs (NSAIDs), physical therapy, and orthopedic measures are used in treatment of less severe cases.

Osteoarthritis, also called **degenerative joint disease (DJD),** is the most common type of connective tissue disease. Cartilage destruction and new bone formation at the edges of joints **(spurs)** are the most common pathologies seen with osteoarthritis. Even though osteoarthritis is less crippling than rheumatoid arthritis, it may result in fusion of two bone surfaces, thereby completely immobilizing the joint. Small, hard nodules may form at the distal interphalangeal joints of the fingers **(Heberden's nodes).**

Gout, a metabolic disease caused by accumulation of uric acid crystals, is characterized by acute arthritis. Although the joint chiefly affected is the big toe, any joint may be involved. Often there is renal involvement. An attack of gout is marked by swelling, inflammation, and extreme pain.

MUSCLES

Myasthenia gravis (MG), a neuromuscular disorder, causes fluctuating weakness of certain skeletal muscle groups (of the eyes, face, and, to a lesser degree, the limbs). It is characterized by destruction of the receptors in the synaptic region that respond to **acetylcholine,** a substance that transmits nerve impulses **(neurotransmitter).** As the disease progresses, the muscle becomes increasingly weaker and may eventually cease to function altogether. Women are affected slightly more often than men. Initial symptoms include a weakness of the eye muscles and difficulty in swallowing **(dysphagia).** Later, the individual has difficulty chewing and talking. Eventually, the muscles of the limbs may become involved.

Muscular dystrophy is a genetic disease characterized by gradual atrophy and weakening of muscle tissue. There are several kinds of muscular dystrophy, none of whose etiology is completely understood. The most common type affects children, boys more often than girls. As muscular dystrophy progresses, the loss of muscle function affects not only skeletal muscle but also cardiac muscle. At present there is no cure for this disease, and most children with muscular dystrophy die before the age of 20 years.

Oncology

Some bone tumors present no problem. Others are exceedingly rare and rapidly become life-threatening. Bone tumors **(osteomas)** can be either benign or malignant. Generally, benign tumors are slow growing and are usually treated by surgical excision. Malignant tumors that arise from bone **(sarcoma)** are rare. They usually develop rapidly and metastasize through lymph channels. Sarcomas are named for the specific tissue that they affect; for example, sarcoma in fibrous connective tissue **(fibrosarcoma),** sarcoma in lymphoid tissue **(lymphosarcoma),** or sarcoma in cartilage **(chondrosarcoma).** A sarcoma that often attacks the shafts rather than the ends of the long bones is called **Ewing's sarcoma.** This highly malignant tumor is found primarily in young men. Included in the treatment of malignant bone tumors are chemotherapy for management of metastasis and radiation when the tumor is radiosensitive.

DIAGNOSTIC, SYMPTOMATIC, AND RELATED TERMS

Term	Meaning
carpal tunnel syndrome (CPT) KAR-păl	painful condition resulting from compression of the median nerve within the carpal tunnel (wrist canal through which the flexor tendons and the median nerve pass)
claudication klăw-dĭ-KĀ-shŭn	lameness, limping
crepitation krĕp-ĭ-TĀ-shŭn	dry, grating sound or sensation caused by bone ends rubbing together, indicating a fracture or joint destruction
electromyography ē-lĕk-trō-mī-ŎG-ră-fē	use of electrical stimulation to record the strength of muscle contraction
exacerbation ĕks-ăs-ĕr-BĀ-shun	increase in severity of a disease or of any of its symptoms
hemarthrosis hĕm-ăr-THRŌ-sĭs	effusion of blood into a joint cavity
multiple myeloma MŬL-tĭ-pl mī-ĕ-LŌ-măh	primary malignant tumor of blood cells usually arising in bone marrow, usually progressive, and generally fatal
phantom limb	illusion, following amputation of a limb, that the limb still exists. The sensation that pain exists in the removed part is known as phantom limb pain
prosthesis PRŎS-thē-sĭs	replacement of a missing part by an artificial substitute, such as an artificial extremity
rickets, rachitis RĬK-ĕts, ră-KĪ-tĭs	form of osteomalacia in children, caused by vitamin D deficiency

DIAGNOSTIC, SYMPTOMATIC, AND OTHER TERMS (Continued)

Term	Meaning
sequestrum sē-KWĔS-trŭm	fragment of necrosed bone that has become separated from surrounding tissue
spondylolisthesis spŏn-dĭ-lō-lĭs-THĒ-sĭs	any forward slipping (subluxation) of a vertebra over the one below it
spondylosis spŏn-dĭ-LŌ-sĭs	degeneration of the cervical, thoracic, and lumbar vertebrae and related tissues; may cause pressure on nerve roots with subsequent pain or paresthesia in the extremities
sprain	tearing of ligament tissue that may be slight, moderate, or complete. A complete tear of a major ligament is especially painful and disabling. Ligamentous tissue does not heal well because of poor blood supply. Treatment consists of surgical reconstruction of the severed ligament
strain	excessive stretching of tissue composing the tendon or muscle, with no serious damage
subluxation sŭb-lŭk-SĀ-shŭn	partial or incomplete dislocation
talipes TĂL-ĭ-pēz	any number of foot deformities, especially those occurring congenitally; clubfoot

Special Procedures

DIAGNOSTIC IMAGING PROCEDURES

Term	Description
arthrography ar-THROG-ră-fē	a series of radiographs taken after injection of a radiopaque substance into a joint cavity, especially the knee or shoulder, in order to outline the contour of the joint
CT scan (bone)	radiograph taken as a camera scans the entire body following injection of a radioactive substance; used to evaluate skeletal involvement related to connective tissue disease
CT scan (joint)	radiograph taken as a camera scan to determine joint damage throughout the entire body; one of the most sensitive studies for early detection of joint disease

DIAGNOSTIC IMAGING PROCEDURES (Continued)

Term	Description
diskography	radiological examination of the intervertebral disk structures in suspected cases of herniated disk
lumbosacral spinal radiography (LS spine) LŬM-bō-sā-krăl SPĪ-năl	radiography of the five lumbar vertebrae and the fused sacral vertebrae, including anteroposterior, lateral, and oblique views of the lower spine. The most common indication for this procedure is lower back pain, to identify or differentiate traumatic fractures, spondylosis, spondylolisthesis, and metastatic tumor
myelography, myelogram MĪ-ĕ-log-ră-fē, MĪ-el-ō-gram	radiography of the spinal cord after injection of a contrast medium; used to identify and study spinal distortions caused by tumors, cysts, herniated intervertebral disks, or other lesions

SURGICAL PROCEDURES

Term	Description
amputation ăm-pū-TĀ-shŭn	partial or complete removal of a limb
arthrocentesis ăr-thrō-sĕn-TĒ-sĭs	puncture of a joint space to remove accumulated fluid
arthroclasia ăr-thrō-KLĀ-zē-ăh	surgical breaking of an ankylosed joint to provide movement
arthroscopy ăr-THRŎS-kŏ-pē	visual examination of a joint, especially the knee; used primarily to detect trauma or lesions and to obtain a biopsy of synovial tissue for microscopic examination. Synovial biopsy may also be obtained by needle or surgical incision
bone grafting bōn GRĂFT-ĭng	implanting or transplanting bone tissue from another part of the body or from another person to serve as replacement for damaged or missing bone tissue
bursectomy bĕr-SĔK-tō-mē	excision of bursa (a padlike sac or cavity found in connective tissue, usually in the vicinity of joints)
closed reduction rē-DŬK-shŭn	treatment of bone fractures by placing the bones in proper position (i.e., reducing the fragments without surgery
laminectomy lăm-ĭ-NĔK-tō-mē	excision of the posterior arch of a vertebra; most often performed to relieve the symptoms of a ruptured intervertebral (slipped) disk

SURGICAL PROCEDURES (Continued)

Term	Description
open reduction rĕ-DŬK-shŭn	treatment of bone fractures by the use of surgery to place the bones in proper position (i.e., reducing the fragments)
sequestrectomy sē-kwĕs-TRĔK-tō-mē	excision of a sequestrum (segment of necrosed bone)
synovectomy sĭn-ō-VĔK-tō-mē	excision of a synovial membrane

PHARMACOLOGY

Medication	Action
anti-inflammatories, antipyretics	non-narcotic analgesics used to relieve pain, fever, and swelling in musculoskeletal inflammatory diseases (e.g., rheumatoid arthritis, gout). The main antirheumatic is aspirin. Prescribed in much larger dosages for arthritis than those used to treat other types of pain. When used for arthritis and gout, these drugs are also called NSAIDs
corticosteroids	major anti-inflammatory drugs used for bone and joint disorders
gold therapy, aurotherapy, chrysotherapy	gold compounds used to treat rheumatoid arthritis
relaxants	drugs that reduce tension and produce relaxation (e.g., muscle relaxants provide therapeutic treatment that specifically relieves muscular tension)

ABBREVIATIONS

Abbreviation	Meaning
AE	above the elbow
AK	above the knee
AP	anteroposterior
BE	below the elbow
BK	below the knee
C1, C2, and so on	first cervical vertebra, second cervical vertebra, and so on

ABBREVIATIONS (Continued)

Abbreviation	Meaning
CDH	congenital dislocation of the hip
CPT	carpal tunnel syndrome
DJD	degenerative joint disease
Fx	fracture
HD	hip disarticulation
HNP	herniated nucleus pulposus (herniated disk)
HP	hemipelvectomy
IM	intramuscular
IS	intracostal space
KD	knee disarticulation
L1, L2, and so on	first lumbar vertebra, second lumbar vertebra, and so on
LAT, lat	lateral
MG	myasthenia gravis
NSAID	nonsteroidal anti-inflammatory drug
Ortho, ORTH	orthopedics
RA	rheumatoid arthritis
SD	shoulder disarticulation
T1, T2, and so on	first thoracic vertebra, second thoracic vertebra, and so on
THA	total hip arthroplasty
THR	total hip replacement
TKA	total knee arthroplasty
TKR	total knee replacement

Case Study

Radiographic Consultation: Injury of Left Wrist and Hand

Left Wrist. Images were obtained with the patient's arm taped to an arm board. There are **fractures** through the **distal shafts** of the **radius** and **ulna.** The radial fracture fragments show approximately 8 **mm** overlap with dorsal displacement of the distal radial fracture fragment. The distal ulnar shaft fracture shows **ventral-lateral angulation** at the fracture **apex.** There is no over-riding at this fracture. No additional fracture is seen. Soft tissue deformity is present, correlating with the fracture sites.

Left Elbow and Left Humerus. Single view of the left elbow was obtained in the lateral projection. **AP** view of the humerus was obtained to include a portion of the elbow. A third x-ray film was obtained but is not currently available for review. There is **lucency** through the distal humerus on the AP view along its medial aspect. It would be difficult to exclude fracture just above the **medial epicondyle.** On the lateral view, there is elevation of the anterior and posterior fat pad. These findings are of some concern. Repeat elbow study is recommended.

Worksheet 5 provides a dictionary and reading application and an analysis of this case study.

Worksheet 1

Use oste/o (bone) to build words meaning:

1. bone cells _____

2. pain in the bones _____

3. disease of the bones and joints _____

4. beginning or formation of bones _____

Use cervic/o (neck) to build words meaning:

5. pertaining to the neck _____

6. pertaining to the neck and arm _____

7. pertaining to the neck and face _____

Use myel/o (bone marrow, spinal cord) to build words meaning:

8. herniation of the spinal cord _____

9. sarcoma of bone marrow (cells) _____

10. softening of the spinal cord _____

11. tumor containing myeloblasts _____

Use stern/o (sternum, breastbone) to build words meaning:

12. pertaining to above the sternum _____

13. resembling the breastbone _____

Use arthr/o (joint) or chondr/o (cartilage) to build words meaning:

14. embryonic cell that forms cartilage _____

15. inflammation of a joint _____

16. inflammation of bones and joints _____

Use pelv/i (pelvis) to build a word meaning:

17. instrument for measuring the pelvis _____

Use my/o (muscle) to build a medical word meaning:

18. tumor containing muscle (tissue) _____

19. hardening of a muscle _____

20. rupture of a muscle _____

Worksheet 2

Build a surgical term meaning:

1. excision of one or more of the phalanges (bones of a finger or toe) _____

2. incision of the thorax (chest wall) _____

3. excision of a vertebra _____

4. binding of a joint _____

5. repair of bones _____

6. repair of muscle (tissue) _____

7. excision of the lamina (part of the vertebral arch) _____

Worksheet 3

Match the following medical words with the definitions in the numbered list.

amputation   rickets
claudication   sequestrum
myasthenia gravis   subluxation
muscular dystrophy   spondylolisthesis
prosthesis   talipes

1. _____ incomplete or partial dislocation

2. _____ softening of the bones caused by a lack of vitamin D

3. _____ slipped vertebrae

4. _____ limping

5. _____ degeneration of the muscles

6. _____ congenital deformity of the foot, which is twisted out of shape or position

7. _____ part of dead or necrosed bone that has become separated from surrounding tissue

8. _____ chronic neuromuscular disorder characterized by weakness manifested in ocular muscles, resulting in bilateral ptosis of the eyelids

9. _____ replacement of a missing limb with an artificial part

Worksheet 4

Special Procedures, Pharmacology, and Abbreviations
Select a term that best describes the statements that follow.

amputation	HNP
arthroclasia	L3
arthrodesis	laminectomy
arthrography	myelography
chrysotherapy	open reduction
corticosteroids	thermography

1. _____ x-ray film of spinal cord after injection of a contrast medium

2. _____ treatment of bone fractures by use of surgery to place bones in proper position

3. _____ oral or injectable gold salts administered to treat rheumatoid arthritis

4. _____ major anti-inflammatory drugs used for bone and joint disorders

5. _____ excision of the posterior arch of a vertebra

6. _____ series of joint radiographs preceded by injection of a radiopaque substance or air into the joint cavity

7. _____ surgical immobilization of a joint

8. _____ partial or complete removal of a limb

9. _____ herniated nucleus pulposus

Worksheet 5

RADIOGRAPHIC CONSULTATION DICTIONARY EXERCISE

Use a medical dictionary or other resource to define the following terms and determine their pronunciation; then practice reading the case study aloud (p. 226).

angulation _____

AP _____

apex _____

distal shafts _____

epicondyle _____

fracture _____

lucency _____

medial _____

mm _____

radiographic _____

radius _____

ulna _____

ventral-lateral _____

ANALYSIS OF RADIOGRAPHIC CONSULTATION: INJURY OF LEFT WRIST AND HAND

1. What is the abbreviation for anteroposterior?

2. What caused the soft tissue deformity?

3. Why was an AP view of the humerus taken?

4. Where are the left wrist fractures located?

5. Did the radiologist take any side views of the left elbow?

Worksheet 6

Label the parts of the bone on the following diagram. To check your answers, refer to Figure 11–1.

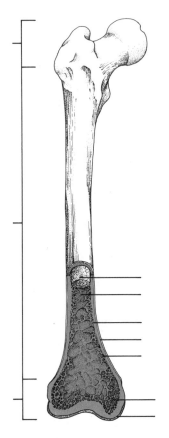

Articular cartilage

Compact bone

Diaphysis

Distal
epiphysis

Endosteum

Marrow

Medullary (marrow)
cavity

Periosteum

Proximal
epiphysis

Spongy bone

Worksheet 7

Label the parts of the skeleton on the following diagram. To check your answers, refer to Figure 11–2.

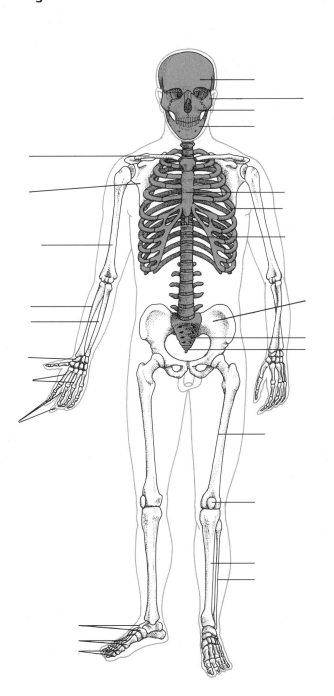

Carpals

Clavicle

Coccyx

Femur

Fibula

Humerus

Mandible

Maxilla

Metacarpals

Metatarsals

Patella

Pelvis

Phalanges

Radius

Ribs

Sacrum

Scapula

Skull (cranium)

Sternum

Tarsals

Tibia

Ulna

Vertebral column

Zygomatic bone

Worksheet 8

Label the muscles and tendons on the following diagram. To check your answers, refer to Figure 11–7A.

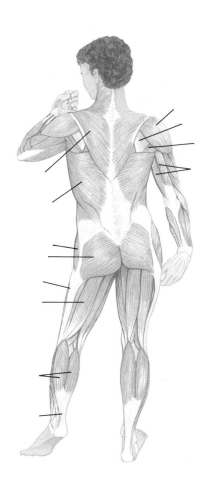

Achilles tendon	Gastrocnemius	Infraspinatus	Trapezius
Biceps femoris	Gluteus medius	Iliotibial band	Teres major
Deltoid	Gluteus maximus	Latissimus dorsi	Triceps

Worksheet 9

Label the muscles on the following diagram. To check your answers, refer to Figure 11–7B.

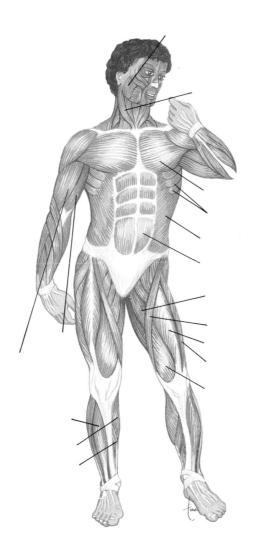

Adductor longus	Masseter	Sartorius	Tibialis anterior
Biceps	Pectoralis major	Serratus anterior	Triceps- lateral head
External oblique	Rectus abdominis	Soleus	Vastus lateralis
Gastrocnemius	Rectus femoris	Sternocleidomastoid	Vastus medialis

Chapter 12

Genitourinary System

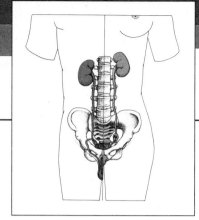

Chapter Outline

Student Objectives
Upon completion of this chapter, you will be able to do the following:

List the macroscopic structures of the urinary system, and describe how they function.

Describe the structure and function of the nephron.

Explain physiological activities involved in the formation of urine.

Identify structures and functions associated with the reproductive process in the male.

Explain the function of the seminal vesicle, prostate, and Cowper's glands.

Identify reproductive structures that also function as part of the urinary system of the male.

Identify combining forms and suffixes related to the genitourinary system.

Identify and discuss pathology related to the genitourinary system.

Student Objectives (Continued)

Identify diagnostic imaging, surgical, clinical and laboratory procedures, and abbreviations related to the genitourinary system.

Discuss pharmacology related to the treatment of disorders associated with the genitourinary system.

Demonstrate your knowledge of the chapter by completing the worksheets.

Anatomy and Physiology

The male and female urinary systems consist of four major structures: two kidneys and ureters, a bladder, and a urethra. This chapter presents information on these structures. In addition, it includes a discussion of the male reproductive system because some of the male reproductive organs also function as urinary structures (Fig. 12–1).

URINARY SYSTEM

The urinary system monitors and regulates the extracellular fluids (plasma, tissue fluid, and lymph) of the body. It filters a variety of substances from plasma. The harmful substances are excreted from the body as urine, and the useful products are returned to the blood.

Some of the harmful products that must be filtered from blood are **nitrogenous wastes** and excess fluid **electrolytes** (sodium, potassium, and calcium). Nitrogenous wastes are products formed when protein is metabolized by the body. Electrolytes are substances that have the ability to carry electrical charges. These are vital to the functioning of the musculoskeletal, cardiovascular, and nervous systems.

Macroscopic Structures

Figure 12–2 illustrates the macroscopic structures of the urinary system. Study and identify each structure as you read the following material.

Two (1) **kidneys,** each about the size of a fist, are located in the retroperitoneal area of the abdominal cavity. A concave medial border gives the kidney its beanlike shape. Near the medial border is an opening, the (2) **hilum (hilus),** where the (3) **renal vein** exits the kidney and the (4) **renal artery** enters the kidney. The renal artery carries blood, laden with waste products, to the microscopic filtering tubules located within the kidney for purification. After the waste products are removed, blood leaves the kidney by way of the renal vein. The waste material, now in the form of urine, passes to a hollow chamber, the (5) **renal pelvis.** This chamber is an enlarged funnel-shaped extension of the (6) **ureter** at the entrance to the kidney. Each ureter is a slender tube about 10 to 12 inches long that carries urine, in peristaltic waves, to the bladder. The (7) **bladder,** an expandable hollow organ, acts as a temporary reservoir for urine. During **voiding** or **micturition,** urine is

Male   Female

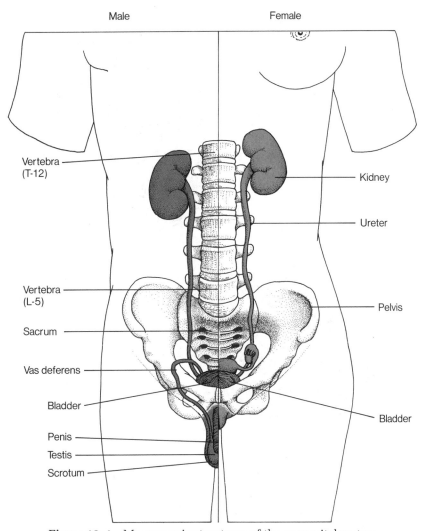

Vertebra
(T-12)

Kidney

Ureter

Vertebra
(L-5)

Pelvis

Sacrum

Vas deferens

Bladder

Bladder

Penis

Testis

Scrotum

Figure 12–1   Macroscopic structures of the urogenital system.

expelled from the bladder through the (8) **urethra,** a membranous tube that terminates at the (9) **urinary meatus.** The length of the urethra is approximately 1.5 inches in women and about 7 inches in men.

Microscopic Structures

Microscopic examination of kidney tissue reveals the presence of approximately 1 million microscopic functional structures called **nephrons.** Nephrons are responsible for maintaining homeostasis by continually adjusting conditions that are necessary for survival. When the level of various products in the blood elevates beyond a normal range, nephrons

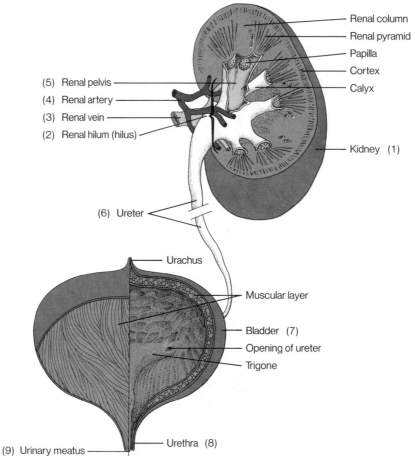

(5) Renal pelvis
(4) Renal artery
(3) Renal vein
(2) Renal hilum (hilus)

Renal column
Renal pyramid
Papilla
Cortex
Calyx

Kidney (1)

(6) Ureter

Urachus

Muscular layer

Bladder (7)
Opening of ureter
Trigone

(9) Urinary meatus
Urethra (8)

Figure 12–2 Macroscopic urinary structures.

selectively remove these products from the blood by producing a substance called urine. This helps re-establish a level that can sustain life. Substances removed by nephrons are nitrogenous wastes, including urea, uric acid, and creatinine, the end products of metabolism. Nephrons also remove excess electrolytes and many other products that exceed the amount tolerated by the body.

Figure 12–3 is an illustration of a nephron. Locate each structure as you read the following material.

Each nephron includes a **renal corpuscle** and a **renal tubule.** The renal corpuscle is composed of a tuft of capillaries called the (1) **glomerulus** and a modified, funnel-shaped end of the renal tubule known as (2) **Bowman's capsule.** This capsule encases the glomerulus. An (3) **afferent arteriole** carries blood to the glomerulus, and a smaller (4) **efferent arteriole** removes it from the glomerulus. As the efferent arteriole passes behind the renal corpuscle, it forms the **peritubular capillaries,** which allow needed products that have been filtered from the blood to re-enter the vascular system.

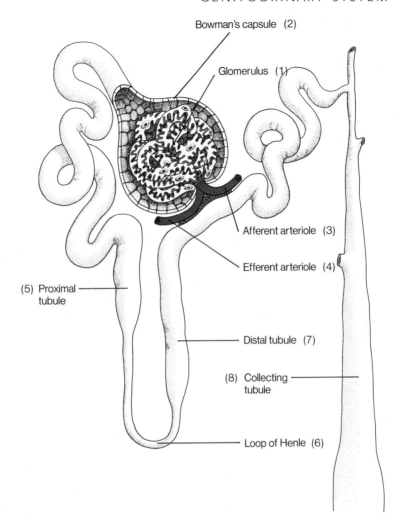

Bowman's capsule (2)

Glomerulus (1)

Afferent arteriole (3)

Efferent arteriole (4)

(5) Proximal tubule

Distal tubule (7)

(8) Collecting tubule

Loop of Henle (6)

Figure 12–3 A nephron.

Each renal tubule consists of four sections: the (5) **proximal tubule;** followed by the narrow (6) **loop of Henle;** then a larger portion, the (7) **distal tubule;** and finally, the (8) **collecting tubule.**

The nephron produces urine by three physiological activities:

- filtration
- reabsorption
- secretion

Filtration takes place in the renal corpuscle. Here, water, electrolytes, sugar, amino acids, and other compounds pass from the blood in the glomerulus into Bowman's capsule. The fluid that is formed is called **filtrate.**

Reabsorption begins as filtrate passes through the four sections of the tubule. As filtrate travels the long and twisted pathway of the tubule, most of the water and some of the electrolytes and amino acids are absorbed by the peritubular capillaries, thus re-entering the circulating blood.

Secretion occurs when specialized cells of the collecting tubules secrete ammonia, uric acid, and other substances directly into the tubule. This process completes urine production.

MALE REPRODUCTIVE SYSTEM

The male reproductive system serves two important functions. First, it produces sperm, the male sex cell, which contains one half of the genetic material necessary to produce a living being. Second, it provides structures necessary to transport and maintain viable sperm. As you read this section, identify the structures in Figure 12–4.

The primary male reproductive organ consists of two (1) **testes** (singular, **testis**), located in an external sac called the (2) **scrotum.** Within the testes are numerous small tubes that twist and coil to form **seminiferous tubules,** which produce sperm, the male sex cell. The testes also secrete testosterone, which develops and maintains secondary sex characteristics. Lying over the superior surface of each testis is a single, tightly coiled tube, the (3) **epididymis.** This structure stores sperm after it leaves the seminiferous tubules. The epididymis is the first duct through which sperm passes after its production in the

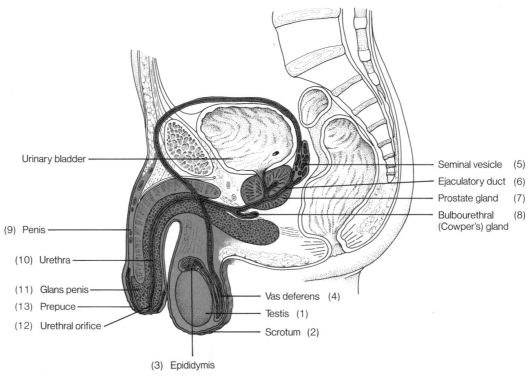

Figure 12–4   The male reproductive system.

testes. Tracing the duct upward, the epididymis forms the (4) **vas deferens (seminal duct** or **ductus deferens)**, a narrow tube that passes through the inguinal canal into the abdominal cavity. The vas extends over the top and down the posterior surface of the bladder, where it joins the (5) **seminal vesicle.** The union of the vas with the duct from the seminal vesicle forms the (6) **ejaculatory duct.**

The seminal vesicle secretes approximately 60 percent of the fluid that is ultimately ejaculated during sexual intercourse **(coitus).** It contains nutrients that support sperm viability. The ejaculatory duct passes at an angle through the (7) **prostate gland,** a triple-lobed organ fused to the base of the bladder. The prostate secretes a thin, alkaline substance that accounts for about 30 percent of the seminal fluid. Its alkalinity helps protect sperm from the acidic environments of both the male urethra and the female vagina. The two pea-shaped (8) **bulbourethral (Cowper's) glands** are located below the prostate and are connected by a small duct to the urethra. Cowper's glands provide an alkaline fluid necessary for sperm viability. The (9) **penis** is the male organ of copulation. It is cylindrical and composed of erectile tissue that encloses the (10) **urethra.** The urethra expels both semen and urine from the body. During ejaculation, the sphincter at the base of the bladder closes. This not only stops the urine from being expelled with the semen, but also prevents semen from entering the bladder.

The enlarged tip of the penis, the (11) **glans penis,** contains the (12) **urethral orifice (meatus).** A movable hood of skin, called (13) **prepuce** or **foreskin,** covers the glans penis.

COMBINING FORMS

Combining Form	Meaning	Example	Pronunciation
Urinary			
cyst/o	bladder	cyst/o/scopy visual examination	sĭs-TŎS-kō-pē
vesic/o		vesic/o/cele herniation	VĔS-ĭ-kō-sēl
glomerul/o	glomerulus	glomerul/o/pathy disease	glō-mĕr-ū-LŎP-ă-thē
nephr/o	kidney	nephr/o/pexy fixation	NĔF-rō-pĕk-sē
ren/o		ren/al pertaining to	RĒ-năl
ureter/o	ureter	ureter/ectasis dilation, expansion	ū-rē-tĕr-ĔK-tăh-sĭs
urethr/o	urethra	urethr/o/plasty surgical repair	ū-RĒ-thrō-plăs-tē
ur/o	urine, urinary	ur/o/lith calculus, stone	Ū-rō-lĭth

COMBINING FORMS (Continued)

Combining Form	Meaning	Example	Pronunciation
Male Reproductive			
andr/o	male	andr/o/logy study	ăn-DRŎL-ō-jē
balan/o	glans penis	balan/o/rrhea flow, discharge	băl-ăn-ō-RĒ-ă
epididym/o	epididymis	epididym/itis inflammation	ĕp-ĭ-dĭd-ĭ-MĪ-tĭs
orch/i		orchi/algia pain	or-kē-ĂL-jē-ă
orchid/o	testes	orchid/itis inflammation	or-kĭ-DĪ-tĭs
orchi/o		orchi/o/rrhaphy suture	or-kē-OR-ră-fē
prostat/o	prostate	prostat/ectomy excision	prŏs-tăh-TĔK-tō-mē
spermat/o	sperm	spermat/o/lysis destruction	spĕr-măt-ŎL-ĭ-sĭs
vas/o	vas deferens, duct, vessel	vas/ectomy excision	văh-SĔK-tō-mē
vesicul/o	seminal vesicle	vesicul/itis inflammation	vĕ-sĭk-ū-LĪ-tĭs
Miscellaneous			
albumin/o	albumin (protein)	albumin/oid resembling	ăl-BŪ-mĭ-noid
bacteri/o	bacteria	bacteri/al pertaining to	băk-TĒ-rē-ăl
crypt/o	hidden	crypt/orchid/ism testes condition	krĭpt-ŎR-kĭd-ĭzm
noct/o	night	noct/uria urine	nŏk-TŪ-rē-ăh
olig/o	scanty	olig/uria urine	ŏl-ĭg-Ū-rē-ăh
py/o	pus	py/osis abnormal condition	pī-Ō-sĭs

SUFFIXES

Suffix	Meaning	Example	Pronunciation
-genesis	forming, producing, origin	spermat/o/<u>genesis</u> sperm	spĕr-măt-ō-GĔN-ĕ-sĭs
-iasis	abnormal condition (produced by something specified)	nephr/o/lith/iasis kidney stone	nĕf-rō-lĭth-Ī-ă-sĭs
-uria	urine	dys/<u>uria</u> painful, difficult	dĭs-Ū-rē-ăh

Pathology

PYELONEPHRITIS

One of the most common forms of kidney disease is **pyelonephritis.** In this disorder, bacteria invade the renal pelvis and kidney tissue, often as a consequence of a bladder infection that has ascended to the kidney via the ureters. When the infection is severe, lesions form in the renal pelvis, causing bleeding. The microscopic examination of urine reveals the following: large quantities of bacteria **(bacteriuria),** white blood cells **(pyuria),** and, when lesions are present, red blood cells **(hematuria).** The onset of the disease is usually acute, with symptoms including chills, fever, nausea, and vomiting.

Pyelonephritis is about eight times more common in females than in males, probably owing to the shorter female urethra. Treatment includes the use of antibiotics.

GLOMERULONEPHRITIS

Any condition that causes the glomerular walls to become inflamed is referred to as **glomerulonephritis.** One of the most common causes of glomerular inflammation is a reaction to the toxins given off by pathogenic streptococci that have recently infected another part of the body, especially the throat. Glomerulonephritis is also associated with autoimmune diseases such as systemic lupus erythematosus, polyarthritis, and scleroderma.

When the glomerular membrane is inflamed, it becomes highly permeable and permits blood cells and protein to enter the filtrate, causing hematuria and proteinuria. In some cases, protein solidifies in the nephron tubules and forms solid masses that take the shape of the tubules in which they develop. These masses are called **casts.** They often pass out of the kidney by way of the urine and may be visible when urine is examined microscopically. Most patients with acute glomerulonephritis associated with a streptococcal infection recover with no residual kidney damage.

NEPHROLITHIASIS

Stones may form in any part of the urinary tract, but most arise in the kidney. They frequently form when dissolved urine salts begin to solidify. As these stones increase in size, they obstruct urinary structures. When they lodge in the ureters they cause intense pulsating pain called **colic.** Because urine is hindered from flowing into the bladder, it refluxes into the renal pelvis and the tubules, causing them to dilate. This distention is called **hydronephrosis.** For calculi that cannot be dislodged or dissolved, ultrasound waves, directed through the skin (**percutaneous ultrasonic lithotripsy** or **extracorporeal shock-wave lithotripsy**), often prove effective.

BLADDER NECK OBSTRUCTION

A blockage of the bladder outlet is referred to as **bladder neck obstruction (BNO).** The obstruction may be caused by an enlarged prostate gland **(prostatic hypertrophy)** or by the presence of an obstructive mass such as a calculus, blood clot, or tumor. The resulting bladder distention may lead to hydronephrosis accompanied by bladder infection **(cystitis).** The patient experiences a need to void but can only void small quantities at a time. This is referred to as retention with overflow. Correction of BNO includes surgery that relieves or removes the obstruction.

BENIGN PROSTATIC HYPERTROPHY

Benign prostatic hypertrophy (BPH), sometimes called **nodular hyperplasia** or **benign prostatic hyperplasia,** is often associated with the aging process. The prostate enlarges and decreases the urethral lumen. Inability to empty the bladder completely may cause cystitis, which may then lead to nephritis. Surgical removal of the prostate may be necessary. The different operative procedures include the removal of the prostate through the perineum **(perineal prostatectomy),** excision through the urethra **(transurethral resection [TUR]),** or excision through an abdominal opening above the pubis and directly over the bladder **(suprapubic prostatectomy).**

CRYPTORCHIDISM

Failure of the testes to descend into the scrotal sac prior to birth is called **cryptorchidism.** In many infants born with this condition, the testes descend spontaneously by the end of the first year. If this does not occur, correction of the disorder involves surgical suspension of the testes **(orchiopexy)** in the scrotum. This procedure is usually done before the child reaches 2 years of age. Because an inguinal hernia often accompanies cryptorchidism, the hernia **(herniorrhaphy)** may be sutured at this time.

ACUTE TUBULAR NECROSIS

Two major causes of **acute tubular necrosis (ATN)** are ischemia and nephrotoxic injury. In ATN, the tubular portion of the nephron is injured through either a decreased blood supply or the presence of toxic substances (usually after ingestion of certain toxic chemical agents). Ischemia may be the result of circulatory collapse, severe hypotension, hemorrhage, dehydration, or other disorders that affect blood supply.

Signs and symptoms of ATN include scanty urine production **(oliguria)** and increased blood levels of calcium **(hypercalcemia).** When tubular damage is not severe, the disorder is reversible.

ONCOLOGY

Carcinoma of the Prostate

The second most common form of cancer in men, and the third leading cause of cancer death, is carcinoma of the prostate. In the United States, the disease is rarely found in men under age 50, but the incidence dramatically increases as the individual grows older. Susceptibility to the disease is influenced, to a large extent, by race, being extremely low in Asians, moderate in whites, and high in blacks.

Symptoms include difficulty in starting and stopping the urinary stream, dysuria, frequency, and hematuria. By the time these symptoms develop and the patient seeks treatment, the disease is quite advanced and long-term survival is not likely.

Like other forms of cancer, prostatic carcinomas are staged and graded to determine metastatic potential, response to treatment, survival, and appropriate forms of therapy.

Metastatic prostatic cancer can usually be arrested by surgical removal of the testes **(bilateral orchiectomy)** and administration of estrogens.

Diagnostic, Symptomatic, and Related Terms

URINARY SYSTEM

Term	Meaning
anuria ăh-NŪ-rē-ăh	absence of urine production
azotemia, uremia ăz-ō-TĒ-mē-ăh, ū-RĒ-mē-ăh	metabolic wastes (urea, creatinine, and uric acid) in the blood
chronic renal failure KRŎ-nĭk RĒ-năl	renal failure that occurs over a period of years, whereby the kidneys lose their ability to maintain volume and composition of body fluids with normal dietary intake; condition is due to deficiency in the total number of functioning nephrons in the kidneys
enuresis, incontinence ĕn-ŭ-RĒ-sĭs, ĭn-KŎN-tĭ-nĕns	involuntary discharge of urine: during the night, nocturnal enuresis; during the day, diurnal enuresis
fistula FĬS-tū-lă	abnormal passage from a hollow organ to the surface, or from one organ to another
frequency FRĒ-kwĕn-sē	voiding at frequent intervals
hesitancy HĔZ-ĭ-tĕn-sē	involuntary delay in initiating urination
nephrotic syndrome nĕ-FRŎT-ĭk	loss of large amounts of plasma protein by way of urine, which results in systemic edema
nocturia, nycturia nŏk-TŪ-rē-ă, nĭk-TŪ-rē-ă	excessive urination during the night

URINARY SYSTEM (Continued)

Term	Meaning
oliguria ŏl-ĭg-Ū-rē-ăh	scanty urine production
urgency ŬR-jĕn-sē	need to void immediately; commonly accompanies frequency in persons with urinary tract infections (UTIs)
urolithiasis ū-rō-lĭ-THĪ-ă-sĭs	presence of stones in any urinary structure; frequently treated by pulverizing the stones with an ultrasonic lithotriptor

MALE REPRODUCTIVE SYSTEM

Term	Meaning
aspermia ăh-SPĔR-mē-ăh	lack of or failure to ejaculate semen
epispadias ĕp-ĭ-SPĀ-dē-ăs	malformation in which the urethra opens on the dorsum of the penis
hydrocele HĪ-drō-sēl	accumulation of serous fluid in a saclike cavity, especially the testes and associated structures
hypospadias hī-pō-SPĀ-dē-ăs	developmental anomaly in the male in which the urethra opens on the underside of the penis, or in extreme cases, on the perineum
impotence ĬM-pō-tĕns	condition characterized by inability to achieve an erection
phimosis fĭ-MŌ-sĭs	stenosis or narrowing of preputial orifice so that the foreskin cannot be pushed back over the glans penis
sterility stĕr-ĬL-ĭ-tē	inability to fertilize the ovum; inability of reproducing an offspring
varicocele VĂR-ĭ-kō-sēl	swelling and distension of veins of the spermatic cord

Special Procedures

Diagnostic Imaging Procedures

Term	Description
cystography sĭs-TŎ-gră-fē	radiography of the urinary bladder using a contrast medium, used to diagnose tumors or defects in the bladder wall, vesicoureteral reflux, stones, or other pathological conditions of the bladder
cystourethrogram sĭs-tŏ-ū-RĒ-thrō-grăm	radiological evaluation of the urinary bladder and urethra following the administration of a contrast medium
intravenous pyelogram (IVP) pī-ĕ-LŌ-grăm excretory urography ĔKS-krē-tō-rē ū-RŎG-ră-fē	series of radiographs taken of the renal calyces, renal pelves, ureters, and urinary bladder after a contrast medium is injected intravenously
nephrotomography, CT scan (kidney) nĕf-rō-tō-MŎG-ră-fē	study visualizing several planes of the kidney, to differentiate solid renal and adrenal tumors from benign renal cysts; performed in conjunction with an IVP
retrograde pyelogram (RP) RĔT-rō-grād pī-ĕ-LŌ-grăm	radiograph of the urinary system via a urinary catheter after introducing a contrast medium, used to locate urinary tract obstructions. The catheter is passed from the urethra, through the urinary bladder, and into the ureters and calyces of the renal pelves while being observed on fluoroscopy

CLINICAL PROCEDURES

Term	Description
cystoscopy sĭs-TŎS-kō-pē	visual examination of urinary bladder with a cystoscope inserted in the urethra; also used to obtain biopsies of tumors or other growths and to remove polyps
hemodialysis hē-mō-dī-ĂL-ĭ-sĭs	removal of chemical substances from the blood by passing it through semipermeable membranous tubes, which are continually bathed by solutions that selectively remove harmful products

CLINICAL PROCEDURES (Continued)

Term	Description
nephroscopy nĕ-FRŎS-kō-pē	visual examination of the kidney(s) using a specialized three-channel endoscope to provide for telescope, fiberoptic light input, and irrigation. The nephroscope is passed through a small incision made in the renal pelvis. Kidney pathology and congenital deformities may be observed
peritoneal dialysis pĕr-ĭ-tŏ-NĒ-ăl dī-ĂL-ĭ-sĭs	removal of toxic substances from the body by perfusing the peritoneal cavity with warm sterile chemical solutions
urethroscopy ū-rē-THRŎS-kō-pē	visualization of the urethra using a urethroscope; used for lithotripsy or for TUR

SURGICAL PROCEDURES

Term	Description
circumcision sĕr-kŭm-SĬZH-ŭn	surgical removal of all or part of the foreskin, or prepuce, of the penis
nephrolithotomy nĕf-rō-lĭth-ŎT-ō-mē	incision of a kidney to remove a stone
nephropexy NĔF-rō-pĕks-ē	fixation of a floating or mobile kidney
orchiectomy ŏr-kē-ĔK-tō-mē	surgical removal of the testes
transurethral resection (TUR) trăns-ū-RĒ-thrăl rē-SĔK-shŭn	procedure to remove prostatic tissue by cauterization or cryosurgery, performed using an endoscope passed through the urethra
urethrorrhaphy ū-rē-THROR-ăf-ē	suture of the urethra, frequently employed to repair a fistula
urethrotomy ū-rē-THRŎT-ō-mē	incision of a urethral stricture

LABORATORY PROCEDURES

Term	Description
blood urea nitrogen (BUN)	test that provides an estimate of kidney function by assessing the nitrogen in blood in the form of urea (increased BUN usually indicates decreased renal function)
semen analysis	test that analyzes a semen sample for volume, sperm count, motility, and morphology; also used to verify sterilization after a vasectomy
urinalysis (UA)	analysis of the chemical composition of urine and microscopic examination for blood cells, bacteria, crystals, and casts

PHARMACOLOGY

Medication	Action
diuretics	agents that promote the secretion of urine
estrogen hormones	hormones used in men to suppress gonadotropic and testicular androgenic hormones; used to treat some prostatic cancers
gonadotropin	hormonal preparation used to raise sperm count in infertility cases
spermicidals	substances that destroy sperm, used within the woman's vagina for contraception
uricosurics	agents that increase the urinary excretion of uric acid; used to treat gout

ABBREVIATIONS

Abbreviation	Meaning
A/G	albumin/globulin ratio
AGN	acute glomerulonephritis
ATN	acute tubular necrosis
BNO	bladder neck obstruction
BPH	benign prostatic hypertrophy; benign prostatic hyperplasia
BUN	blood urea nitrogen

ABBREVIATIONS (Continued)

Abbreviation	Meaning
cysto	cystoscopic examination
ESL	extracorporeal shock-wave lithotripsy
GU	genitourinary
IVP	intravenous pyelogram
KUB	kidney, ureter, bladder
pH	hydrogen ion concentration
RP	retrograde pyelogram
TUR, TURP	transurethral resection (for prostatectomy)
UA	urinalysis
UTI	urinary tract infection
VCU, VCUG	voiding cystourethrogram

Case Study

Operative Report

Preoperative and Postoperative Diagnosis. Hematuria with left **ureterocele** and uretero-cele **calculus**

Operation. Cystoscopy, transurethral incision of ureterocele, extraction of stone and **cystolithotripsy**

Anesthesia. General

Procedure. The patient was prepped and draped and placed in the **lithotomy position.** The **urethra** was **calibrated** with ease, using a #26 French Van Buren **sound.** A #24 **resectoscope** was inserted with ease. The **prostate** and **bladder** appeared normal, except for the presence of a left **ureterocele;** this was incised longitudinally and a large calculus was extracted from the ureterocele. There was minimal bleeding and no need for **fulguration.** The stone was crushed with the Storz stone-crushing instrument, and the fragments were **evacuated.** The bladder was emptied and the procedure terminated.

Worksheet 5 provides a dictionary and reading application and an analysis of this case study.

Worksheet 1

Use nephr/o (kidney) to build a medical word meaning:

1. stone in the kidney _____

2. specialist in the study of the kidney _____

3. abnormal condition of pus in the kidney _____

4. abnormal condition of water in the kidney _____

Use pyel/o (renal pelvis) to build a medical word meaning:

5. dilation of the renal pelvis _____

6. disease of the renal pelvis _____

Use ureter/o (ureter) to build a medical word meaning:

7. dilation of the ureter _____

8. calculus in the ureter _____

9. enlargement of the ureter _____

Use cyst/o (bladder) to build a medical word meaning:

10. inflammation of the bladder _____

11. instrument to view the bladder _____

Use vesic/o (bladder) to build a medical word meaning:

12. herniation of the bladder _____

13. pertaining to the bladder and prostate _____

Use urethr/o (urethra) to build a medical word meaning:

14. narrowing or stricture of the urethra _____

15. an instrument to incise the urethra _____

Use ur/o (urine, urinary) to build a medical word meaning:

16. x-ray of urinary (structures) _____

17. disease of the urinary (tract) _____

Use the suffix -uria (urine) to build a medical word meaning:

18. blood in the urine _____

19. difficult or painful urination _____

20. scanty urination _____

Use orchid/o or orchi/o (testes) to build a medical word meaning:

21. disease of the testes _____

22. pain in the testes _____

Use vesicul/o (seminal vesicle) to build a medical word meaning:

23. disease of the seminal vesicle _____

Use prostat/o (prostate) to build a medical word meaning:

24. discharge from the prostate _____

Use balan/o (glans penis) to build a medical word meaning:

25. discharge from the glans penis _____

Worksheet 2

Build a surgical term meaning:

1. removal of the vas deferens _____

2. suturing of the urethra _____

3. surgical repair of ureter and renal pelvis _____

4. removal of the kidney and its ureter _____

5. excision of a stone from the bladder _____

6. surgical repair of the bladder _____

7. surgical connection between the kidney and the bladder _____

8. removal of the prostate _____

9. incision for removal of a stone in the prostate _____

10. removal of the testes _____

Worksheet 3

Match the following medical terms with the definitions in the numbered list:

anuria   hypospadias

aspermia   impotence

incontinence   oliguria

epispadias   urgency

frequency   urolithiasis

hypertension   varicocele

1. _____ involuntary discharge of urine

2. _____ scanty urine production

3. _____ malformation in which the urethra opens on the dorsum of the penis

4. _____ condition characterized by the inability to achieve an erection

5. _____ swelling and distension of the veins of the spermatic cord

6. _____ male developmental anomaly in which the urethra opens on the underside of the penis

7. _____ presence of stones in the urinary system

8. _____ voiding at frequent intervals either in small or large amounts

9. _____ lack of or failure to ejaculate semen

10. _____ the need to void immediately

Worksheet 4

SPECIAL PROCEDURES, PHARMACOLOGY, AND ABBREVIATIONS

Match the following medical terms with the definitions in the numbered list.

blood urea nitrogen (BUN)

circumcision

cystography

cystoscopy

diuretics

estrogenic hormones

gonadotropins

nephrotomography

pH

intravenous pyleogram (IVP)

retrograde pyelogram (RP)

semen analysis

spermicidal preparations

urethroscopy

uricosuric agents

urinalysis (UA)

UTI

1. _____ use of a radiopaque dye administered intravenously to visualize the urinary structures, especially the structures of the kidney

2. _____ one of the most widely used laboratory tests that provides information on the urinary structures as well as other body systems

3. _____ test that determines kidney function by assessing its ability to remove urea

4. _____ drugs that increase the excretion of uric acid by the kidney, used in the treatment of gout

5. _____ hormonal preparations used to raise sperm count in cases of infertility

6. _____ hydrogen ion concentration

7. _____ removal of all or part of the foreskin, or prepuce

8. _____ increase the production of urine

9. _____ substances that destroy sperm

10. _____ analysis of volume, sperm count, motility, and morphology, usually performed as part of an infertility work-up

11. _____ detailed x-ray examination of the urinary structures via catheter after contrast medium is introduced

12. _____ study visualizing several planes of the kidney

13. _____ hormonal agents used to treat prostate cancer

14. _____ procedure that permits visualization of the urethra, often used for lithotripsy or TUR

15. _____ radiographic procedure that involves the introduction of a contrast medium into the bladder to visualize this structure

Worksheet 5

OPERATIVE REPORT DICTIONARY EXERCISE

Use a medical dictionary or other resource to define the following terms and to determine their pronunciation; then practice reading the case study aloud (p. 252).

bladder _____

calculus _____

calibrated _____

cystolithotripsy _____

cystoscopy _____

evacuated _____

fulguration _____

hematuria _____

lithotomy position _____

prostate _____

resectoscope _____

sound _____

transurethral _____

ureterocele _____

urethra _____

ANALYSIS OF OPERATIVE REPORT

1. Why did the doctor perform a cystoscopy?

2. What size of urethral sound was used?

3. Why is a sound used?

4. In what direction did the urologist cut the uretherocele?

5. Did the urologist need to use fulguration? If no, why?

Worksheet 6

Label the following figure, and compare your answers with Figure 12–2.

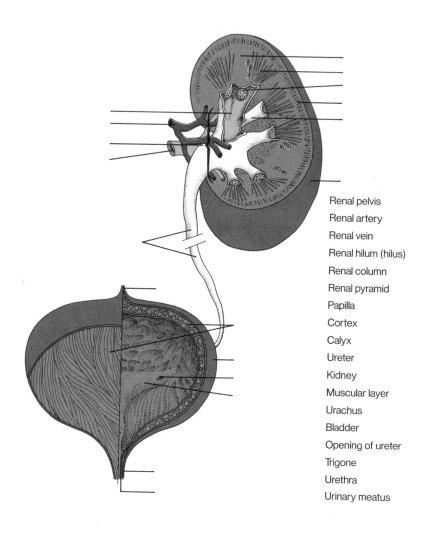

Renal pelvis
Renal artery
Renal vein
Renal hilum (hilus)
Renal column
Renal pyramid
Papilla
Cortex
Calyx
Ureter
Kidney
Muscular layer
Urachus
Bladder
Opening of ureter
Trigone
Urethra
Urinary meatus

Worksheet 7

Label the following figure, and compare your answers with Figure 12–3.

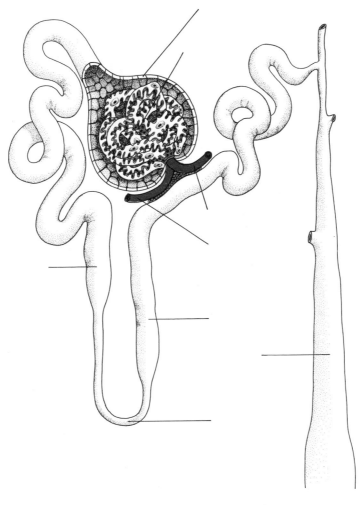

| Afferent arteriole | Collecting tubule | Efferent arteriole | Loop of Henle |
| Bowman's capsule | Distal tubule | Glomerulus | Proximal tubule |

Worksheet 8

Label the following figure, and compare your answers with Figure 12–4.

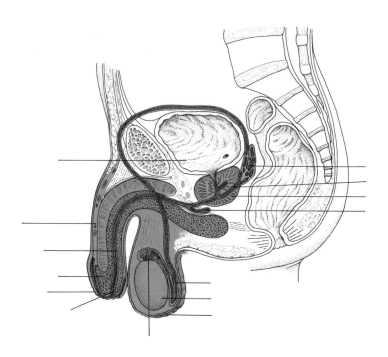

Bulbourethral (Cowper's) gland	Prepuce	Urethra
Ejaculatory duct	Prostate gland	Urethral orifice
Epididymis	Seminal vesicle	Urinary bladder
Glans penis	Scrotum	Vas deferens
Penis	Testis	

Chapter 13

Female Reproductive System

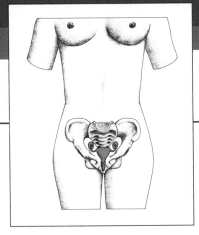

Chapter Outline

Student Objectives

Upon completion of this chapter, you will be able to do the following:

List the organs of the female reproductive system.

Describe the position and function of each organ.

Explain the series of events associated with maturation of the ovum.

Describe the condition and stages of pregnancy.

Student Objectives (Continued)

Identify combining forms and suffixes associated with the female reproductive system.

Identify and discuss pathology related to the female reproductive system.

Identify diagnostic imaging, endoscopic, surgical and laboratory procedures, and abbreviations related to the female reproductive system.

Explain pharmacology related to treatment of female reproductive disorders.

Demonstrate your understanding of the chapter by completing the worksheets.

Anatomy and Physiology

The female reproductive system (Fig. 13–1) consists of internal and external organs of reproduction (Fig. 13–2). The internal, or essential, organs of reproduction are the (1) **ovaries,** (2) **fallopian tubes (oviducts, uterine tubes),** (3) **uterus,** and (4) **vagina.** The external genitalia include the (5) **labia majora,** (6) **labia minora,** (7) **clitoris,** and (8) **Bartholin's glands.** The combined structures of the external genitalia are known as the **vulva.**

INTERNAL ORGANS OF REPRODUCTION

Ovaries

Refer the Figure 13–3 as you read the following material. The (1) **ovaries** are almond-shaped glands located in the pelvic cavity, one on each side of the uterus, which produce the ovum (egg), the female reproductive cell, and various hormones.

Two hormones secreted by the ovaries, estrogen and progesterone, are responsible for the menstrual cycle and menopause. In addition, both hormones prepare the uterus for implantation of the fertilized egg, help maintain pregnancy, and promote growth of the placenta. Estrogen and progesterone also play an important role in development of secondary sex characteristics (see Chapter 14).

Fallopian Tubes

Two (2) **fallopian tubes (oviducts, uterine tubes)** extend laterally from superior angles of the uterus. Fingerlike projections, (3) **fimbriae,** create wavelike currents (peristalsis) in fluid surrounding the ovary to pull the ovum into the uterine tube. If the egg unites with a spermatozoon, the male reproductive cell, fertilization or conception takes place. If conception does not occur, the ovum disintegrates within 48 hours.

Uterus and Vagina

The (4) **uterus** contains and nourishes the embryo from the time the fertilized egg is implanted until the fetus is born. It is a muscular, hollow, pear-shaped structure located

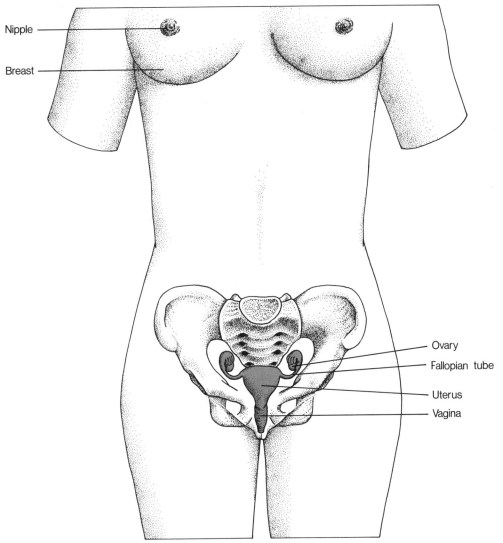

Figure 13–1 Anterior view of the female reproductive system.

in the pelvic area between the bladder and rectum. The uterus is normally in a position of anteflexion (bent forward) and consists of three parts: the (5) **fundus,** which is the upper-rounded part; the (6) **body,** which is the central part; and the (7) **cervix,** also called the neck of the uterus or **cervix uteri,** which is the inferior constricted portion that opens into the vagina.

The (8) **vagina** is a muscular tube that extends from the cervix to the exterior of the body. Its lining consists of mucous membrane folds that give the organ an elastic quality. During sexual excitement, the vaginal orifice is lubricated by secretions from (9) **Bartholin's glands.** Besides serving as the organ of sexual intercourse and receptor of semen, the vagina discharges menstrual flow. The vagina also acts as a passageway for the delivery of the fetus.

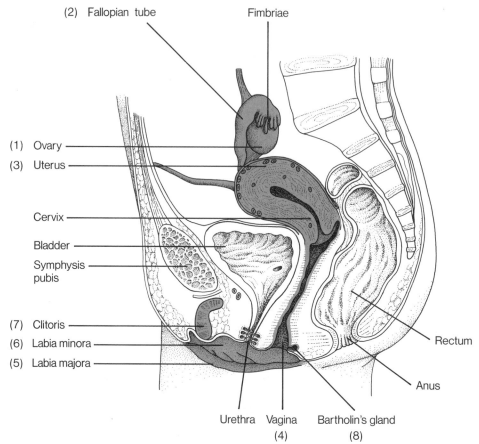

Figure 13–2 Lateral view of the female reproductive system.

MENSTRUAL CYCLE

Menarche, the initial menstrual period, occurs at puberty (about 13 years of age) and continues approximately 40 years, except during pregnancy. The menstrual cycle consists of approximately 28 days and can be described in terms of three phases: menstrual phase, follicular phase, and luteal phase.

Menstrual Phase

The loss of the functional layer of endometrium is known as menstruation. Menstruation may last 2 to 8 days, with an average of 3 to 6 days. Secretion of the follicle-stimulating hormone (FSH) increases, and several ovarian follicles begin to develop.

Follicular Phase

The FSH stimulates the ovarian follicles to develop and stimulates secretion of estrogen by the ovaries. Secretions of the luteinizing hormone (LH) work with FSH to bring about

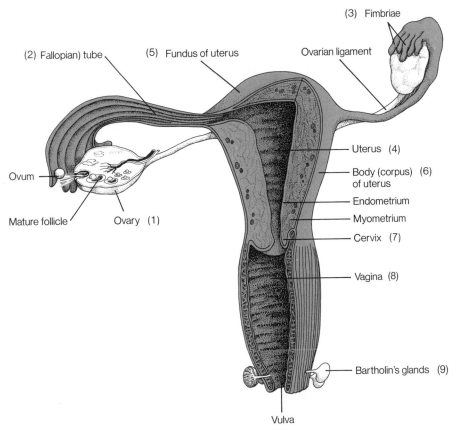

(3) Fimbriae

(2) Fallopian) tube

(5) Fundus of uterus

Ovarian ligament

Ovum

Mature follicle

Ovary (1)

Uterus (4)

Body (corpus) (6)
of uterus

Endometrium

Myometrium

Cervix (7)

Vagina (8)

Bartholin's glands (9)

Vulva

Figure 13–3   Female reproductive organs.

final maturation of the follicle and trigger its rupture a day or two later. This phase ends with ovulation, when a sharp increase in LH ruptures a mature ovarian follicle.

Luteal Phase

After ovulation, the empty graafian follicle is stimulated by LH to become a new structure, the corpus luteum. The corpus luteum secretes increasing quantities of estrogen and progesterone. If the ovum is not fertilized, another menstrual cycle is initiated by a decrease in secretions of progesterone and estrogen.

PREGNANCY

During pregnancy, the uterus changes its shape, size, and consistency. The peritoneal covering becomes enlarged, and there is an enormous increase in muscle mass. The vaginal canal elongates as the uterus rises in the pelvis. The mucosa thickens, secretions increase, and the vascularity and elasticity of both the cervix and vagina become more pronounced.

The average pregnancy **(gestation)** lasts approximately 9 months and is followed by childbirth **(parturition).** Up to the third month of pregnancy, the product of conception is referred to as the embryo. From the third month to the time of birth, the unborn offspring is referred to as the fetus.

Pregnancy also causes enlargement of the breasts, sometimes to the point of painfulness. Many other changes occur throughout the body to accommodate the development and birth of the fetus.

Toward the end of gestation, the myometrium begins to contract weakly at irregular intervals. At this time the full-term fetus is usually positioned head down within the uterus (Fig. 13–4).

LABOR AND BIRTH

Labor is the physiological process by which the fetus is expelled from the uterus. Labor occurs in three stages. The first is the **stage of dilation,** which begins with uterine contractions and terminates when there is complete dilation (10 cm) of the cervix. The second is the **stage of expulsion.** This is the time from complete cervical dilation to birth of the baby. The last is the **placental stage,** or afterbirth. It begins shortly after childbirth, when the uterine contractions discharge the placenta from the uterus.

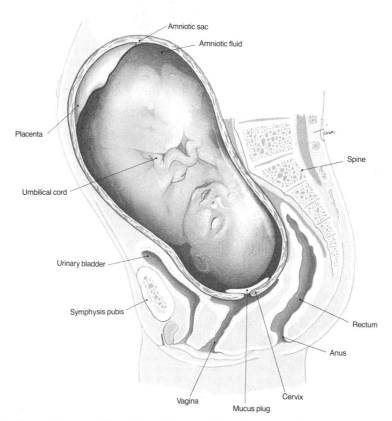

Figure 13–4 Full-term fetus positioned head down within the uterus. (From Scanlon, VC and Sanders, T: Essentials of Anatomy and Physiology, ed 2. FA Davis, Philadelphia, 1995, p 493, with permission.)

MENOPAUSE

Menopause is the cessation of ovarian activity and diminished hormone production that occurs at about 50 years of age. Menopause is usually diagnosed if absence of menses **(amenorrhea)** has persisted for 1 year. The period of time in which symptoms of approaching menopause occur is also known as **change of life** or **climacteric.**

Many women experience hot flashes and vaginal drying and thinning **(vaginal atrophy)** as estrogen levels fall. Although **estrogen therapy replacement (EST)** is still controversial, it is used to treat vaginal atrophy and porous bones **(osteoporosis),** and is believed to play a role in prevention of heart attacks. Restraint in prescribing estrogens for long periods in all menopausal women arises from concern that there is an increased risk that long-term usage will induce neoplastic changes in estrogen-sensitive aging tissue.

COMBINING FORMS

Combining Form	Meaning	Example	Pronunciation
amni/o	amnion (amniotic sac)	amni/o/centesis _____ puncture	ăm-nē-ō-sĕn-TĒ-sĭs
cervic/o	neck, cervix uteri (neck of uterus)	cervic/itis _____ inflammation	sĕr-vĭ-SĪ-tĭs
colp/o	vagina	colp/o/rrhapy _____ suture	kŏl-PŎR-ă-fē
vagin/o	vagina	vagin/itis _____ inflammation	văj-ĭn-Ī-tĭs
episi/o	vulva	episi/o/tomy _____ incision	ĕ-pĭz-ē-ŎT-ō-mē
vulv/o	vulva	vulv/ectomy _____ excision	vŭl-VĔK-tō-mē
galact/o	milk	galact/o/rrhea _____ flow	gă-lăk-tō-RĒ-ăh
lact/o	milk	lact/o/gen/ ic _____ production relating to	lăk-tō-JĔN-ĭk
gynec/o	woman, female	gynec/o/logy _____ study of	gī-nĕ-KOL-ō-jē
hyster/o	uterus, womb	hyster/ectomy _____ excision	hĭs-tĕr-ĔK-tō-mē
uter/o	uterus, womb	intra/uter/ine within pertaining to	ĭn-tră-Ū-tĕr-ĭn
metr/o	uterus, womb	metr/o/rrhea _____ discharge	mē-trō-RĒ-ă
labi/o	lip	labi/al _____ pertaining to	LĀ-bē-ăl

COMBINING FORMS (Continued)

Combining Form	Meaning	Example	Pronunciation
lapar/o	abdomen	lapar/o/scopy visual examination	lăp-ăr-ŎS-kō-pē

mamm/o
 	
mast/o
	breast	mamm/ary
		        relating to
		gynec/o/mast/ia
		female noun
		                ending
			MĂM-ă-rē
			
			gī-nē-kō-MĂS-tē-ăh

men/o	menses, menstruation	men/o/rrhagia bursting forth	mĕn-ō-RĀ-jē-ăh
nat/a	birth	post/nat/al after pertaining to	pōst-NĀ-tăl

oophor/o
ovari/o
	ovary	oophor/itis
		          inflammation
		ovari/o/cele
		             herniation
			ō-ŏf-ō-RĪ-tĭs
			
			ō-VĀ-rē-Ō-sēl

perine/o	perineum	perine/al pertaining to	pĕr-ĭ-NĒ-ăl
salping/o	fallopian tubes, oviducts, uterine tubes	salping/o/rrhaphy suture	săl-pĭng-GOR-ă-fē

SUFFIXES

Suffix	Meaning	Example	Pronunciation
-arche	beginning	men/arche menses, menstruation	mĕn-ĂR-kē
-gravida	pregnancy	multi/gravida many	mŭl-tĭ-GRĂV-ĭ-dă
-para	to bear (offspring)	nulli/para none	nŭh-LĬP-ăh-răh
-gravida	fallopian tubes, oviducts,	Hem/o/Salpinx	mul-ti-GRAV-i-da
-salpinx	fallopian tubes, oviducts, uterine tubes	hem/o/salpinx blood	hē-mō-SĂL-pĭnks
-tocia	childbirth, labor	dys/tocia difficult, painful	dĭs-TŌ-sē-āh

Pathology

MENSTRUAL DISTURBANCES

Menstrual disturbances are usually caused by hormonal dysfunctions or pathological conditions of the uterus and may produce a variety of symptoms.

Menstrual pain and tension **(dysmenorrhea)** may be the result of uterine contractions, a pathological growth, or general chronic disorders such as anemia, fatigue, diabetes, or tuberculosis. The female hormone estrogen is used to treat dysmenorrhea and also to regulate menstrual abnormalities.

Irregular uterine bleeding between menstrual periods **(metrorrhagia)** of after menopause is usually symptomatic of some disease, often benign or malignant uterine tumors. Consequently, early diagnosis and treatment is warranted. Metrorrhagia is probably the most significant form of menstrual dysfunction.

Profuse or prolonged bleeding during regular menstruation **(menorrhagia** or **hypermenorrhea)** may, during early life, be caused by endocrine disturbances. However, in later life, it is usually due to inflammatory diseases, tumors, or emotional disturbances, which also affect bleeding.

PREMENSTRUAL SYNDROME

Premenstrual syndrome (PMS) occurs several days before the onset of menstruation and ends a short time after. A great number of symptoms involving almost every organ have been attributed to PMS. The direct cause of PMS is unknown, but the most common manifestations are irritability, emotional tension, anxiety, mood changes (especially depression), headaches, breast tenderness with or without swelling, and water retention, which may be sufficient enough to cause edema. The reason most individuals with PMS seek medical assistance is related to mood change.

TOXIC SHOCK SYNDROME

Toxic shock syndrome (TSS) or septic shock is caused by one or more toxins produced by certain strains of the bacterium *Staphylococcus aureus.* TSS usually occurs in young menstruating women, most of whom use vaginal tampons for menstrual protection. TSS is characterized by high fever, cerebral manifestations (confusion, syncope, headache), and skin rash. The bacterial toxins may migrate from the infection site (i.e., the vagina) into the blood, triggering a widespread inflammatory response that leads to peripheral vasodilation, impaired cellular metabolism, and septic shock.

ENDOMETRIOSIS

Endometriosis is the presence of functioning endometrial tissue outside the uterus. Such **ectopic** (out-of-place) tissue or implants are usually confined to the pelvic area but may appear anywhere in the body. Like normal endometrial tissue, the ectopic endometrium responds to hormonal fluctuations of the menstrual cycle.

PELVIC INFECTIONS

Pelvic inflammatory disease (PID) is an acute, subacute, recurrent, or chronic condition of the oviducts and ovaries with adjacent tissue involvement. It includes inflammation of the cervix **(cervicitis),** uterus **(endometritis),** fallopian tubes **(salpingitis),** and ovaries **(oophoritis).** PID can extend to connective tissue lying between the broad ligaments **(parametritis).** If left untreated, PID may cause infertility and may lead to potentially fatal septicemia, pulmonary emboli, and shock.

VAGINAL INFECTIONS

An inflammation of the vagina **(vaginitis)** occurs when organisms such as *Escherichia coli,* staphylococci, and streptococci invade the vagina. The normal whitish vaginal discharge **(leukorrhea),** which usually occurs in slight amounts, becomes more profuse and yellowish in vaginitis. It is not uncommon for vaginitis to be accompanied by urethritis because of the proximity of the urethra to the vagina.

Candidiasis, a vaginal fungal infection caused by *Candida albicans,* is characterized by a curdy or cheeselike discharge and extreme itching **(pruritus).** Because the organism thrives in an environment rich in carbohydrates, it is commonly seen in patients with poorly controlled diabetes. Also, patients who have been receiving steroid therapy or antibiotics often develop a *Candida* infection. Antifungal agents **(mycostatics)** that suppress the growth of fungi are used to treat this disease.

SEXUALLY TRANSMITTED DISEASES

Sexually transmitted diseases (STDs), also called venereal diseases (VDs), are contagious diseases acquired as a result of sexual activity with an infected individual. In the United States the frequency of STDs is regarded as an epidemic and includes gonorrhea, syphilis, chlamydia, genital herpes, and a complex array of infections and clinical syndromes that make up a new generation of STDs of which the newest and most serious is acquired immunodeficiency syndrome (AIDS) (see Chapter 10).

Gonorrhea is caused by infection with the bacterium *Neisseria gonorrhoeae* and involves the mucosal surface of the genitourinary tract, rectum, and pharynx. This disease may be acquired through sexual intercourse and through orogenital and anogenital contacts between members of the opposite sex and between members of the same sex.

Some women do not experience pain or manifest overt clinical symptoms **(asymptomatic)** until the disease has spread to the ovaries **(oophoritis)** and uterine tubes **(salpingitis),** causing PID. The most common symptom of gonorrhea in women is a greenish-yellow cervical discharge. An untreated pregnant woman with gonorrhea may transmit the disease to the eyes of her newborn during vaginal delivery, which may result in blindness. Men with this disease suffer inflammation of the urethra **(urethritis),** which may cause painful urination **(dysuria),** along with a discharge of pus. If left untreated, the disease may infect the bladder **(cystitis)** and inflame the joints **(arthritis).** In addition, sterility may result from formation of scars that close the reproductive tubes of both sexes. Both sex partners must be treated because the infection can recur.

Syphilis, although less common than gonorrhea, is the more serious of the two diseases. It is caused by infection with the bacterium *Treponema pallidum*. Syphilis is a chronic infectious multisystemic disease acquired through sexual contact or at birth **(congenitally)**. A primary sore **(chancre)** develops at the point where the bacteria entered the body. The chancre is an ulcerated sore with hard edges that contains contagious organisms for 10 days to 3 months. In pregnancy, the fetus is infected from the mother by way of the placenta. The vast majority of cases are contracted through sexual activity; the danger of transmission is greatest in the early stage of syphilis. If left untreated, the end result is blindness, insanity, and eventual death.

Genital herpes, which causes red blisterlike sores, is the most common infectious genital ulceration in the United States. The fluid in the blisters is highly infectious. Most genital herpes infections are caused by the herpes simplex virus (HSV) type 2 and is transmitted primarily through direct sexual contact. Individuals with herpes infection may have only one episode or may have repeated attacks. There seems to be a greater incidence of cervical cancer and miscarriages in individuals with this disease. Genital herpes is also associated with the danger of seriously infecting children during childbirth. In men, lesions appear on the glans, foreskin, or penile shaft.

Chlamydia, caused by infection with the bacterium *Chlamydia trachomatis,* is the most prevalent and among the most damaging of all STDs seen in the United States. In men, chlamydial infections cause urethritis with a whitish discharge from the penis. In women, chlamydial infections cause an inflammation of the cervix uteri **(cervicitis)** with a mucopurulent discharge and an alarming increase in pelvic infections. These complications contribute significantly to the increase in the number of women who experience ectopic pregnancies. In pregnant women, transmission of chlamydia to the fetus can result in substantial newborn morbidity. In both sexes, chlamydia has been associated with many other health problems.

Trichomoniasis, caused by the protozoan *Trichomonas vaginalis,* is now known to be one of the most common causes of sexually transmitted lower genital tract infections. It is more commonly found in women and causes **vaginitis, urethritis,** and **cystitis.**

UTERINE TUMORS

About 30 to 40 percent of all women develop myomatous or fibroid tumors of the uterus **(leiomyomas)** that are benign. These benign tumors develop slowly between the ages of 25 and 40, and often enlarge in response to fluctuating endocrine stimulation after this period. Some persons with this type of tumor experience no symptoms. When symptoms are present, the most common is menorrhagia. Other symptoms are due to pressure on surrounding organs: pain, backache, constipation, and urinary symptoms. In addition, such tumors often cause metrorrhagia and even sterility.

Treatment of uterine fibroid tumors frequently depends on their size and location. If the patient plans to have children, treatment is as conservative as possible. As a rule, large tumors that produce pressure symptoms should be removed. Usually, the uterus is removed **(hysterectomy),** but the ovaries are preserved. If the tumor is small, a myomectomy may be performed to remove it. However, when the tumor is producing excessive bleeding, both the uterus and the tumor are excised.

ONCOLOGY

Cervical Cancer

Cancer of the cervix, a malignancy of the female reproductive system, most often affects women who are 40 to 49 years of age. Statistics indicate that infection owing to sexual activity has some relationship to the incidence of cervical cancer. First coitus at a young age, large number of sex partners, infection with certain sexually transmitted viruses, and frequent intercourse with men whose previous partners had cervical cancer are all associated with increased risk of developing cervical cancer.

A cytological examination known as a Papanicolaou test (Pap smear) can detect cervical cancer before the disease becomes clinically evident. Abnormal cervical cytology routinely calls for colposcopy, which can detect the presence and extent of preclinical lesions requiring biopsy and histologic examination. Treatment of cervical cancer consists of surgery, radiation, and/or chemotherapy. If left untreated, the cancer will eventually metastasize and lead to death.

Diagnostic, Symptomatic, and Related Terms

FEMALE REPRODUCTIVE SYSTEM

Term	Meaning
adnexa ăd-NĔK-să	accessory parts of a structure (adnexa uteri are the ovaries and fallopian tubes)
atresia ăh-TRĒ-zē-ăh	congenital absence or closure of a normal body opening
choriocarcinoma kō-rē-ō-kăr-sĭ-NŌ-măh	malignant neoplasm of the uterus or at the site of an ectopic pregnancy. Although its actual cause is unknown, this rare tumor may occur following pregnancy or abortion
corpus luteum KŎR-pŭs LOO-tē-ŭm	ovarian scar tissue that results from rupturing of a follicle during ovulation. This small yellow body produces progesterone following ovulation
dyspareunia dĭs-pă-RŪ-nē-ăh	occurrence of pain during sexual intercourse
endocervicitis ĕn-dō-sĕr-vĭ-SĪ-tĭs	inflammation of mucous lining of the cervix uteri; usually chronic, often due to infection, and accompanied by cervical erosion
fibroids, fibromyoma uteri FĪ-broids, fĭ-brō-mī-Ō-măh	benign uterine tumors that are composed of muscle and fibrous tissue; leiomyomas. Myomectomy or hysterectomy may be indicated if the fibroids grow too large, causing symptoms such as metrorrhagia, pelvic pain, or menorrhagia

FEMALE REPRODUCTIVE SYSTEM (Continued)

Term	Meaning
gynecology gī-nĕ-KŎL-ō-jē	study of the female reproductive system, including the breasts
infertility ĭn-fĕr-TĬL-ĭ-tē	inability or diminished ability to produce offspring
menarche mĕn-ĂR-kē	beginning of the menstrual function
perineum pĕr-ĭ-NĒ-ŭm	region between the vulva and anus that constitutes the pelvic floor
pyosalpinx pī-ō-SAL-pingks	pus in the fallopian tube
puberty PŪ-bĕr-tē	period during which secondary sex characteristics begin to develop and the capability of sexual reproduction is attained
vaginismus văj-ĭn-ĬZ-mŭs	painful spasm of the vagina from contraction of the muscles surrounding the vagina

OBSTETRICS

Term	Meaning
abruptio placentae ăb-RŬP-shē-ō plăh-SĔN-tăh	premature separation of a normally situated placenta
abortion ă-BOR-shŭn	termination of pregnancy before the embryo or fetus is capable of surviving outside the uterus
amnion ĂM-nē-ŏn	innermost membrane enclosing the developing fetus; the transparent sac that holds the fetus suspended in amniotic fluid
breech presentation	common abnormality of delivery in which the fetal buttocks or feet present rather than the head
Down's syndrome, trisomy 21 dŏwnz SĬN-drōm	preferred terms for mongolism. A congenital condition characterized by physical malformations and some degree of mental retardation. Trisomy of chromosome 21 usually occurs in 1 of 700 live births.
dystocia dĭs-TŌ-sē-ă	difficult labor; may be produced by either the large size of the fetus or the small size of the pelvic outlet

OBSTETRICS (Continued)

Term	Meaning
eclampsia ĕ-KLĂMP-sē-ăh	most serious form of toxemia of pregnancy, manifested by high blood pressure, edema, convulsions, renal dysfunction, proteinuria, and, in severe cases, coma
ectopic pregnancy ĕk-TŎP-ĭk PRĔG-năn-sē	pregnancy in which the fertilized ovum does not reach the uterine cavity but instead becomes implanted on any tissue other than the lining of the uterine cavity (e.g., fallopian tube, ovary, abdomen, or even the cervix uteri). In a tubal pregnancy, as the fertilized ovum increases in size, the tube becomes more and more distended until, about 4 to 6 weeks after conception, it ruptures and the fertilized ovum is discharged into the abdominal cavity.
gestation jĕs-TĀ-shŭn	pregnancy; the 9-month period of time from conception to birth
gravida GRĂV-ĭ-dă	pregnant woman; may be followed by numbers, indicating number of pregnancies (i.e., gravida 1, 2, 3, 4 or I, II, III, IV, and so on)
hydrocephalus hī-drō-SĔF-ăh-lŭs	enlargement of the cranium caused by accumulation of fluid within the ventricles of the brain
kernicterus kĕr-NĬK-tĕr-ŭs	extremely serious condition involving mental retardation, jaundice, and brain damage by excessive bilirubin (hyperbilirubinemia)
multigravida mŭl-tĭ-GRĂV-ĭ-dăh	pregnant woman who has been pregnant one or more times previously
multipara mŭl-TĬP-ăh-răh	woman who has delivered more than one viable offspring
obstetrician ŏb-stĕ-TRĬSH-ăn	physician who specializes in the branch of medicine dealing with pregnancy, labor, and the puerperium
obstetrics ŏb-STĔT-rĭks	specialty concerned with pregnancy and delivery of the fetus
para PĂR-Ă	woman who has delivered one viable offspring; para may be followed by numbers, indicating number of deliveries (i.e., para 1, 2, 3, 4 or I, II, III, IV, and so on)
parturition păr-tū-RĬSH-ŭn	act or process of giving birth to a child
pelvimetry pĕl-VĬM-ĕ-trē	measurement of the pelvic dimensions or proportions; helps determine whether or not the fetus can be delivered by the normal route

OBSTETRICS (Continued)

Term	Meaning
placenta previa plă-SĔN-tăh PRE-vē-ăh	condition in which the placenta is attached near the cervix and ruptures prematurely, with spotting as the early symptom. Prevention of hemorrhage may necessitate a cesarean section
primigravida prī-mĭ-GRĂV-ĭ-dăh	woman during her first pregnancy
primipara prī-MĬP-ăh-răh	woman who has delivered one viable offspring
puerperium pū-ĕr-PĒ-rē-ŭm	period of 42 days following childbirth and expulsion of the placenta and membranes, during which the reproductive organs usually return to normal
viable	capable of living outside of the uterus

Special Procedures

DIAGNOSTIC IMAGING PROCEDURES

Term	Description
hysterosalpingography, hysterosalpingogram hĭs-tĕr-ō-săl-pĭn-GŎG-ră-fe	radiography of the uterus and oviducts after a contrast medium is injected into those organs; used to determine pathology in the uterine cavity, evaluate tubal patency, and determine the cause of fertility problems
ultrasonography, ultrasonogram	noninvasive technique in which ultrasonic echoes are recorded as they strike organs or tissues of different densities, producing an image or photograph of the patient; used to evaluate the female reproductive system as well as the fetus in the obstetric patient

ENDOSCOPIC PROCEDURES

Term	Description
colpomicroscopy kŏl-pō-mī-KRŎS-kō-pē	use of optical instruments designed to permit three-dimensional views of stained or unstained cervical epithelium in situ (in position, localized); provides visual access to suspicious tissue areas, even though biopsy is often required for accurate diagnosis
laparoscopy, peritoneoscopy lăp-ăr-ŌS-kō-pe, pĕr-ĭ-tō-nē-ŎS-kō-pē	visual examination of the abdominal cavity after a small incision of the abdominal wall to admit a laparoscope; used to examine the ovaries or fallopian tubes and to perform gynecological sterilization

SURGICAL PROCEDURES

Term	Description
amniocentesis ăm-nē-ō-sĕn-TĒ-sĭs	transabdominal puncture of the amniotic sac to remove amniotic fluid. The material obtained is cultured in order to make biochemical and cytological studies
cesarean birth, C-section sē-SĀR-ē-ăn	incision of the abdomen and uterus to remove the fetus; most commonly used in the event of cephalopelvic disproportion, presence of sexually transmitted disease organisms in the birth canal, fetal distress, and breech presentation
colpectomy, vaginectomy kŏl-PĔK-tō-mē, văj-ĭn-ĔK-tō-mē	excision of the vagina
colpocleisis kŏl-pō-KLĪ-sĭs	surgical closure of the vaginal canal
colpoperineoplasty, colpoperineorrhaphy kŏl-pō-pĕr-ĭ-NĒ-ō-plăs-tē, kŏl-pō-pĕr-ĭ-nē-ŎR-ăh-fē	plastic surgery of the vagina and perineum
conization kŏn-ĭ-ZĀ-shŭn	excision of a cone of tissue (e.g., mucosa of the cervix) for histologic examination; uses cold knife blade or laser so as to preserve histologic characteristics

SURGICAL PROCEDURES (Continued)

Term	Description
cryosurgery, cryocautery krī-ō-SĔR-jĕr-ē, krī-ō-KĂW-tĕr-ē	process of freezing tissue to destroy cells; used for chronic cervical infections and erosions because offending organisms may be entrenched in cervical cells and glands. Process destroys these infected areas, and in the healing process, normal cells are replenished. May also be used when a patient shows atypical or possible malignancy, as seen on a Pap smear.
dilatation and curettage (D&C) dĭl-ă-TĀ-shŭn, kū-rē-TĂHZH	widening of the cervical canal with a dilator and the scraping of the uterine endometrium with a curette; used for cytological examination of tissue, to control abnormal uterine bleeding, and as a therapeutic measure for incomplete abortion. Because this procedure usually is performed under anesthesia and requires surgical asepsis, it is done in the operating room
episiotomy ĕ-pĭz-ē-ŎT-ō-mē	incision of perineum from the vaginal orifice, usually done to facilitate childbirth
episiorrhaphy ĕ-pĭz-ē-ŎR-āh-fē	suturing of a lacerated perineum
hymenotomy hī-mĕn-ŎT-ō-mē	incision of the hymen
hysterectomy hĭs-tĕr-ĔK-tō-me	excision of the uterus. Abdominal: excision of the uterus through an abdominal incision. Vaginal: excision of the uterus through the vagina. Total abdominal hysterectomy (TAH): excision of the uterus, including the cervix, through an abdominal incision
myomectomy mī-ō-MĔK-tō-mē	excision of a myomatous tumor, generally uterine
salpingo-oophorectomy săl-pĭng-gō-ō-ŏf-ō-RĔK-tō-mē	excision of an ovary and fallopian tube, usually identified as right (R), left (L), or bilateral
tubal ligation TŪ-băl lī-GĀ-shŭn	ligating (tying) the uterine tubes to prevent pregnancy; sterilization surgery

LABORATORY PROCEDURES

Test	Description
chorionic villus sampling (CVS)	a sample of chorionic villi is obtained using a catheter inserted into the cervix and into the outer portion of the membranes surrounding the fetus; used to detect chromosomal abnormalities and fetal biochemical disorders
endometrial biopsy, endometrial smear	used in screening high-risk patients for endometrial cancer, performed during the gynecological examination. Following the administration of a small amount of anesthetic, a thin, hollow curette is used to remove endometrial tissue for laboratory analysis
Papanicolaou test, Pap smear	simple smear method of examining exfoliative cells; used most commonly to detect cervical cancer but may be used for tissue specimens from any organ; usually obtained during a routine pelvic examination

PHARMACOLOGY

Medication	Action
estrogen hormones	used in oral contraceptives and as a replacement hormone in the treatment of menopause; its long-term, continued use increases the risk of endometrial carcinoma
oral contraceptives, "the pill"	taken to prevent ovulation; almost 100% effective when taken according to instructions
oxytocins	stimulate the uterus to contract, thus inducing labor; also used to rid the uterus of an unexpelled placenta or a fetus that has died
spermicidals	destroy sperm; used within the vagina for contraceptive purposes; 85% effective for birth control; available in the form of jellies, creams, and foams, and do not require a prescription

ABBREVIATIONS

Maternal/Gynecological and Other

ABBREVIATION	MEANING
AB	abortion
AI	artificial insemination
CPD	cephalopelvic disproportion
D&C	dilatation and curettage
DC	discharge
DUB	dysfunctional uterine bleeding
Dx	diagnosis
EDC	estimated date of confinement
EST	estrogen therapy replacement
FH	family history
FSH	follicle-stimulating hormone
GC	gonorrhea
Gyn	gynecology
HSV	herpes simplex virus
IUD	intrauterine device
IVF	in vitro fertilization
LH	luteinizing hormone
LMP	last menstrual period
lt, L	left
MH	marital history
OCPs	oral contraceptive pills
PAP	papanicolau
PID	pelvic inflammatory disease
PMP	previous menstrual period
PMS	premenstrual syndrome
R/O	rule out
rt, R	right
STD	sexually transmitted diseases

ABBREVIATIONS (Continued)

Maternal/Gynecological and Other

ABBREVIATION	MEANING
TSS	toxic shock syndrome
VD	venereal disease

Fetal-Obstetric

CS, C-section	cesarean section
CVS	chorionic villus sampling
CWP	childbirth without pain
DOB	date of birth
FEKG	fetal electrocardiogram
FHR	fetal heart rate
FHT	fetal heart tone
FTND	full-term normal delivery
HSG	hysterosalpingography
HCG	human chorionic gonadotropin
IUGR	intrauterine growth rate, intrauterine growth retardation
NB	newborn
OB	obstetrics
TAH	total abdominal hysterectomy
UC	uterine contractions
XX	female sex chromosomes
XY	male sex chromosomes

Case Study

Primary Herpes I Infection

A family practice resident, aged 24 years, started having some sore areas around the **labia,** both rt and lt side. She stated that the last few days she started having a brownish **DC.** She has **pruritus** and pain of her **vulvar** area with adenopathy and fever at pm, and blisters. Apparently her partner had a cold sore and they had oral **genital** sex.

Has been using condoms since last seen in April. **LMP** 5/15/xx. She has not missed any **OCPs.** Patient has what looks like herpes lesions and ulcers all over vulva and **introitus** area. Rt labia appears as an ulcerlike lesion; it appears to be almost like an infected follicle. **Speculum** inserted, a brown DC noted. **GC** screen, **chlamydia** screen, and general culture obtained from that. Wet prep revealed **monilial** forms. Viral culture obtained from the ulcerlike lesion on the right.

Dx: Primary herpes I infection; will R/O other infectious etiologies.

Worksheet 5 provides a dictionary exercise and an analysis of this case study.

Worksheet 1

Use gynec/o (woman, female) to build a medical word meaning:

1. disease (specific to) women _____

2. study (of diseases) of the female _____

3. physician who specializes in diseases of the female _____

Use cervic/o (neck, cervix uteri) to build a medical word meaning:

4. inflammation of the cervix uteri and vagina _____

5. pertaining to the cervix uteri and bladder _____

Use colp/o (vagina) to build a medical word meaning:

6. instrument used to examine the vagina _____

7. visual examination of the vagina _____

Use vagin/o (vagina) to build a medical word meaning:

8. inflammation of the vagina _____

9. relating to the vagina _____

10. abnormal condition of a vaginal fungus _____

11. related to the vagina and the labia _____

Use hyster/o (uterus) to build a medical word meaning:

12. myoma of the uterus _____

13. disease of the uterus _____

14. radiography of the uterus and oviducts _____

Use metr/o (uterus) to build a medical word meaning:

15. hemorrhage from the uterus _____

16. inflammation around the uterus _____

Use uter/o (uterus) to build a medical word meaning:

17. herniation of the uterus _____

18. relating to the uterus and cervix _____

19. pertaining to the uterus and rectum _____

20. pertaining to the uterus and bladder _____

Use oophor/o (ovary) to build a medical word meaning:

21. inflammation of an ovary _____

22. pain in an ovary _____

23. inflammation of an ovary and oviduct _____

Use salping/o (fallopian tube) to build a medical word meaning:

24. herniation of a fallopian tube _____

25. radiography of the uterine tubes _____

Worksheet 2

Build a surgical term meaning:

1. fixation of (a displaced) ovary _____

2. suture of a displaced ovary (to the pelvic wall) _____

3. surgical repair of the vagina _____

4. excision of the uterus and ovaries _____

5. surgical repair of the vagina and perineum _____

6. suturing the perineum _____

7. excision of the uterus, oviducts, and ovaries _____

8. puncture of the amnion (amniotic sac) _____

Worksheet 3

Match the following medical terms with the definitions in the numbered list.

atresia	dystocia	LMP
corpus luteum	gestation	primipara
Down's syndrome	hydrocephalus	pruritus vulvae
D&C	laparomyitis	pyosalpinx

1. _____ accumulation of pus in a uterine tube

2. _____ woman who has had one pregnancy that has resulted in a viable offspring

3. _____ pregnancy; 40 weeks in human beings

4. _____ last menstrual period

5. _____ enlargement of the cranium caused by abnormal accumulation of cerebrospinal fluid within the ventricles of the brain

6. _____ yellow glandular mass in the ovary formed by an ovarian follicle that has matured and discharged its ovum

7. _____ difficult labor or childbirth

8. _____ congenital absence or closure of a normal body opening

9. _____ trisomy 21

10. _____ intense itching of the external female genitalia

Worksheet 4

SPECIAL PROCEDURES, PHARMACOLOGY, AND ABBREVIATIONS

Choose the following words that best describe the following statements:

amniocentesis

chorionic villus sampling

colpocleisis

contraceptives

CPD

cryosurgery

D&C

estrogens

hysterosalpingography

laparoscopy

oxytocin

Pap smear

spermicidals

tubal ligation

total abdominal hysterectomy (TAH)

ultrasonography

1. _____ cervical scrapings to detect cancerous cells in the mucus of the uterus and cervix

2. _____ radiography of the uterus and oviducts after a contrast medium is injected into those organs

3. _____ transabdominal puncture of the amniotic sac to remove amniotic fluid for biochemical and cytological studies

4. _____ destroying cells by the process of freezing tissue

5. _____ surgical closure of the vaginal canal

6. _____ widening of the cervical canal with a dilator and scraping the uterine endometrium with a curette

7. _____ excision of the entire uterus, including the cervix through an abdominal incision.

8. _____ tying the uterine tubes to prevent pregnancy; sterilization surgery

9. _____ cephalopelvic disproportion

10. _____ small incision in the abdominal wall that permits examination of the abdominal cavity to determine abnormalities

11. _____ agents that destroy sperm, used within the vagina for contraceptive purposes

12. _____ noninvasive ultrasound technique used to evaluate the female genital tract and fetus in the obstetric patient

13. _____ test to detect chromosomal abnormalities that can be done earlier than amniocentesis

14. _____ replacement hormones used during menopause to ease discomforts as the production of natural hormones decreases

15. _____ agent used to induce labor and to rid uterus of unexpelled placenta or fetus that has died

Worksheet 5

PRIMARY HERPES I INFECTION DICTIONARY EXERCISE

Use a medical dictionary or other resource to define the following terms and to determine their pronunciation; then practice reading the case study aloud (p. 283).

chlamydia _____

DC _____

Dx _____

GC _____

genital _____

herpes _____

introitus _____

labia _____

LMP _____

monilial _____

OCPs _____

Primary herpes I _____

pruritus _____

speculum _____

vulvar _____

ANALYSIS OF PRIMARY HERPES I INFECTION

1. Did the patient have any discharge? If so, describe it.

2. What type of discomfort was she experiencing around the vulvar area?

3. Has she been taking her oral contraceptive pills regularly?

4. Where was the viral culture obtained from?

5. Even though her partner used a condom, how do you think she became infected with herpes?

Worksheet 6

Label the diagram. To check you answers, refer to Figure 13–2.

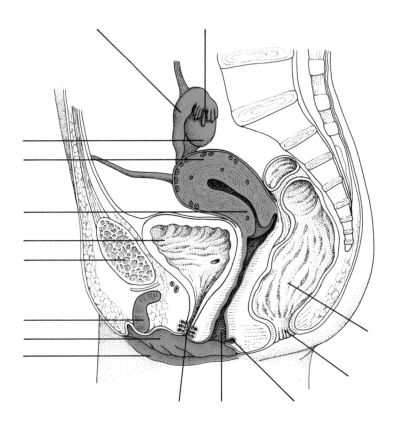

Anus	Fallopian tube	Rectum
Bartholin's gland	Fimbriae	Symphysis pubis
Bladder	Labia major	Urethra
Cervix	Labia minor	Uterus
Clitoris	Ovary	Vagina

Worksheet 7

Label the diagram. To check your answers, refer to Figure 13–3.

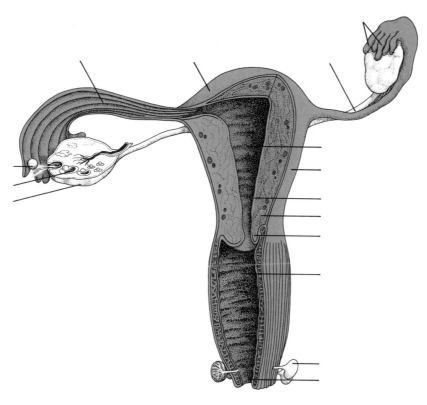

Fallopian tube	Fundus of uterus	Body (corpus) of uterus
Ovum	Vulva	Endometrium
Mature follicle	Uterus	Myometrium
Ovary	Fimbriae	Vagina
Cervix	Ovarian ligament	Bartholin's glands

Chapter 14

Endocrine System

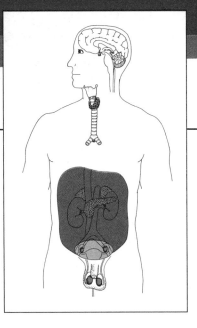

Chapter Outline

Student Objectives

Upon completion of this chapter, you will be able to do the following:

List the glands of the endocrine system.

Describe the function of each endocrine gland.

Differentiate between endocrine and exocrine glands.

Identify the principal hormones secreted by the endocrine glands and briefly explain their function.

Identify the combining forms and suffixes of the endocrine system.

Identify and discuss pathology related to the endocrine system.

Identify diagnostic imaging, surgical and laboratory procedures, and abbreviations related to the endocrine system.

Explain pharmacology related to the treatment of endocrine disorders.

Demonstrate your knowledge of the chapter by completing the worksheets.

Anatomy and Physiology

The endocrine system and the nervous system work together to regulate many intricate activities of the body. Their functions are closely related because they strive to maintain **homeostasis** (the state of equilibrium in the internal environment of the body).

The glands of the endocrine system produce specific effects on body functions by slowly releasing chemical substances called hormones into the bloodstream (Table 14–1). In contrast, the nervous system is designed to act instantaneously through the transmission of electrical impulses to specific body locations. The nervous system is covered in Chapter 15.

Included in the endocrine system are a number of ductless glands located in various parts of the body (Fig. 14–1), which release their secretions directly into blood vessels. These glands are not to be confused with exocrine glands such as the sweat and oil glands of the skin, which release their secretions externally through ducts.

This chapter discusses the function of the **pituitary, thyroid, parathyroid, adrenals, pancreas,** and **pineal glands.** The functions of the other endocrine glands are discussed in the following chapters: Chapter 10, blood and lymph (thymus); Chapter 12, genitourinary (testes); and Chapter 13, female reproductive system (ovaries).

Table 14–1   **Definition and Characteristics of Hormones**

Hormones are chemical substances produced by specialized cells of the body.
Hormones are released slowly in minute amounts directly into the bloodstream.
Hormones are produced primarily by the endocrine glands.
Most hormones are inactivated or excreted by the liver and kidneys.

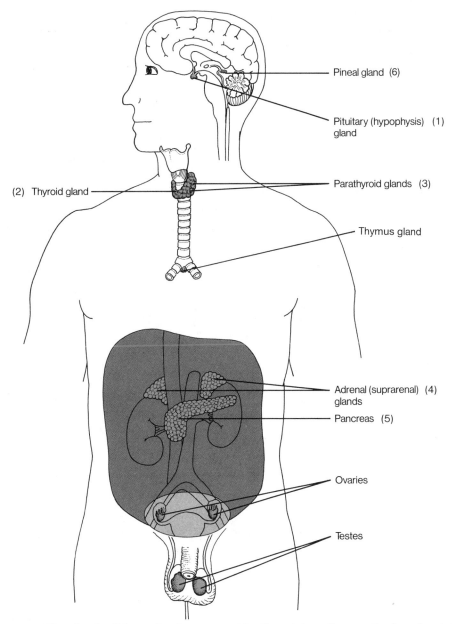

Figure 14–1   The glands of the endocrine system (ductless, internally secreting) are located in various parts of the body.

PITUITARY GLAND

Refer to Figure 14–1 as you read the following material. The (1) **pituitary gland,** or **hypophysis,** is no larger than a pea and is located at the base of the brain. It is known as the "master gland" because it regulates many body activities and stimulates other glands to secrete their own specific hormone.

Table 14–2 **Hormones of the Pituitary Gland**

Gland	Hormone	Function(s)
Adenohypophysis (anterior lobe)	Growth hormone (GH)	Stimulates bone and body growth
	Thyroid-stimulating hormone (TSH), or thyrotropin	Controls secretions of hormones from the thyroid gland
	Prolactin	Promotes growth of breast tissue Stimulates milk production after birth
	Adrenocorticotropic hormone (ACTH)	Stimulates secretions by the adrenal cortex, especially cortisol
	Follicle-stimulating hormone (FSH)	Stimulates development of eggs in the ovaries Stimulates secretion of estrogen in females Stimulates production of sperm cells in the testes
	Luteinizing hormone (LH), or interstitial cell-stimulating hormone (ICSH) in males	Promotes the secretion of sex hormones in both males and females Plays a role in the release of the egg cell in females
Neurohypophysis (posterior lobe)	Antidiuretic hormone (ADH)	Decreases volume of urine excreted Increases volume of water reabsorbed in kidney
	Oxytocin	Causes contraction of the uterus during labor and childbirth Stimulates milk secretion

The gland consists of two distinct portions: an anterior lobe (adenohypophysis) and a posterior lobe (neurohypophysis). Both lobes secrete hormones, which are summarized in Table 14–2.

THYROID GLAND

The (2) **thyroid gland** is the largest gland of the endocrine system. An H-shaped organ located in the neck just below the larynx, this gland is composed of two fairly large lobes that are separated by a strip of tissue called an **isthmus.**

The function of the thyroid gland is to produce, store, and release **thyroxine (T_4)** and **triiodothyronine (T_3),** the major thyroid hormones. Both T_3 and T_4 regulate metabolism and are responsible for energy level. They increase the rate of oxygen consumption and thus the rate at which carbohydrates, proteins, and fats are metabolized. In addition, both hormones work with the growth hormone (GH) and stimulate activity in the nervous system. Refer to Table 14–3 for a summary of hormones of the thyroid gland.

Table 14–3 **Hormones of the Thyroid Gland**

Hormone	Function(s)
Thyroxine and triiodothyronine	Regulates metabolism of the body Increases energy production from all food types Increases rate of protein synthesis
Calcitonin	Decreases the reabsorption of calcium and phosphate from bones to blood

PARATHYROID GLANDS

The (3) **parathyroid glands** consist of at least four separate glands located on the posterior surface of the lobes of the thyroid gland. The only hormone known to be secreted by the parathyroid glands is parathyroid hormone (PTH). PTH helps regulate homeostasis of calcium by stimulating three target organs: bones, intestines, and kidneys (Table 14–4).

Because of PTH stimulation, calcium and phosphates are released from bones, increas-

Table 14–4 **Hormone of the Parathyroid Glands**

Hormone	Function(s)
Parathyroid hormone (PTH)	Stimulates the reabsorption of calcium and phosphate from bone to blood Stimulates the conservation of calcium by the kidneys Stimulates the absorption of calcium by the intestine

The effect of PTH release is to raise levels of calcium, which in turn inhibits further PTH release

ing concentration of these substances in blood. Thus, calcium that is necessary for the proper functioning of body tissues is available in the bloodstream. At the same time, PTH enhances the absorption of calcium and phosphates from foods in the intestine, and this action also produces a rise in the blood levels of calcium and phosphates. PTH causes the kidneys to conserve blood calcium and to increase the excretion of phosphates in the urine.

ADRENAL GLANDS

The (4) **adrenal glands** are paired organs covering the superior surface of the kidneys. Because of their location, the adrenal glands are also known as **suprarenal glands.** Each adrenal gland is structurally and functionally differentiated into two sections: the outer **adrenal cortex,** which makes up the bulk of the gland, and the inner **adrenal medulla.** Although these regions are not sharply divided, they represent distinct glands that secrete different hormones. Steroids (Table 14–5) are secreted by the adrenal cortex. Cells of the adrenal medulla secrete two closely related hormones, epinephrine (adrenaline) and norepinephrine (noradrenaline) Table 14–6).

Adrenal Cortex

The hormones of the adrenal cortex, steroids (corticosteroids), are essential to life. In fact, in the absence of cortical secretions, death usually occurs within a week unless extensive electrolyte therapy (controlled levels of sodium, potassium, and calcium levels) is provided.

Histologically, the cortex is subdivided into three zones, each of which has a different cellular arrangement and secretes different groups of hormones.

1. **Mineralocorticoids** help regulate water and mineral salts (also called electrolytes) that are retained in the body. One of the major mineralocorticoids is **aldosterone.** Like all hormones of the adrenal cortex, aldosterone is a steroid. This hormone acts mainly through the kidneys to maintain homeostasis of sodium and potassium. More specifically, aldosterone causes the kidneys to conserve sodium and to excrete potassium. At the same time, it promotes water conservation and reduces urine output.
2. **Glucocorticoids** influence the metabolism of carbohydrates, fats, and proteins. The glucocorticoid with the greatest activity is **cortisol.** It helps to regulate the concentration of glucose in the blood, protecting against low blood sugar levels between meals. Cortisol also stimulates the breakdown of fats in adipose tissue and releases fatty acids into the blood. The increase in fatty acids causes many cells to use relatively less glucose.

Table 14–5 **Hormones of the Adrenal Cortex**

Hormone	Function(s)
Aldosterone	Regulates the amount of salts in the body
Cortisol	Regulates the metabolism of carbohydrates, proteins, and fats
Androgens	Maintain secondary sex characteristics

Table 14–6   **Hormones of the Adrenal Medulla**

Hormone	Function(s)
Epinephrine (adrenaline)	Increases heart rate and force of contraction
	Dilates bronchial tubes
	Increases conversion of glycogen to glucose in the liver
	Increases use of fats for energy
Norepinephrine (noradrenaline)	Raises blood pressure and constricts vessels

3. **Gonadocorticoids** (sex hormones) affect sexual characteristics. Although the sex hormones are primarily male type (adrenal androgens), small quantities of female hormones (adrenal estrogens and progesterone) are also present. The normal functions of these hormones are not clear, but they may supplement the supply of sex hormones from the gonads and stimulate early development of the reproductive organs. Also, there is some evidence that the adrenal androgens play a role in controlling the female sex drive. Refer to Table 14–5 for a summary of adrenal cortex hormones.

Adrenal Medulla

Epinephrine (adrenaline) and norepinephrine (noradrenaline) are two closely related hormones secreted by the adrenal medulla. The effects of the medullary hormones resemble those of the sympathetic nervous system. The adrenal medulla, like the rest of the sympathetic nervous system, is not essential to life, but it is important because it stimulates the responses necessary to meet emergencies. Refer to Table 14–6 for a summary of adrenal medulla hormones.

PANCREAS (ISLETS OF LANGERHANS)

Continue to refer to Figure 14–1 as you read the following material.

The (5) **pancreas** lies inferior to the stomach in a bend of the duodenum. It functions both as an exocrine and endocrine gland. A large pancreatic duct runs through the gland, carrying enzymes and other exocrine digestive secretions from the pancreas to the small intestine (see Chapter 7). The pancreas has groups of cells called islets of Langerhans, which produce endocrine secretions. There are two kinds of cells in the islets: A cells (alpha cells), which produce glucagon and constitute about 25% of the islet cells; and B cells (beta cells), which produce insulin and constitute about 75% of the islet cells. Both of these hormones, glucagon and insulin, play an important role in the proper metabolism

Table 14–7   **Hormones of the Pancreas**

Hormone	Function(s)
Insulin	Lowers blood sugar by promoting the movement of glucose to the body cells
Glucagon	Increases blood sugar by stimulating the liver to convert glycogen to glucose

of sugars and starches in the body. Refer to Table 14–7 for a summary of pancreatic hormones.

PINEAL GLAND

The (6) **pineal gland,** which is shaped like a pine cone, is attached to the posterior part of the third ventricle of the brain. Although the exact functions of this gland have not been established, there is evidence that it secretes melatonin hormone. It is believed that melatonin may inhibit the activities of the ovaries. When melatonin production is high, ovulation is blocked, and there may be a delay in puberty development. The pineal gland starts to degenerate at about 7 years of age; in the adult, it consists mostly of fibrous tissue.

COMBINING FORMS

Combining Form	Meaning	Example	Pronunciation
acr/o	extremity	<u>acr</u>/o/megaly enlargement	ăk-rō-MĔG-ă-lē
adren/o adrenal/o	adrenal glands	<u>adren</u>/al relating to <u>adrenal</u>/ism condition	ăd-RĒ-năl ă-DRĔN-ăl-ĭzm
andr/o	male	<u>andr</u>/o/gen forming, producing, origin	ĂN-drō-jĕn
calc/o	calcium	hypo/<u>calc</u>/emia under, blood below	hī-pō-kăl-SĒ-mē-ăh
gluc/o glyc/o	sugar, sweetness	<u>gluc</u>/o/genesis producing hyper/<u>glyc</u>/emia excessive blood	gloo-ko-JĔN-ĕ-sĭs hī-pĕr-glī-SĒ-mē-ăh
gonad/o	sex glands	hypo/<u>gonad</u>/ism below condition, state of being	hī-pō-GŌ-năd-ĭzm
home/o	same, alike	<u>home</u>/o/stasis standing still	hō-mē-ō-STĀ-sĭs
parathyroid/o	parathyroid glands	<u>parathyroid</u>/ectomy excision	păr-ăh-thī-roi-DĔK-tō-mē
pancreat/o	pancreas	<u>pancreat</u>/itis inflammation	păn-krē-ă-TĪ-tĭs

COMBINING FORMS (Continued)

Combining Form	Meaning	Example	Pronunciation
somat/o	body	somat/ic pertaining to	sō-MĂT-ĭc
thym/o	thymus	thym/o/lysis destruction	thī-MŎL-ĭ-sĭs

thyr/o
 	
 thyroid/o
	thyroid	thyr/o/toxic/ osis
		     poison abnormal
		            condition
		 thyroid/ectomy
		      excision
			thī-rō-tŏks-ĭ-KŌ-sĭs
			
			 thī-roid-ĔK-tō-mē

SUFFIXES

Suffix	Meaning	Example	Pronunciation
-crine	secrete	endo/crine within	ĔN-dō-krīn (or) krĭn
-dipsia	thirst	poly/dipsia many, much	pŏl-ē-DĬP-sē-ăh
-phagia	eating, swallowing	poly/phagia many, much	pŏl-ē-FĀ-jē-ăh
-trophy	nourishment, development	a/ trophy without	ĂT-rō-fē
-toxic	poison	thyr/o/toxic thyroid	thī-rō-TŎKS-ĭk
-uria	urine	poly/uria much	pŏl-ē-Ū-rē-ăh
-physis	growth	adeno/hypo/physis gland under	ăd-ē-nō-hī-PŎF-ĭ-sĭs
-tropin	stimulate	somat/o/tropin body	sō-măt-ō-TRŌ-pĭn

Pathology

Disorders of the endocrine system are based on underproduction **(hyposecretion)** or over-production **(hypersecretion)** of hormones. In general, hyposecretion is treated by the use of hormones in drug therapy replacement. Hypersecretion is generally treated by surgery. Most hormone deficiencies result from genetic defects in the glands, surgical removal of the glands, or production of poor-quality hormones.

PITUITARY DISORDERS

Hypersecretion or hyposecretion of growth hormone (GH) leads to body-size abnormalities. Abnormal variations of antidiuretic hormone (ADH) secretions lead to disorders in the composition of the blood and marked electrolyte imbalance. Some pituitary disorders are summarized in Table 14–8.

THYROID DISORDERS

Thyroid gland disorders are common and may develop at any time during life. They may be the result of a developmental problem, injury, disease, or dietary deficiency. One form of hypothyroidism that develops in infants is called **cretinism.** If not treated, this disorder leads to mental retardation, impaired growth, low body temperatures, and abnormal bone formation. Usually these symptoms do not appear at birth because the infant has received thyroid hormones from the mother's blood during fetal development.

When hypothyroidism develops during adulthood, it is known as **myxedema.** The characteristics of this disease are edema, low blood levels of T_3 and T_4, mental retardation, weight gain, and sluggishness.

Hyperthyroidism results from excessive secretions of T_3, T_4, or both. Two of the most common disorders of hyperthyroidism are **Graves' disease** and **toxic goiter.** Graves' disease is considerably more prevalent and is characterized by an elevated metabolic rate, abnormal weight loss, excessive perspiration, muscular weakness, and emotional instability. Also, the eyes are likely to protrude **(exophthalmos)** because of edematous swelling in the tissues behind them. At the same time, the thyroid gland is likely to enlarge, producing goiter.

It is believed that toxic goiter may occur because of excessive release of thyroid-stimulating hormone (TSH) from the anterior lobe of the pituitary gland. Overstimulation by TSH causes thyroid cells to enlarge and secrete extra amounts of hormones. Treatment for this condition may involve drug therapy to block the production of thyroid hormones or surgical removal of all or part of the thyroid gland. Another method for treating this disorder is to administer a sufficient amount of radioactive iodine to destroy the thyroid secretory cells.

PARATHYROID DISORDERS

As with the thyroid gland, dysfunction of the parathyroids is usually characterized by excessive hormone secretion **(hyperparathyroidism)** or inadequate hormone secretion **(hypoparathyroidism).**

Table 14–8 **Pituitary Disorders**

Disorder	Hormone	Source	Hyposecretion or Hypersecretion	Possible Cause	Effects
Acromegaly	GH	Anterior lobe	Hypersecretion as an adult	Primary tumor after puberty	Disproportionate increase in size of bones of face, hands, and feet
Diabetes insipidus	ADH	Posterior lobe	Hyposecretion	Damage to the hypothalamus	Failure of kidneys to reabsorb needed salts and water
Giantism	GH	Anterior lobe	Hypersecretion during childhood	Pituitary tumor before puberty	Abnormal overgrowth of body
High levels of ADH in blood	ADH	Posterior lobe	Hypersecretion	Pituitary tumor, head injury	Excessive sodium, water retention in the body
Pituitary dwarfism, hypopituitary dwarfism	GH	Anterior lobe	Hyposecretion during childhood	Congenital deficiency or destruction of GH-producing cells	Small but well-proportioned body; sexual immaturity

Hypoparathyroidism can result from an injury or from surgical removal of the glands, sometimes in conjunction with thyroid surgery. The primary effect of hypoparathyroidism is the lowering of the blood calcium level. The decreased calcium **(hypocalcemia)** lowers the electrical threshold and causes neurons to depolarize more easily, and the number of nerve impulses to increase. This results in muscle twitches and spasms, causing a condition called **tetany.**

Hyperparathyroidism is most often caused by a benign tumor. The resulting increase in PTH secretion leads to demineralization of bones **(osteitis fibrosa cystica),** making them porous **(osteoporosis)** and highly susceptible to fracture and deformity. When this condition is the result of a benign glandular tumor **(adenoma)** of the parathyroid, the tumor is removed. Treatment may also include orthopedic surgery to correct severe bone deformities. An excess of PTH also causes calcium to be deposited in the kidneys. When the disease is generalized and all bones are affected, this disorder is known as **von Recklinghausen's disease.** Renal symptoms and kidney stones **(nephrolithiasis)** may also develop.

DISORDERS OF THE ADRENAL GLANDS

Adrenal Medulla

No specific diseases can be traced directly to a deficiency of hormones from the medulla. However, medullary tumors sometimes cause excess secretions. The most common disorder is in the form of a neoplasm known as **pheochromocytoma,** which produces excessive amounts of epinephrine and norepinephrine. Most of these tumors are encapsulated and benign. These hypersecretions produce stress, fear, palpitations, headaches, visual blurring, muscle spasms, and sweating. The usual form of treatment consists of administration of antihypertensive drugs and surgery.

Adrenal Cortex

Addison's disease, a relatively uncommon chronic disorder caused by a deficiency of cortical hormones, results when the adrenal cortex is destroyed. It is caused by atrophy of the adrenals, probably the result of some autoimmune process in which circulating adrenal antibodies slowly destroy the gland. Ninety percent of the gland is usually destroyed before clinical signs of adrenal insufficiency appear. Hypofunction of the adrenal cortex interferes with the body's ability to handle internal and external stress. In severe cases, the disturbance of sodium and potassium metabolism may be marked by depletion of sodium and water through urination, resulting in severe chronic dehydration. Other clinical manifestations include muscular weakness, anorexia, gastrointestinal symptoms, fatigue, hypoglycemia, hypotension, low blood sodium **(hyponatremia),** and high serum potassium **(hyperkalemia).** If treatment for this condition begins early, usually with adrenocortical hormone therapy, the prognosis is excellent. If untreated, the disease will continue a chronic course with progressive but relatively slow deterioration. In some patients, the deterioration may be rapid.

Cushing's syndrome, caused by hypersecretion of the adrenal cortex, results in excessive production of glucocorticoids. This overactivity is commonly due to an abnormal growth of the adrenal cortices. It may also be caused by a tumor arising in the cortex of one of the adrenal glands, a pituitary tumor, or excessive administration of cortisone.

Symptoms include rapidly developing adiposity of the face ("moon-face") and neck, purple striae on the skin, fatigue, high blood pressure, and excessive hair growth in unusual places **(hirsutism),** especially in females. Treatment is partial removal of the adrenal gland **(adrenalectomy)** or removal of the tumor.

PANCREATIC DISORDERS

Diabetes mellitus (DM), in its two forms, is by far the most common pancreatic disorder. **Type I diabetes,** also known as **insulin-dependent diabetes mellitus (IDDM),** occurs mostly in children and adolescents (juvenile onset) and may be associated with a genetic predisposition for the disorder. It is characterized by destruction of beta cells of the islets of Langerhans with complete insulin deficiency in the body. Treatment includes injection of insulin in order to maintain a normal level of glucose in the blood.

    Type II diabetes, also known as **non–insulin-dependent diabetes mellitus (NIDDM),** is distinctively different from type I. Its onset is usually later in life (maturity onset), and risk factors include a family history of diabetes and obesity. Even though insulin is produced, the insulin cannot exert its effects on cells because of the body's insensitivity to insulin. Treatment includes medications that stimulate the release of pancreatic insulin and improve the body's sensitivity to insulin **(oral hypoglycemic agents),** weight reduction, and diet. Clinical manifestations of both forms are summarized in Tables 14–9 and 14–10.

    Diabetes is characterized by numerous complications, such as upsets in carbohydrate metabolism as well as disturbances in protein and fat metabolism. There is a rise in the concentration of blood sugar **(hyperglycemia).** Some of the glucose, along with electrolytes (particularly sodium), is excreted in the urine **(glycosuria),** causing excessive urination **(diuresis),** dehydration, and thirst **(polydipsia).** Sodium and potassium losses result in muscle weakness and fatigue. Because glucose cannot enter the cells, cellular starvation results. This leads to hunger and an increased appetite **(polyphagia).** Unless treatment is initiated, ketoacidosis, which appears in advanced stages of hyperglycemia, will develop.

    Ketoacidosis, also referred to as diabetic acidosis or diabetic coma, may develop over several days or weeks. It can be caused by too little insulin, failure to follow a prescribed diet, physical or emotional stress, or undiagnosed diabetes. Low blood sugar **(hypoglycemia)** occurs when the level of insulin in the blood is out of proportion to that of available

---

Table 14–9   **Clinical Manifestations of Insulin-Dependent Diabetes***

Insulin-dependent diabetes is characterized by the sudden appearance of:

    Constant urination (polyuria) and glycosuria
    Abnormal thirst (polydipsia)
    Unusual hunger (polyphagia)
    The rapid loss of weight
    Irritability
    Obvious weakness and fatigue
    Nausea and vomiting

Any one of these signals can indicate diabetes. Children usually exhibit dramatic, sudden symptoms and must receive prompt treatment.

*From American Diabetes Association, New York.

Table 14–10 **Clinical Manifestations of Non–Insulin-Dependent Diabetes***

Non–insulin-dependent diabetes may include any of the signs of insulin-dependent diabetes or:

Drowsiness
Itching
A family history of diabetes
Blurred vision
Excessive weight
Tingling, numbness, pain in the extremities
Easily fatigued
Skin infections and slow healing of cuts and scratches, especially of the feet

Many adults may have diabetes with none of these symptoms. The disease is often discovered during a routine physical examination.

*From American Diabetes Association, New York.

glucose. Hyperinsulinism may also be due to a tumor involving the islet cells, but similar symptoms occur if a person with diabetes receives too large a dosage of insulin. In either case, the condition is referred to as insulin shock. Treatment includes administering glucose intravenously, which usually brings the patient out of shock within a few minutes.

Longstanding diabetes is a leading cause of blindness, as it causes diabetic retinopathy. Diabetes in pregnant women **(gestational diabetes)** usually subsides after the child is born **(parturition).**

ONCOLOGY

Pancreatic Cancer

Most carcinomas of the pancreas arise as epithelial tumors **(adenocarcinomas)** and make their presence known by obstruction and local invasion. Because the pancreas is richly supplied with nerves, pain is a prominent feature of pancreatic cancer, whether it arises in the head, the body, or the tail of the organ.

The prognosis of this tumor is poor, with only a 2-percent survival rate for 5 years. Pancreatic cancer is the fourth leading cause of cancer deaths in the United States. The highest incidence is among people 60 to 70 years of age. The etiology is unknown, but cigarette smoking, exposure to occupational chemicals, a diet high in fats, and heavy coffee intake are associated with an increased incidence of pancreatic cancer.

Pituitary Tumors

Pituitary tumors are not really malignancies, but because their growth is invasive, they are considered neoplastic and are usually treated as such. Initial signs and symptoms include headache, blurred vision, and often times, personality changes, dementia, and seizures. Tomography, skull x-rays, pneumonoencephalography, angiography, and CT scans assist in diagnosis. Depending on size of the tumor and its location, different treatment modalities are employed. Some of these treatments include surgical removal, radiation, or a combination of both.

Thyroid Cancer

There are a variety of thyroid cancers, classified according to the specific tissue that is affected. In general, however, all share many predisposing factors, including radiation, prolonged TSH stimulation, familial disposition, and chronic goiter. The malignancy usually begins with a painless, often hard nodule, or a nodule in the adjacent lymph nodes accompanied with an enlarged thyroid. When the tumor is excessively large, it frequently destroys thyroid tissue, which results in symptoms of hypothyroidism. Sometimes the tumor stimulates the production of thyroid hormone, resulting in symptoms of hyperthyroidism. Treatment includes surgical removal, radiation, or both.

DIAGNOSTIC, SYMPTOMATIC, AND RELATED TERMS

Term	Meaning
acromegaly ăk-rō-MĔG-ă-lē	disease characterized by enlarged features, particularly the face and hands, the result of oversecretion of the pituitary growth hormone after puberty
diuresis dī-ū-RĒ-sĭs	increased excretion of urine, as occurs in diabetes mellitus; can also be early sign of chronic interstitial nephritis
glucagon GLOO-kă-gŏn	hormone secreted by the pancreatic alpha cells that increases blood glucose concentration
glucose GLOO-kōs	simple sugar
glucosuria, glycosuria gloo-kō-SŪ-rē-ăh, GLĪ-kō-sū-rē-ăh	presence of glucose in the urine; abnormal amount of sugar in the urine
hirsutism hĕr-SOOT-ĭzm	abnormal hairiness, especially in women
homeostasis hō-mē-ō-STĀ-sĭs	state of equilibrium in the internal environment of the body
hypercalcemia hī-pĕr-kăl-SĒ-mē-ăh	excessive amount of calcium in the blood
hyperkalemia hī-pĕr-kă-LĒ-mē-ăh	excessive amount of potassium in the blood, most often due to defective renal excretion
hyponatremia hī-pō-nă-TRĒ-mē-ăh	abnormal condition of low sodium in the blood
obesity ō-BĒ-sĭ-tē	excessive accumulation of fat in the body
pheochromocytoma fē-ō-krō-mō-sī-TŌ-măh	small chromaffin cell tumor, usually located in the adrenal medulla

DIAGNOSTIC, SYMPTOMATIC, AND RELATED TERMS (Continued)

Term	Meaning
virile VĬR-ĭl	masculine; having characteristics of a man, especially copulative powers
virilism VĬR-ĭl-ĭzm	masculinization in a woman; development of male secondary sex characteristics in the woman

Special Procedures

DIAGNOSTIC IMAGING PROCEDURES

Term	Description
thyroid echogram (ultrasound examination of thyroid)	valuable for distinguishing cystic from solid nodules. If the nodule is found to be purely cystic and fluid filled, it is aspirated and surgery is avoided. However, if the nodule has a mixed or solid appearance, carcinoma is a likely possibility and surgery is usually necessary. A nonfunctioning thyroid nodule can be evaluated with the use of reflected sound waves
CT scan (pancreas, thyroid, adrenal glands)	used to detect disease in soft body tissues, such as the pancreas, thyroid, and adrenal glands; may also involve the use of radiographic contrast media

SURGICAL PROCEDURES

Term	Description
microneurosurgery of pituitary gland mī-krō-nū-rō-SĔR-jĕr-ē pĭ-TŪ-ĭ-tār-ē	microdissection of a tumor using a binocular surgical microscope for magnification
parathyroidectomy păr-ăh-thī-roi-DĔK-tō-mē	excision of one or more of the parathyroid glands, usually done to control hyperparathyroidism
pinealectomy pĭn-ē-ăl-ĔK-tō-mē	removal of the pineal body
thymectomy thī-MĔK-tō-mē	excision of the thymus gland

SURGICAL PROCEDURES (Continued)

Term	Description
partial thyroidectomy thī-roi-DĔK-tō-mē	method of choice for removal of a fibrous nodular thyroid
subtotal thyroidectomy thī-roi-DĔK-tō-mē	removal of most of the thyroid to relieve hyperthyroidism

LABORATORY PROCEDURES

Test	Description
radioactive iodine uptake (RAIU) test	used to measure thyroid function. Radioactive iodine is administered orally, and its uptake into the thyroid is measured
serum glucose tests	used to determine adjustments in insulin dosages and to determine hypoglycemia and hyperglycemia
fasting blood sugar (FBS)	measures circulating glucose level after a 12-hour fast
glucose tolerance test (GTT)	performed by giving a certain amount of glucose (sugar) orally or intravenously, drawing blood samples at specified intervals, and determining the blood glucose level in each sample; most often used to assist in the diagnosis of diabetes or other disorders that affect carbohydrate metabolism
insulin tolerance test	determines insulin levels in serum (blood). Insulin is administered and blood glucose is measured at regular intervals. In hypoglycemia, the glucose levels may be lower and slower to return to normal
protein-bound iodine (PBI)	test that measures the concentration of thyroxine in a blood sample; result furnishes an index of thyroid activity
thyroxine iodine test (T_4)	evaluates thyroid function; amount of iodine associated with the thyroxine in the sample is measured using several laboratory procedures
total calcium	measures calcium to detect bone and parathyroid disorders: hypercalcemia can indicate primary hyperparathyroidism; hypocalcemia can indicate hypoparathyroidism

PHARMACOLOGY

Medication	Action
antihyperlipidemics	lower cholesterol levels in the bloodstream; help prevent atherosclerosis (fatty build-up in the blood vessels)
corticosteroids	replacement hormones for adrenal insufficiency (Addison's disease); widely used to suppress inflammation, control allergic reactions, reduce rejection in transplantation, and treat some cancers
insulin	major drug for treating diabetes; administered by injection to lower blood glucose (sugar) level
oral hypoglycemics	used with certain types of diabetes mellitus patients, mainly those who are overweight and have developed the condition as adults. These drugs are unrelated to insulin and are used in cases where the pancreas is already producing some insulin. Their effect is to stimulate the pancreas to secrete more insulin and make the body cells more receptive to the action of insulin
vasopressin	controls diabetes insipidus and subsequent polyuria due to ADH deficiency; replaces pituitary ADH and promotes reabsorption of water in the kidneys

ABBREVIATIONS

Abbreviation	Term
ACTH	adrenocorticotropic hormone
ADH	antidiuretic hormone (vasopressin)
DI	diabetes insipidus; diagnostic imaging
DM	diabetes mellitus
ECF	extracellular fluid
FBS	fasting blood sugar
FSH	follicle-stimulating hormone
GH	growth hormone
GTT	glucose tolerance test
ICF	intracellular fluid
ICSH	interstitial cell-stimulating hormone
IDDM	insulin-dependent diabetes mellitus

ABBREVIATIONS (Continued)

Abbreviation	Term
LDL	low-density lipoproteins
LH	luteinizing hormone
MSH	melanocyte-stimulating hormone
NIDDM	non–insulin-dependent diabetes mellitus
NPH	neutral protamine Hagedorn (insulin)
PBI	protein-bound iodine
PGH	pituitary growth hormone
PTH	parathyroid hormone
RAI	radioactive iodine
RAIU	radioactive iodine uptake
T_3	triiodothyronine
T_4	thyroxine
TSH	thyroid-stimulating hormone

Case Study

Hyperparathyroidism and Diabetes Mellitus

A 66-year-old former blackjack dealer is under evaluation for **hyperparathyroidism.** Surgery evidently has been recommended, but there is confusion as to how urgent this is. She has a 14-year history of **type I diabetes mellitus,** a history of shoulder pain, osteoarthritis of the spine, and peripheral vascular disease with claudication. She states her 548-pack-year smoking history ended 3.5 years ago. Her first knowledge of parathyroid disease was about 3 years ago when laboratory findings revealed an elevated calcium level. This subsequently led to the diagnosis of hyperparathyroidism. She was further evaluated by an **endocrinologist** in the Lake Tahoe area, who determined that she also had **hypercalciuria,** although there is nothing to suggest a history of kidney stones.

Impression. Hyperparathyroidism and hypercalciuria, probably a **parathyroid adenoma.**

Worksheet 5 provides a dictionary and reading application and an analysis of this case study.

Worksheet 1

Use glyc/o (sugar) to build a medical word meaning:

1. condition of excessive sugar in the blood _____

2. condition of deficiency of sugar in the blood _____

3. formation of glycogen _____

Use pancreat/o (pancreas) to build a medical word meaning:

4. inflammation of the pancreas _____

5. destruction of the pancreas _____

6. any pancreatic disease _____

Use thyr/o or thyroid/o (thyroid) to build a medical word meaning:

7. inflammation of the thyroid gland _____

8. enlargement of the thyroid _____

Worksheet 2

Build a surgical term meaning:

1. excision of the thyroid _____

2. incision of thyroid cartilage _____

3. excision of a parathyroid gland _____

4. removal of the adrenal _____

5. excision of the adrenal glands on both sides _____

Worksheet 3

Match the following words with the definitions in the numbered list.

Addison's disease   exophthalmic goiter   insulin

cretinism   hirsutism   myxedema

diuresis   hyperkalemia   pheochromocytoma

tetany   hypokalemia   virile

1. _____ having characteristics of a man; masculine

2. _____ hypothyroidism that develops after puberty

3. _____ increased excretion of urine

4. _____ excessive growth of hair or the presence of hair in unusual places, especially in women

5. _____ hypothyroidism that develops in an infant

6. _____ hormone produced by B cells (beta cells) of the pancreas

7. _____ disease resulting from deficiency in the secretion of adrenocortical hormones

8. _____ a condition marked by protrusion of the eyeballs, increased heart action, enlargement of the thyroid gland, weight loss, and nervousness

9. _____ excessive amount of potassium in the blood

10. _____ small chromaffin cell tumor, usually located in the adrenal medulla

Worksheet 4

SPECIAL PROCEDURES, PHARMACOLOGY, AND ABBREVIATIONS

Choose the word(s) that best describes the following statements:

antihyperlipidemics	RAIU
corticosteroids	T_3
FBS	T_4
insulin	thyroid echogram
RAI	toxicosis
serum glucose test	vasopressin

1. _____ measures circulating glucose level after a 12-hour fast

2. _____ test based on the ability of the thyroid gland to trap and retain iodine, and provides an indirect measure of thyroid activity

3. _____ replacement hormones for adrenal insufficiency

4. _____ drug that controls diabetes insipidus and subsequent polyuria due to ADH deficiency

5. _____ ultrasound examination of the thyroid

6. _____ thyroxine

7. _____ major drug that lowers glucose level and is administered by injection

8. _____ diagnostic test to determine hypoglycemia, hyperglycemia, and determine adjustments of insulin dosages

9. _____ lowers cholesterol levels in the bloodstream

10. _____ radioactive iodine

11. _____ triiodothyronine

Worksheet 5

HYPERPARATHYROIDISM AND DIABETES MELLITUS DICTIONARY EXERCISE

Use a medical dictionary or other resource to define the following terms and determine their pronunciation; then practice reading the case study aloud (p. 311).

adenoma _____

type I diabetes mellitus _____

endocrinologist _____

hypercalciuria _____

hyperparathyroidism _____

parathyroid _____

ANALYSIS OF HYPERPARATHYROIDISM AND DIABETES MELLITUS

1. Referring to Figure 14–1, designate the location of the parathyroid glands.

2. How many parathyroid glands are there?

3. What is an adenoma?

4. What body system was involved in her condition?

5. Define endocrinologist.

6. What is hypercalciuria?

7. If she smoked 548 packs of cigarettes a year, how many packs did she smoke in an average day?

Worksheet 6

Label the diagram. To check your answers, refer to Figure 14–1.

Pineal gland

Pituitary (hypophysis) gland

Thyroid gland

Parathyroid glands

Adrenal (suprarenal) glands

Pancreas

Ovaries

Testes

Thymus gland

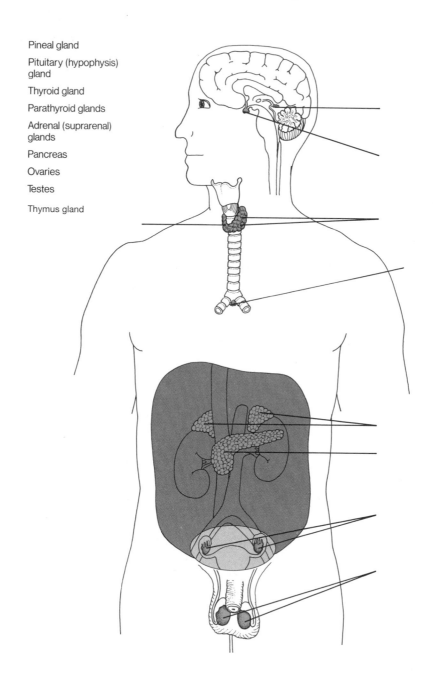

Chapter 15

Nervous System

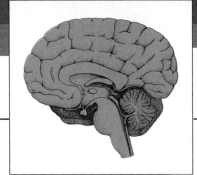

Chapter Outline

Student Objectives
Upon completion of this chapter, you will be able to do the following:

List and briefly describe the subdivisions of the nervous system.

Describe the structure and functions of neurons.

List and briefly describe the functions of four types of neuroglial cells.

Describe the function of four major parts of the brain.

Discuss the structure and function of the spinal cord.

Student Objectives (Continued)

List the three meninges and describe their function.

Identify combining forms, suffixes and prefixes related to the nervous system.

Identify and discuss pathology related to the nervous system.

Define diagnostic and symptomatic terms related to the nervous system.

Identify diagnostic imaging, surgical, clinical and laboratory procedures, and abbreviations related to the nervous system.

Discuss pharmacology related to the treatment of the nervous system.

Demonstrate your knowledge of the chapter by completing the worksheets.

Anatomy and Physiology

The nervous system is one of the most complicated systems of the body (Fig. 15–1). Along with the endocrine system, it controls many bodily activities. The nervous system senses changes in both the internal and external environments, interprets these changes, and then coordinates appropriate responses in order to maintain homeostasis.

SUBDIVISIONS OF THE NERVOUS SYSTEM

Figure 15–2 illustrates the subdivisions of the nervous system. Refer to this figure as you read the following paragraphs. The nervous system includes the **central nervous system (CNS)**, consisting of the brain and the spinal cord, and the **peripheral nervous system (PNS)**, consisting of all other neural elements of the body. The PNS includes 12 pairs of **cranial nerves**, which emerge from the base of the skull, and 31 pairs of **spinal nerves**, which emerge from the spinal cord. All of these nerves consist of fibers that may be **sensory** or **motor**, or a mixture of both. Sensory nerves receive impulses from the sense organs, including the eyes, ears, nose, tongue, and skin, and transmit them to the CNS. Because they conduct impulses *toward* the CNS, they are also known as **afferent nerves.**

Motor nerves, which conduct impulses *away from* the CNS, are known as **efferent nerves.** Motor impulses travel primarily to muscles, causing them to contract, or to glands, causing them to secrete.

Nerves composed of both sensory and motor fibers are called **mixed nerves.** An example of a mixed nerve is the facial nerve. When the facial nerve transmits an impulse to the face for smiling or frowning, it functions as a motor nerve. When it transmits a taste impulse from the tongue to the brain, it functions as a sensory nerve. Cranial nerves may be sensory, motor, or mixed; but all spinal nerves are mixed nerves.

Spinal nerves have two points of attachment to the spinal cord, an anterior root and a posterior root. The anterior root contains motor fibers and the posterior root contains sensory fibers. These two roots unite to form the spinal nerve.

Functionally, the PNS is subdivided into two specialized systems: the **somatic nervous system (SNS)** and the **autonomic nervous system (ANS).** The SNS primarily innervates (supplies with nerves) skeletal muscles. The movement it produces is controlled consciously or voluntarily by the individual. Examples of voluntary activities include

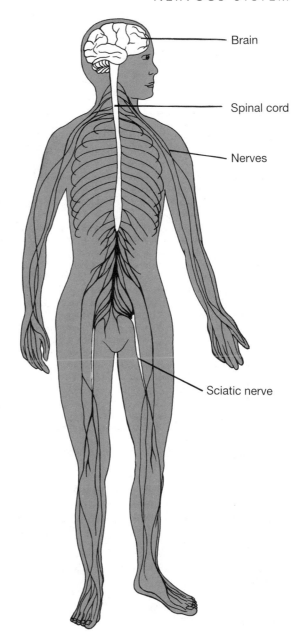

Figure 15–1   The nervous system.

walking, talking, and playing tennis. However, the ANS sends impulses to glands, smooth muscles, and cardiac muscles. This system is considered involuntary, as it operates without conscious control. Examples of autonomic activities include digestion, heart contraction, and vasoconstriction.

The ANS is further subdivided into the **sympathetic** and **parasympathetic** systems. To a large extent, these subdivisions each oppose the action of the other, although in certain instances, they may exhibit independent action. In general, sympathetic nerve fibers produce vasoconstriction, increased heart rate, elevated blood pressure, and slowing

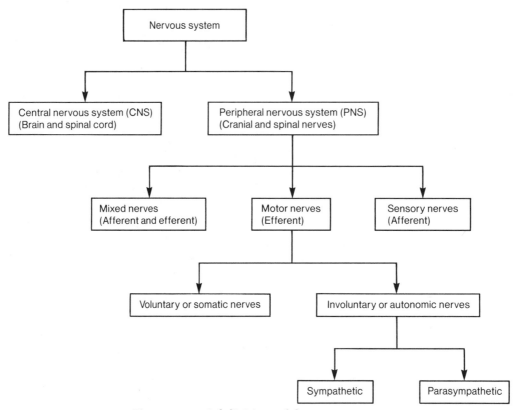

Figure 15–2 Subdivisions of the nervous system.

of gastrointestinal activity. The parasympathetic system generally transmits impulses that bring about vasodilation, a slower heart rate, a decrease in blood pressure, and a return to normal gastrointestinal activity. Sympathetic functions are evident in "fight or flight" situations. Blood flow increases in skeletal muscles to prepare an individual to either fight or run away from a threatening situation. When danger passes, more blood is directed to internal organs. This time of "rest and relaxation" is dominated by the parasympathetic division.

NERVOUS TISSUE

In spite of its complexity, the nervous system is composed of two principal types of nerve cells: **neurons** and **neuroglia.** Neurons are responsible for impulse conduction. Neuroglia function primarily as connecting and supporting tissue and play an important role in the reaction of the nervous system to injury and infection.

Neurons

Figure 15–3 illustrates a sensory neuron transmitting an impulse to a motor neuron. Refer to this illustration as you read the following material.

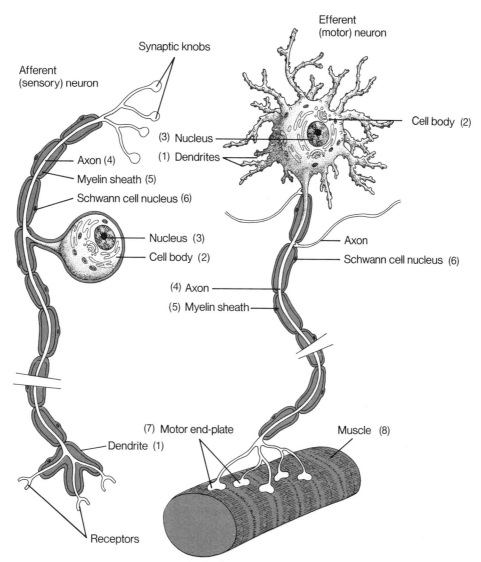

Figure 15–3 Schematic representation of a sensory neuron (*left*) transmitting an impulse to the central nervous system, and a motor neuron (*right*) transmitting an impulse from the central nervous system.

Neurons consist of three major structures:

- (1) **dendrites,** the branching cytoplasmic projections that receive impulses and transmit them to the cell body
- (2) **cell body,** the structure containing the (3) **nucleus**
- (4) **axon,** the long single projection that transmits the impulse from the cell body

Many axons in both the PNS and the ANS possess a white, lipoid covering called a (5) **myelin sheath.** This wrapping acts as an electrical insulator that reduces the possibility of an impulse stimulating adjacent nerves. It also accelerates impulse transmission through the axon. The myelin on axons in the brain and spinal cord gives these structures a white appearance and constitutes the white matter of the CNS. Unmyelinated fibers, dendrites, and nerve cell bodies make up the gray matter of the brain and spinal cord.

On peripheral nerves, the myelin sheath is formed by a neuroglial cell called a Schwann cell that wraps tightly around the axon. The (6) **Schwann cell nucleus** is pushed to the outer surface to form a thin cellular membrane called **neurolemma,** or **neurolemmal sheath.** The neurolemmal sheath permits a damaged axon to regenerate. Because neurolemma is not found in the CNS, severed CNS nerves cannot regenerate. Therefore, function of severed nerves is permanently lost unless alternate neural pathways are established.

Neurons are not continuous with one another. Instead, a small space, known as a **synapse,** is found between the axon of one neuron and the dendrite or cell body of another. In order for an impulse to travel along a nerve path, it must cross the synapse. This transmission is facilitated by chemical substances called **neurotransmitters** released at the synaptic knobs of the axon. Neurotransmitters initiate an impulse in the dendrite of the next neuron, and thus, impulses travel through neural pathways. The (7) **motor end-plates** attach to (8) **muscle** fibers. Upon stimulus by the motor neuron, the muscle contracts.

Neuroglia

The term **neuroglia** literally means "nerve glue." It was once believed that neuroglia served only a supporting role for neurons, but it is now known that neuroglia cells perform many functions.

Astrocytes, as their name suggests, are star-shaped neuroglia. They form tight sheaths around the capillaries of the brain. These sheaths keep large molecules from entering the brain and constitute the phenomenon called the **blood-brain barrier.** However, small molecules such as water, carbon dioxide, oxygen, and alcohol readily pass from blood vessels through the barrier and enter the interstitial spaces of the brain. Researchers must take the blood-brain barrier into consideration when developing drugs for treatment of brain disorders.

Oligodendrocytes, also called oligodendroglia, help in the development of myelin on neurons of the CNS.

Microglia, the smallest of the neuroglia, possess phagocytic properties and may become very active during times of infection.

Ependyma are ciliated cells that line fluid-filled cavities of the CNS, especially the ventricles of the brain. They assist in cerebrospinal fluid (CSF) circulation.

BRAIN

In addition to being one of the largest organs of the body, the brain is also the most complex in structure and function. It integrates almost every physical and mental activity of the body. This organ is also the center for memory, emotion, thought, judgment, reasoning, and consciousness. It is composed of four major structures:

- cerebrum
- cerebellum
- diencephalon
- brain stem

In order to develop a better understanding of the anatomy of the brain, refer to Figure 15–4 as you read the following material.

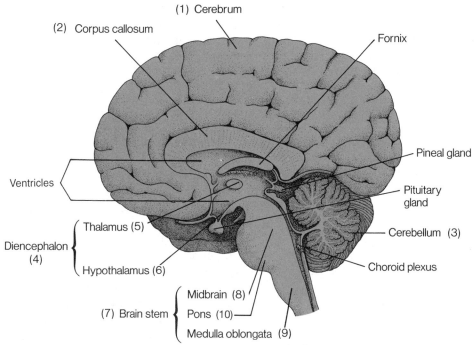

Figure 15–4 Sections of the brain.

The (1) **cerebrum** is the largest and uppermost portion of the brain. It consists of two hemispheres divided by a deep longitudinal fissure, or groove. The fissure does not completely separate the hemispheres. A structure called the (2) **corpus callosum** joins these hemispheres, permitting communication between the right and left sides of the brain. Each hemisphere is divided into five lobes. Four of these lobes are named for the bones that lie directly above them (frontal, parietal, temporal, and occipital). The fifth lobe, the insula (not shown in figure) is hidden from view and can be seen only upon dissection.

The cerebral surface consists of numerous folds, or convolutions, called **gyri.** They are separated by furrows or fissures called **sulci.** A thin gray layer called the **cerebral cortex** covers the entire cerebrum. It is composed of millions of cell bodies, which are responsible for its gray color.

The remainder of the cerebrum is composed primarily of white matter (myelinated axons). Major functions of the cerebrum include sensory perception and interpretation, muscular movement, and the emotional aspects of behavior and memory.

The second largest part of the brain, the (3) **cerebellum,** occupies the posterior portion of the brain. All functions of the cerebellum are concerned with movement. When the cerebrum initiates muscular movement, the cerebellum coordinates and refines it. The cerebellum also aids in maintaining equilibrium and balance.

The (4) **diencephalon,** is composed of many smaller structures, two of which are the (5) **thalamus** and the (6) **hypothalamus.** The thalamus receives all sensory stimuli except olfactory. It processes and transmits them to the cerebral cortex. In addition, the thalamus receives impulses from the cerebrum and relays them to efferent nerves. The hypothalamus integrates autonomic nerve impulses and regulates certain endocrine functions.

The (7) **brain stem** completes the last major section of the brain. It is composed of three structures: the (8) **midbrain** (mesencephalon), separating the cerebrum from the brain stem; the (9) **medulla oblongata,** which attaches to the spinal cord; and (10) the **pons,** or "bridge," connecting the midbrain to the medulla. In general, the brain stem serves as a pathway for impulse conduction between the brain and spinal cord. The brain stem serves as the origin for 10 of the 12 pairs of cranial nerves and controls respiration, blood pressure, and heart rate. This section is sometimes called the primary brain because it is the site where life begins and ends.

SPINAL CORD

The spinal cord transmits sensory impulses from different parts of the body to the brain and also transmits motor impulses from the brain to muscles and organs of the body. The sensory nerve tracts are called **ascending tracts** because the direction of the impulse is upward. Conversely, motor nerve tracts are called **descending tracts** because they carry impulses in a downward direction to muscles and organs. A cross-section of the spinal cord reveals an inner gray area composed of cell bodies and dendrites, with a white outer area composed of myelinated tissue of the ascending and descending tracts.

The entire spinal cord is located within the spinal cavity of the vertebral column. Thirty-one pairs of spinal nerves exit between the intervertebral spaces almost throughout the entire length of the spinal column. Unlike the cranial nerves, which have specific names, the spinal nerves are known by the region of the vertebral column from which they exit. Refer to Chapter 11, Musculoskeletal System, for the divisions of the vertebral column.

MENINGES

Both the brain and the spinal cord receive limited protection from three coverings called **meninges** (singular, **meninx**). The outermost coat, the **dura mater,** is tough and fibrous, composed primarily of connective tissue. Beneath the dura mater is a cavity called the **subdural space,** filled with serous fluid. The next layer of the meninges is the **arachnoid.** As its name suggests, the arachnoid has a spider-web appearance. A **subarachnoid space,** which contains CSF, provides additional protection for the brain and spinal cord by acting as a shock absorber. Finally, the innermost layer, the **pia mater,** contains numerous blood vessels and lymphatics that nourish the underlying tissues.

Cerebrospinal fluid circulates around the spinal cord and brain and through spaces called **ventricles,** located within the inner portion of the brain. This colorless fluid contains proteins, glucose, urea, salts, and some white blood cells. It provides nutritive substances to the CNS. Normally, CSF is absorbed as rapidly as it is formed, maintaining a constant fluid volume. Any interference with absorption results in a collection of fluid in the brain, a condition called hydrocephalus.

COMBINING FORMS

Combining Form	Meaning	Example	Pronunciation
cerebr/o	cerebrum	cerebr/o/malacia softening	sĕr-ĕ-brō-mă-LĀ-shē-ăh
crani/o	cranium (skull)	crani/o/tomy incision	krā-nē-ŎT-ō-mē
encephal/o	brain	encephal/o/tomy incision	ĕn-sĕf-ă-LŎT-ō-mē
gli/o	glue, neuroglia	gli/oma tumor	glī-Ō-mă
kinesi/o	movement	kinesi/o/logy study	kĭ-nē-sē-Ŏl-ō-jē
mening/o	meninges	mening/o/cyte cell	mĕ-NĬNG-gō-sīt
myel/o	spinal cord, bone marrow	myel/o/gram record	MĪ-ĕ-lō-grăm
narc/o	stupor, numbing	narc/o/tic pertaining to	năr-KŎ-tĭk
neur/o	nerve, nervous system	neur/algia pain	nū-RĂL-jē-ă
thalam/o	thalamus, chamber	thalam/ectomy excision	thăl-ĕm-ĔK-tō-mē
ton/o	tone, tension, pressure	ton/o/meter instrument for measuring	tōn-ŎM-ĕ-ter
ventricul/o	ventricle (of heart or brain)	ventricul/o/stomy forming an opening	vĕn-trĭk-ū-LŎS-tō-mē

SUFFIXES

Suffix	Meaning	Example	Pronunciation
-algesia -algia	pain	an/algesia without syn/algia together	ăn-ăl-JĒ-zē-ăh
-esthesia	feeling, sensation	hyper/esthesia excessive	hī-pĕr-ĕs-THĒ-zē-ă

SUFFIXES (Continued)

Suffix	Meaning	Example	Pronunciation
-lepsy	seizure	narco/lepsy stupor, numbing	NĂR-kō-lĕp-sē
-phasia	speech	tachy/phasia rapid	tăk-ē-FĀ-zē-ăh

PREFIXES

Prefix	Meaning	Example	Pronunciation
a-, an-	not, without	a/phasia speech	ăh-FĀ-zē-ăh
brady-	slow	brady/kinesia movement	brăd-ē-kĭ-NĒ-sē-ăh

Pathology

BELL'S PALSY

Bell's palsy is a facial paralysis caused by a functional disorder of the seventh cranial nerve and any or all of its branches. It may be unilateral, bilateral, transient, or permanent. Symptoms include weakness (**asthenia**) and numbness of the face, distortion of taste perception, facial disfigurement, and facial spasms. The cornea becomes dry owing to the lack of the blink reflex, often leading to corneal infections (**keratitis**). Speech difficulties (**dysphasia**) and pain behind the ear or in the face are also symptomatic of this disease.

Anti-inflammatory drugs and the application of heat help promote circulation. Spontaneous recovery can be expected in about 3 to 5 weeks.

CEREBROVASCULAR DISEASE

Cerebrovascular disease (CVD) refers to any functional abnormality of the cerebrum caused by disorders of the blood vessels that vascularize the brain. These disorders include hemorrhage, an impairment of cerebral circulation due to hardening of blood vessels (**arteriosclerosis**), cerebral thromboses, or emboli. Both hemorrhage and occlusion may lead to stroke (**cerebral vascular accident [CVA]; apoplexy**). During a CVA, blood supply is decreased (**ischemia**) or absent. If the CVA is mild, the individual may experience a brief "blackout," blurred vision, or dizziness and may not be aware of the "minor stroke" (**transient ischemic attack [TIA]**). In more serious cases, signs and symptoms include weakness in one half of the body (**hemiparesis**), paralysis in one half of the body (**hemiplegia**), inability to speak (**aphasia**), lack of muscular coordination (**ataxia**), stupor, or coma. Treatment involves speech, physical, and/or occupational therapy.

SEIZURE DISORDERS

Chronic or recurring seizure disorders are called **epilepsies.** These disorders involve electrical disturbances (**dysrhythmias**) in the brain, which result in abnormal, recurrent, and uncontrolled electrical discharges. Causes of epilepsy include brain injury, congenital anomalies, metabolic disorders, brain tumors, vascular disturbances, and genetic disorders.

Epilepsies are characterized by sudden bursts of abnormal electrical activity in neurons, resulting in temporary changes in brain function. These bursts may be mild and cause only slight changes in the level of consciousness, motor control, and sensory perception, or they may be severe and cause spastic, involuntary muscle contractions (**convulsions**) and, occasionally, loss of consciousness. Different classifications of epilepsy are based on the location and duration of changes in electrical activity in the brain. Two major types of epilepsies include petit mal and grand mal.

In **petit mal epilepsy** there are brief episodes (10 to 30 seconds) in change of level of consciousness. The seizures are frequently characterized by eye or muscle flutterings, mouth movement, and, occasionally, loss of muscle tone. If untreated, seizures can recur as often as 100 times a day.

In **grand mal seizures,** there is a loss of consciousness, with firm and violent (**tonic**) spasms, followed by episodes that alternate between muscular rigidity and relaxation (**clonic**) spasms, involuntary convulsive movements, labored breathing, tongue biting, and incontinence.

Diagnosis and evaluation often rely on measuring brain waves (**electroencephalography [EEG]**) to locate the affected area of the brain. Epilepsy can often be effectively controlled by antiepileptic medications.

PARKINSON'S DISEASE

Parkinson's disease, also called "shaking palsy," is a progressive neurological disorder affecting the portion of the brain responsible for controlling movement. As neurons degenerate, the patient develops a nodding of the head, slowness of movement (**bradykinesia, hypokinesia**), tremors, stiffness of large joints, and a shuffling gait. Muscle rigidity causes facial expressions to appear fixed and masklike. The eyes are unblinking. Sometimes the patient exhibits "pill rolling," in which he or she inadvertently rubs the thumb against the index finger.

In patients with Parkinson's disease, dopamine, a neurotransmitter that facilitates the transmission of impulses at synapses, is lacking in the brain. Management involves the administration of L-dopa, which can cross the blood-brain barrier. L-dopa is converted in the brain to dopamine. This treatment, however, only reduces the symptoms.

MULTIPLE SCLEROSIS

Multiple sclerosis (MS) is a progressive degenerative disease of the CNS. MS is characterized by inflammation, hardening, and, finally, loss of myelin (**demyelination**) throughout the spinal cord and brain. As myelin deteriorates, the transmission of electrical impulses from one neuron to another is impeded. In effect, the conduction pathway develops "short circuits."

Signs and symptoms include tremors, muscle weakness, and slowness of movement.

Occasionally, visual disturbances exist. During remissions, symptoms temporarily disappear, but progressive hardening of myelin areas leads to other attacks.

Ultimately, most voluntary motor control is lost and the patient becomes bedridden. Death occurs anywhere from 7 to 30 years after the onset of the disease. Young adults, usually women, between the ages of 20 and 40 years are the most frequent victims of MS. The etiology of the disease is uncertain, but autoimmune disease or a slow virus infection is believed to be the most probable cause.

TAY-SACHS DISEASE

Tay-Sachs disease is a genetic disorder resulting from an enzyme deficiency at birth. The lack of the enzyme hexosaminidase causes an accumulation of lipid substances in the cells of the CNS, which distends and destroys them.

The Tay-Sachs gene occurs most frequently in descendants of the Ashkenazic Jews of Eastern Europe. The afflicted child develops normally until the age of 4 to 8 months. After this time, the infant shows progressive deterioration in physiological activities, becomes paralyzed and blind, and is no longer able to eat. Inevitably the child dies. Because there is no known cure, treatment is supportive in nature. A simple blood test can identify carriers of this gene.

ONCOLOGY

Intracranial tumors can arise from any structure within the cranial cavity including the pituitary, pineal region, cranial nerves, and the arachnoid and pia mater (**leptomeninges**). However, most intracranial tumors originate directly in brain tissue. In addition, all of these tissues may be the site of metastatic spread from primary malignancies that occur outside of the nervous system. Metastatic tumors of the cranial cavity tend to exhibit growth characteristics similar to those of the primary malignancy but tend to grow more slowly than the parent tumor. Metastatic tumors of the cranial cavity are usually easier to remove than primary intracranial tumors.

Primary intracranial tumors are often classified according to histologic type and include those that originate in neurons and those that develop in glial tissue.

The signs and symptoms of intracranial neoplasms include headaches, especially upon arising in the morning, during coughing episodes, and upon bending or sudden movement. Occasionally the optic nerve swells (**papilledema**) in the back of the eyeball owing to increased intracranial pressure. Often there are personality changes, which include depression, anxiety, and irritability.

Computed tomography (CT) scans and magnetic resonance imaging (MRI) help establish a diagnosis but are not definitive. Surgical removal relieves pressure and confirms or rules out malignancy. Even after surgery, most intracranial neoplasms require radiation therapy (RT) as a second line of treatment. Chemotherapy, when added to RT, provides the best chance for survival and quality of life.

DIAGNOSTIC, SYMPTOMATIC, AND RELATED TERMS

Term	Meaning
agnosia ăg-NŌ-zē-ăh	loss of comprehension of auditory, visual, or other sensations even though the sensory sphere is intact
asthenia ăs-THĒ-nē-ăh	weakness or debility
ataxia ă-TĂK-sē-ăh	lack of muscular coordination in the execution of voluntary movement
aura AW-ră	premonitory awareness of an approaching physical or mental disorder; peculiar sensation that precedes epileptic seizures
clonic spasm KLŎN-ik spăzm	alternate contraction and relaxation of muscles
cerebrospinal otorrhea sĕr-ē-brō-SPĪ-năl ō-tō-RE-ăh	escape of CSF through the ear as a result of trauma to the head
closed head trauma TRAW-mă	traumatic injury to the head, in which the dura mater remains intact and brain tissue is not exposed. The injury site may occur at the impact site where the brain hits the inside of the skull (coup), or at the rebound site where the opposite side of the brain strikes the skull (contra coup)
coma KŌ-măh	abnormally deep unconsciousness with absence of voluntary response to stimuli
concussion kŏn-KŬSH-ŭn	injury (usually to the brain) resulting from impact with an object
Guillain-Barré syndrome gwĕ-YĀN BĂR-rā SĬN-drōm	acute polyneuritis with progressive muscular weakness of extremities; most commonly occurs in people aged 30 to 50 years; spontaneous and complete recovery in about 95% of cases
Huntington's chorea HŬNT-ĭng-tŭnz kō-RĒ-ă	inherited disease of the CNS that usually has its onset in people between 30 and 50 years of age. This disease is characterized by quick, involuntary movements, speech disturbances, and mental deterioration
lethargy LĔTH-ăr-jē	abnormal activity or lack of response to normal stimuli; sluggishness
neuritis nū-RĪ-tĭs	inflammation of nerve(s) usually associated with a degenerative process

DIAGNOSTIC, SYMPTOMATIC, AND RELATED TERMS (Continued)

Term	Meaning
paraplegia păr-ăh-PLĒ-jē-ăh	paralysis of the lower portion of the trunk and both legs
paresis PĂR-ē-sĭs/pă-RĒ-sĭs	partial or incomplete paralysis
paresthesia păr-ĕs-THĒ-zē-ăh	sensation of numbness, prickling, or tingling; heightened sensitivity
quadriplegia kwŏd-rĭ-PLĒ-jē-ăh	paralysis of all four extremities and usually the trunk
Reye's syndrome RĪZ SĬN-drōm	acute encephalopathy and fatty infiltration of the liver and possibly pancreas, heart, kidney, spleen, and lymph nodes; usually seen in children younger than 15 years of age who had an acute viral infection. The mortality may be as high as 80%. The use of aspirin by children experiencing chickenpox or influenza may induce Reye's syndrome
sciatica sī-ĂT-ĭ-kă	severe pain in the leg along the course of the sciatic nerve felt at the base of the spine, down the thigh, and radiating down the leg, because of a compressed nerve
syncope SĬN-kō-pē	fainting
transient ischemic attack (TIA) TRAN-zē-ĕnt ĭs-KĒ-mĭk	temporary interference with blood supply to the brain lasting from a few minutes to a few hours

Special Procedures

DIAGNOSTIC IMAGING PROCEDURES

Term	Description
cerebral angiography, cerebral arteriography	visualization of the cerebral vascular system after injection of radiopaque dye into the carotid or vertebral artery to visualize abnormalities of the cerebrovascular circulation, vascular tumors, aneurysms, and occlusions. Abscesses, nonvascular tumors, and hematomas are often identified because they distort the normal vascular image

DIAGNOSTIC IMAGING PROCEDURES (Continued)

Term	Description
CT scan (cranial)	procedure that provides a 3-dimensional visual "slice" of the cranial contents; relatively safe; helps differentiate intracranial pathologies such as tumors, cysts, edema, hemorrhage, and cerebral aneurysms
echoencephalography	ultrasound technique used to study the intracranial structures of the brain, and especially to diagnose conditions that cause a shift in the midline structures of the brain
myelography	radiography of the spinal cord after injection of a contrast medium
positron emission tomography (PET) scan	technique that produces cross-sectional images of brain by using radioactive substances. Radioactive substances emit positrons, which form images of the brain, used to measure regional cerebral blood flow, blood volume, oxygen uptake, glucose transport and metabolism, and locate neurotransmitter receptors

SURGICAL PROCEDURES

Term	Description
cordotomy kor-DŎT-ō-mē	surgical sectioning of part of the spinal cord
cryosurgery krī-ō-SĔR-jer-ē	technique of exposing tissues to extreme cold, sometimes used to destroy portions of the brain (e.g., the thalamus)
stereotaxy STĔR-ē-ō-tăk-sē	precise method of locating and destroying deep-seated brain structures using 3-dimensional coordinates generated by CT scan
sympathectomy sĭm-păh-THĔK-tō-mē	excision or resection of part of the SNS pathways
thalamotomy thăl-ăh-MŎT-ō-mē	partial destruction of the thalamus to treat psychosis or intractable pain
tractotomy trăk-TŎT-ō-mē	transection of a nerve tract in the brain stem or spinal cord, sometimes used to relieve intractable pain

SURGICAL PROCEDURES (Continued)

Term	Description
trephination trĕf-ĭ-NĀ-shŭn	cutting a circular opening into the skull to reveal brain tissue and decrease intracranial pressure
vagotomy vā-GŎT-ō-mē	interruption of the function of the vagus nerve to relieve peptic ulcer

CLINICAL AND LABORATORY PROCEDURES

Term	Description
cisternal puncture	spinal puncture through the dura mater, at the base of the brain, to extract spinal fluid for laboratory testing or to inject medications
electroencephalography (EEG)	recording of electric activity in the brain by placing electrodes on the skull; produces graphic tracing called an electroencephalogram
electromyogram	graphic recording of muscle contractions as a result of electrical stimulation
spinal puncture, spinal tap, CSF analysis	needle puncture of the spinal cavity to extract spinal fluid for diagnostic purposes, to introduce anesthetic agents into the spinal canal, or to remove fluid to allow other fluids (e.g., radiopaque substances) to be injected

PHARMACOLOGY

Medication	Action
analgesics	reduce or relieve pain (e.g., aspirin, codeine, morphine)
anticonvulsants	prevent or reduce the severity of epileptic or other convulsive seizures
antidepressants	alleviate mental depression
hypnotics	induce sleep or hypnosis
opiates	narcotic drugs that contain opium or its derivatives; used as a analgesic, as a hypnotic, and to control diarrhea and spasmodic conditions
psychotropic drugs	alter psychic function, behavior, or experience; often used in management of psychotic disorders

PHARMACOLOGY (Continued)

Medication	Action
sedatives	exert a soothing or tranquilizing effect by depressing CNS activity; tend to cause lassitude and reduced mental activity
tranquilizers	calm anxiety or agitation, without decreasing level of consciousness

ABBREVIATIONS

Abbreviation	Term
ANS	autonomic nervous system
AVMs	arteriovenous malformations
CNS	central nervous system
CP	cerebral palsy
CSF	cerebrospinal fluid
CT scan	computed tomography scan
CVA	cerebrovascular accident
CVD	cerebrovascular disease
EEG	electroencephalogram
EMG	electromyogram
HNP	herniated nucleus pulposus (herniated disk)
LP	lumbar puncture
MRI	magnetic resonance imaging
MS	multiple sclerosis
PET	positron emission tomography
PNS	peripheral nervous system
R/O	rule out
RT	radiation therapy
SAH	subarachnoid hemorrhage
SNS	somatic nervous system
TIA	transient ischemic attack

Case Study

Subarachnoid Hemorrhage

History of Present Illness. The patient is a 61-year-old woman with a history of developing sudden onset of "extremely severe headaches" while swimming. She had associated neck pain, **occipital** pain, nausea, and vomiting.

A **CT scan** was obtained that showed blood in the **cisterna subarachnoidalis** consistent with subarachnoid hemorrhage. The patient also had mild acute **hydrocephalus.** Neurologically, the patient was found to be within normal limits. A **cerebral angiogram** was performed and no **aneurysm** was noted. The patient was hospitalized on 7/5/xx. On 7/7/xx, she had sudden worsening of her headache associated with nausea and vomiting. Also she was noted to have **meningismus** on examination. A **lumbar puncture** was performed in order **R/O** possible rebleed. At the time of the lumbar puncture, **CSF** in four tubes was read as consistent with recurrent subarachnoid hemorrhage. An **MRI** was performed without evidence of an aneurysm.

Disposition. On 7/16/xx, the patient underwent repeat **angiogram,** which again showed no aneurysm. The patient was deemed stable for discharge on 7/16/xx.

Activity. She was instructed to avoid any type of activity that could result in raised pressure in the head (i.e., **Valsalva maneuvers** associated with constipation, coughing, sneezing, or vomiting). The patient was advised that she should undergo no activity more vigorous than walking.

Discharge Diagnosis. Subarachnoid hemorrhage.

Worksheet 5 provides a dictionary and reading application and an analysis of this case study.

Worksheet 1

Use encephal/o (brain) to build a medical word meaning:

1. disease of the brain _____

2. herniation of the brain _____

Use cerebr/o (cerebrum) to build a medical word meaning:

3. pertaining to the cerebrum and spinal cord _____

4. abnormal condition of hardening of the cerebrum _____

5. disease of the cerebrum _____

Use crani/o (cranium, skull) to build a medical word meaning:

6. herniation (through the) cranium _____

7. softening of the cranium _____

8. condition of hardening of the skull _____

9. instrument for measuring the skull _____

Use neur/o (nerve) to build a medical word meaning:

10. embryonic nerve (cell) _____

11. nerve pain _____

12. specialist in the study of the nervous system _____

Use myel/o (spinal cord) to build a medical word meaning:

13. radiograph of the spinal cord _____

14. herniation of the spinal cord _____

15. paralysis of the spinal cord _____

Use mening/o (meninges) to build a medical word meaning:

16. herniation of the meninges _____

17. herniation of the meninges and spinal cord _____

Use the suffix -plegia (paralysis) to build a medical word meaning:

18. paralysis of one half (of the body) _____

19. paralysis of four (limbs) _____

Use the suffix -lepsy (seizure) to build a medical word meaning:

20. seizure of sleep _____

Use the suffix -algesia (pain) to build a medical word meaning:

21. without pain _____

Use the suffix -phasia (speech) to build a medical word meaning:

22. difficult speech _____

23. lacking or without speech _____

Use the suffix -trophy (nourishment) to build a medical word meaning:

24. excessive nourishment _____

25. lacking nourishment _____

Worksheet 2

Build a surgical term meaning:

1. destruction of a nerve _____

2. incision of the skull _____

3. surgical repair of the skull _____

4. suture of a nerve _____

5. incision of the brain _____

6. incision of the thalamus _____

Worksheet 3

Match the following words with the definitions in the numbered list.

asthenia

aura

coma

concussion

contusion

Huntington's chorea

lethargy

paraplegia

Reye's syndrome

sciatica

transient ischemic attack

tremor

1. _____ head injury resulting from an impact with an object

2. _____ abnormally deep unconsciousness

3. _____ inherited disease of the CNS, characterized by quick involuntary movements, speech disturbances, and mental deterioration

4. _____ premonitory awareness of an approaching mental disorder; the peculiar sensation that precedes an epileptic seizure

5. _____ paralysis of the lower portion of the trunk and both legs

6. _____ severe pain felt at the base of the spine and down the thigh to the leg, owing to a compressed nerve

7. _____ temporary interference with blood supply to the brain

8. _____ acute encephalopathy seen in children, often associated with the use of aspirin to relieve symptoms of chickenpox or influenza

9. _____ sluggishness, abnormal inactivity

10. _____ weakness or debility

Worksheet 4

SPECIAL PROCEDURES, PHARMACOLOGY, AND ABBREVIATIONS

Match the following words with the definitions in the numbered list.

analgesic

cerebral angiography

cisternal puncture

computed tomography (CT)

cordotomy

cryosurgery

echoencephalography

electromyogram

laminectomy

myelography

pneumoencephalograph

SAH

syncope

tranquilizer

trephination

TIA

1. _____ visualization of the cerebrovascular system after injection of a radiopaque dye into the vertebral or carotid artery

2. _____ technique of destroying tissue by exposure to extreme cold; frequently used in brain surgery

3. _____ cutting a circular opening into the skull

4. _____ spinal puncture through the dura mater to extract spinal fluid

5. _____ graphic recording of muscular contraction owing to electrical stimulation

6. _____ medication that reduces or relieves pain

7. _____ calms anxiousness or agitation without decreasing level of consciousness

8. _____ excision of vertebral posterior arch to relieve pressure on spinal nerves

9. _____ assessment of the ventricles and subarachnoid spaces following withdrawal of CSF fluid and injection of air or gas via a lumbar puncture

10. _____ fainting

11. _____ provides a three-dimensional slice of the cranial contents

12. _____ ultrasound technique used to study the brain

13. _____ surgical sectioning of part of the spinal cord

14. _____ x-ray examination of the spinal cord after injection of a contrast medium

15. _____ subarachnoid hemorrhage

Worksheet 5

SUBARACHNOID HEMORRHAGE DICTIONARY EXERICSE

Use a medical dictionary or other resource to define the following terms and to determine their pronunciation; then practice reading the case study aloud (p. 334).

aneurysm _____

angiogram _____

cerebral angiogram _____

cisterna subarachnoidalis _____

CSF _____

CT scan _____

hydrocephalus _____

lumbar puncture _____

meningismus _____

MRI _____

occipital _____

R/O _____

subarachnoid hemorrhage _____

Valsalva maneuvers _____

ANALYSIS OF SUBARACHNOID HEMORRHAGE

1. In what part of the head did the patient feel pain?

2. List the radiological tests performed on the patient and the finding each provided.

3. How does meningismus differ from meningitis?

4. Did the lumbar puncture rule out or confirm a second subarachnoid hemorrhage?

5. Which two tests ruled out an aneurysm?

6. What is the Valsalva maneuver?

Worksheet 6

Label the following figure. To check your answers, refer to Figure 15–4.

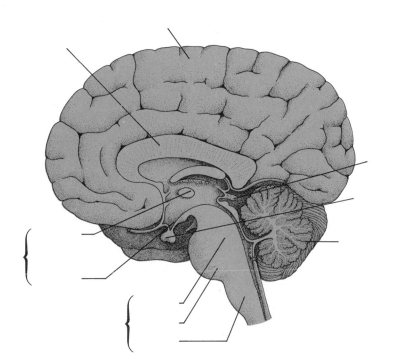

Corpus callosum

Cerebrum

Pineal gland

Cerebellum

Diencephalon

Thalamus

Hypothalamus

Pituitary
gland

Brain stem

Midbrain

Pons

Medulla oblongata

Chapter 16

Special Senses

Chapter Outline

Student Objectives

Upon completion of this chapter, you will be able to do the following:

Identify major structures and functions of the eye.

List and describe accessory structures associated with the eye.

Identify major structures and functions of the ear.

Explain the physiology of hearing.

Describe the structures and functions of the ear that are related to the sense of equilibrium.

Identify combining forms, suffixes, and prefixes related to the special senses.

Identify and discuss pathology related to the special senses.

Student Objectives (Continued)

Identify clinical and surgical procedures and abbreviations related to the special senses.

Discuss pharmacology related to the treatment of eye and ear disorders.

Demonstrate your knowledge of the chapter by completing the worksheets.

Anatomy and Physiology

The special senses include taste, smell, sight, hearing, and equilibrium. The senses of taste and smell have been covered in previous chapters. This chapter presents information on the eye, the sense organ for sight, and the ear, the sense organ for hearing and equilibrium.

THE EYE

The eye (Fig. 16–1) is a globe-shaped organ composed of three distinct layers. Its outermost layer, the (1) **sclera,** is a tough fibrous tissue that serves as a protective shield for more sensitive structures beneath. The sclera is also known as the white of the eye. A highly vascular middle layer, the (2) **choroid,** provides the blood supply for the entire eye. It contains pigmented cells that prevent extraneous light from entering the inside of the eye. The innermost layer of the eye, the (3) **retina,** is composed of nerve endings that are responsible for the reception and transmission of light impulses.

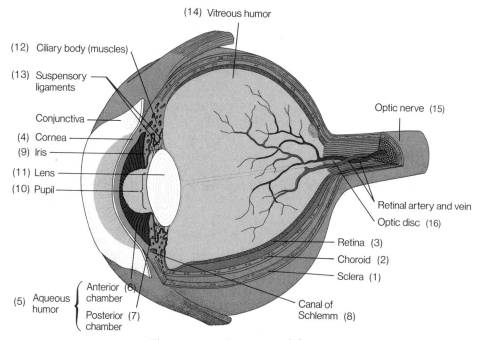

Figure 16–1 Structures of the eye.

A specialized portion of the sclera, the (4) **cornea,** passes in front of the lens. Rather than being opaque, it is transparent, allowing light to enter the interior of the eye. The cornea is one of the few body structures that does not contain capillaries.

One of the two major humors, or fluids, of the eye is the (5) **aqueous humor.** The iris divides the aqueous humor into two small chambers, the (6) **anterior chamber** and the (7) **posterior chamber.** Aqueous humor is continually produced in the posterior chamber and drained from the eye by way of a small opening called the (8) **canal of Schlemm,** located near the anterior chamber. A colored contractile membrane, the (9) **iris,** functions as a sphincter. Its perforated center is the (10) **pupil.** By changing its size, the pupil regulates the amount of light entering the eye. As environmental light increases, the pupil constricts; as light decreases, the pupil dilates.

The (11) **lens** is located behind the posterior chamber. This crystalline structure is held between the (12) **ciliary body (muscles)** by the (13) **suspensory ligaments.** As these muscles relax or contract, they alter the shape of the lens, making it thicker or thinner, respectively. This enables light rays to focus on the retina, a process called **accommodation.**

The second major humor of the eye is the (14) **vitreous humor.** This clear, jellylike fluid occupies the entire orbit of the eye behind the lens. The vitreous humor, lens, and aqueous humor are the refractive structures of the eye. They bend light rays, focusing them sharply on the retina. If any one of these structures does not function properly, vision is impaired.

The retina is an extremely delicate eye membrane. It is continuous with the optic nerve and has two types of visual receptors, **rods** and **cones.** Rods function in dim light, producing black-and-white vision. Cones function in bright light, producing color vision.

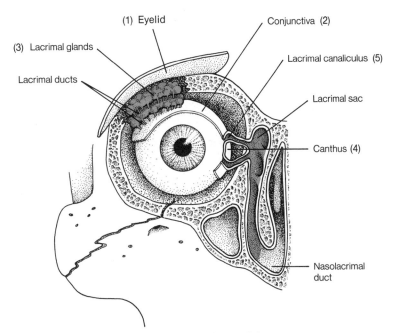

Figure 16–2   The front of the eye.

Rods and cones contain chemicals called **photopigments.** As light strikes the photopigments, a chemical change occurs that stimulates rods and cones. The impulses they produce are transmitted through the (15) **optic nerve** to the brain, where they are interpreted as vision.

Both the optic nerve and blood vessels of the eye enter the eyeball at the (16) **optic disc.** Its center is referred to as the **blind spot** because the area has neither rods nor cones.

Six muscles control the movement of the eye: the superior, inferior, lateral, and medial rectus muscles and the superior and inferior oblique muscles. These muscles are coordinated to move both eyes in a synchronized manner.

Refer to Figure 16–2 as you read the following paragraphs.

Two movable folds of skin constitute the (1) **eyelids,** each with eyelashes that protect the front of the eye. A thin mucous membrane called the (2) **conjunctiva** lines the inner surface of the eyelids and the cornea. Lying superior and to the outer edge of each eye are the (3) **lacrimal glands,** which produce tears that bathe and lubricate the eyes. The tears collect at the inner edges of the eyes, the (4) **canthi** (singular, **canthus**), and pass through pinpoint openings, the (5) **lacrimal canaliculi** (singular, **canaliculus**), to the mucous membranes that line the inside of the nose.

THE EAR

The ear is the sense organ receptor for hearing and equilibrium. Hearing is a function of the cochlea, whereas equilibrium is controlled by the semicircular canals and vestibule.

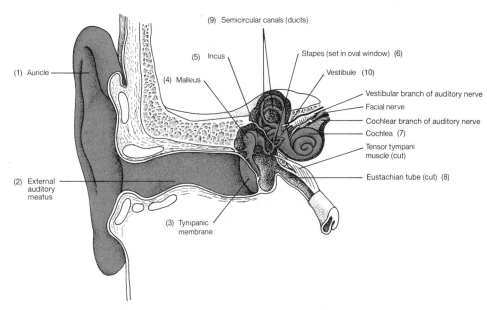

Figure 16–3   Outer, middle, and inner ear structures as shown in a frontal section through the right temporal bone.

Hearing

The ear consists of three major sections: the outer or **external ear,** the middle ear or **tympanic cavity,** and the inner ear or **labyrinth.** Each of these sections transmits sound waves, but in different ways. The external ear conducts sound waves through air; the middle ear, through bone; and the inner ear, through fluid. This series of transmissions plays an integral part in hearing.

Refer to Figure 16–3 and identify the following structures associated with hearing.

An (1) **auricle** (or **pinna**), collects waves traveling through air and channels them to the (2) **external auditory meatus** (ear canal). This canal is a slender tube lined with glands that produce a waxy secretion called **cerumen.** Its stickiness prevents tiny foreign particles from entering the deeper areas of the canal. A flat membranous structure, the (3) **tympanic membrane (tympanum,** or eardrum) is drawn over the end of the ear canal. Sound waves that enter the ear canal strike against the tympanum, causing it to vibrate. The tympanic vibrations are picked up by three tiny articulating bones called **ossicles,** located in the middle ear. These bones, the (4) **malleus** (hammer), the (5) **incus** (anvil), and the (6) **stapes** (stirrups) are responsible for transmitting sound waves through the middle ear. These ossicles form a chain that stretches from the inner surface of the tympanum to a snail-shaped structure, the (7) **cochlea,** located in the inner ear. The cochlea is filled with fluid. Lining its inner surface are tiny nerve endings called the **hairs of Corti.** A membrane-covered opening on the external surface of the cochlea, the **oval window,** is the place of attachment for the stapes. Transmission of sound along the ossicles in the middle ear causes the stapes to exert a gentle pumping action against the oval window. The pumping action forces the cochlear fluid to move. Disturbance of the fluid stimulates the hairs of Corti, generating impulses that are transmitted to the brain by way of the auditory nerve, where they are interpreted as sound.

The (8) **eustachian tube** connects the middle ear to the pharynx. Its purpose is to equalize pressure on the outer and inner surfaces of the eardrum. When sudden pressure changes occur, pressure can be equalized on either side of the tympanic membrane by deliberately swallowing.

Equilibrium

Besides the cochlea, the inner ear contains the (9) **semicircular canals** and the (10) **vestibule.** The vestibule joins the cochlea and the semicircular canals. The inner ear is sometimes referred to as the labyrinth because of its complicated mazelike design. Complex structures located in this maze are responsible for maintaining a sense of equilibrium. Both **static** and **dynamic equilibrium** are provided by these structures. Static equilibrium refers to the orientation of the body relative to gravity. It allows an individual to maintain posture and orientation while at rest. Dynamic equilibrium refers to maintaining body position in response to movement.

COMBINING FORMS

Combining Form	Meaning	Example	Pronunciation
EYE			
ambly/o	dull, dim	ambly/opia vision	ăm-blē-Ō-pē-ăh
aque/o	water	aque/ous pertaining to	Ā-kwē-ŭs

blephar/o	eyelid	blephar/o/ptosis
		    prolapse, downward
		    displacement
			blĕf-ă-rō-TŌ-sĭs

choroid/o	choroid	choroid/o/pathy disease	kō-roy-DŎP-ă-thē
corne/o	cornea	corne/itis inflammation	kor-nē-Ī-tĭs

kerat/o	cornea, horny tissue	kerat/o/meter
		    instrument for
		    measuring
			kĕr-ă-TŎM-ĕ-tĕr

cycl/o	ciliary body	cycl/o/plegia paralysis	sī-klō-PLĒ-jē-ăh
dacry/o	tear, lacrimal sac	dacry/o/stenosis narrowing	dăk-rē-ō-stĕn-Ō-sĭs
irid/o	iris	irid/o/plegia paralysis	ĭr-ĭd-ō-PLĒ-jē-ăh

ophthalm/o	eye	ophthalm/o/logist
		    specialist in the
		    study of
			ŏf-thăl-MŎL-ō-jĭst

ocul/o		ocul/o/nas/ al nose pertaining to	ŏk-ū-lō-NĀ-săl
opt/o	vision, eye	opt/ic pertaining to	ŎP-tĭk
phac/o	lens	phac/o/cele herniation	FĀK-ō-sēl
presby/o	old age	presby/opia vision	prĕz-bē-Ō-pē-ăh
pupill/o	pupils	pupill/o/scopy examination	pū-pĭl-ŎS-kō-pē
core/o		core/o/plasty surgical repair	KŌ-rē-ō-plăs-tē

COMBINING FORMS (Continued)

Combining Form	Meaning	Example	Pronunciation
EYE			
retin/o	retina	retin/o/pathy 　　　　disease	rĕt-ĭn-ŎP-ă-thē
scler/o	sclera, hardening	scler/ectomy 　　excision	sklĕ-RĚK-tō-mē
EAR			
audi/o	hearing	audi/o/logy 　　　study of	aw-dē-ŎL-ō-jē
labyrinth/o	labyrinth, inner ear	labyrinth/itis 　　　　inflammation	lāb-ĭ-rĭn-THĪ-tĭs
ot/o	ear	ot/o/rrhea 　　discharge	ō-tō-RĒ-ăh
salping/o	eustachian tube, oviduct	salping/itis 　　　inflammation	săl-pĭn-JĪ-tĭs
staped/o	stapes	staped/ectomy 　　excision	stā-pĕ-DĔK-tō-mē
tympan/o	tympanic membrane, eardrum	tympan/o/centesis 　　　　puncture	tĭm-pă-nō-sĕn-TĒ-sĭs
myring/o		myring/o/tomy 　　　incision	mĭr-ĭn-GOT-ō-mē

SUFFIXES

Suffix	Meaning	Example	Pronunciation
-opia	vision	dipl/opia double	dĭp-LŌ-pē-ăh
-tropia	turning	hyper/tropia excessive	hī-pĕr-TRŌ-pē-ăh

PREFIXES

Prefix	Meaning	Example	Pronunciation
eso-	inward	<u>eso</u>/tropia turn	ĕs-ō-TRŌ-pē-ăh
exo-	outward	<u>exo</u>/trop/ic turn pertaining to	ĕks-ō-TRŌ-pĭk

Pathology

ERRORS OF REFRACTION

An error of refraction, also called **ametropia,** exists when light rays fail to focus sharply on the retina. This may be due to a defect in the lens, cornea, or the shape of the eyeball. If the eyeball is too long, the image falls in front of the retina, causing nearsightedness, or **myopia** (Fig. 16–4). Correction is made using a concave lens. In farsightedness **(hyperopia, hypermetropia)** which is the opposite of myopia, the eyeball is too short and the image falls behind the retina. A form of farsightedness is **presbyopia,** a defect associated with the aging process. The onset usually occurs between 40 and 45 years of age. The individual can see distant objects clearly but cannot see near objects in proper focus. Correction involves the use of a convex lens.

In another form of ametropia called **astigmatism,** the cornea or lens has a defective curvature. This causes light rays to diffuse over a large area of the retina, rather than being focused sharply on a given point. Corrective lenses that compensate for the imperfect curvature of the cornea or lens are used for astigmatism.

CATARACTS

Cataracts are opacities that form on the lens or on the capsule containing the lens. These opacities are frequently produced by protein that slowly builds up until vision is lost. The only effective treatment is removal of the lens or capsule.

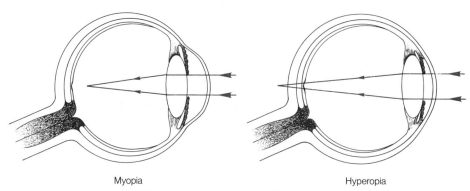

Myopia   Hyperopia

Figure 16–4   Myopia and hyperopia.

Several techniques may be employed for cataract removal. In one method, a super-cooled metal probe **(cryoprobe)** is placed on the cataract. The cataract bonds to the cold probe, and the cataract and lens are gently lifted from the eye. This method of treatment is known as **intracapsular extraction.** It is usually the method of choice when the cataract develops as a result of old age **(senescent** or **senile cataract).**

Cataracts found in children are usually a result of genetic defects or maternal rubella during the first trimester of pregnancy. In children and young adults, the surgery of choice is **extracapsular extraction.** Both the cortex and lens are removed, but the posterior lens capsule is retained.

In **phacoemulsion,** the capsule is fragmented using ultrasonic vibrations. Prognosis is good in most patients, with vision improvement in 95 percent of all patients.

GLAUCOMA

Glaucoma is characterized by increased pressure within the eyeball **(intraocular pressure)** caused by the failure of aqueous humor to drain from the eye through a tiny duct called the canal of Schlemm. The increased pressure on the optic nerve destroys it, and vision is permanently lost.

Medications that cause the pupils to constrict **(miotics)** permit aqueous humor to escape from the eye, thereby relieving pressure. If miotics are ineffective, surgery may be necessary. Surgery for glaucoma includes **paracentesis** of the cornea; excision of a small portion of the iris **(partial iridectomy);** or separation of the iris from its attachment **(iridodialysis, coredialysis).**

Glaucoma is diagnosed by using an instrument that measures the internal pressure of the eye **(tonometer).** This procedure should be performed in all patients older than 35 years of age during routine eye examinations.

STRABISMUS

Strabismus is a condition in which the eyes turn from the normal position so that they deviate in different directions. If the eyes turn outward **(exotropia),** causing a divergent squint, the individual is said to be wall-eyed. If the eyes turn toward each other **(esotropia),** causing a convergent squint, the individual is said to be cross-eyed. Strabismus may be due to poor vision, unequal ocular muscle tone, or an oculomotor nerve lesion.

In children, strabismus is associated with "lazy eye syndrome" **(amblyopia).** Vision is suppressed in one eye so that the child uses only the other eye for vision. The suppression of vision in the "lazy" eye is usually due to extreme nearsightedness **(unilateral myopia)** or to double vision that develops because of strabismus.

Methods of treatment include corrective lenses, eye exercises to correct vision **(orthoptic training),** and surgery **(strabotomy)** in which the ocular tendons are cut.

RETINITIS PIGMENTOSA

Retinitis pigmentosa, a chronic progressive disease, results in degeneration of the retina and atrophy of the optic nerve. In all forms of this disease, the retinal rods deteriorate and the pigmented layer of the retina undergoes irreversible change. This genetic disorder usually occurs before adulthood, beginning with night blindness and loss of peripheral vision. In some cases, cataracts form, in addition to choroidal sclerosis and glaucoma. Ultimately, this disorder leads to complete blindness, usually before a person is 50 years of age. There is no known cure for retinitis pigmentosa.

OTITIS MEDIA

Otitis media is an inflammation of the middle ear. It is found most commonly in infants and young children, especially in the presence of an upper respiratory infection (URI). Symptoms may include earache, draining of pus from the ear **(otopyorrhea),** or rupturing of the eardrum **(tympanorrhexis, myringorrhexis).** Treatment consists of bed rest, medications to relieve pain **(analgesics),** and antibiotics. Occasionally, an incision of the eardrum **(myringotomy, tympanotomy)** may be necessary to relieve pressure and promote draining of pus from the middle ear.

Recurrent episodes of otitis media may cause scarring of the tympanic membrane, causing hearing loss. If left untreated, otitis media may lead to infection of the mastoid process **(mastoiditis)** or inflammation of brain tissue near the middle ear **(otoencephalitis).**

OTOSCLEROSIS

Otosclerosis is characterized by an abnormal hardening **(ankylosis)** of spongy bone around the oval window. This decreases the ability of the stapes to move the oval window, causing hearing loss. Occasionally, the individual perceives a ringing sound **(tinnitus)** within the ear. Surgical correction involves the removal of the stapes **(stapedectomy)** and reconstruction of the oval window.

ONCOLOGY

Two major neoplastic diseases account for more than 90 percent of all primary intraocular diseases: **retinoblastoma,** found primarily in children, and **melanoma,** found primarily in adults.

Most retinoblastomas tend to be familial. The cell involved is the retinal neuron. Vision is impaired, and in about 30 percent of the patients, the disease is found in both eyes **(bilateral).** Treatment usually involves the removal of the affected eye(s) **(enucleation),** followed by radiation.

Intraorbital melanoma frequently arises in the pigmented cells of the choroid. Sometimes, however, it may originate in the iris or ciliary body. The disease is usually asymptomatic until there is a hemorrhage into the anterior chamber. Any discrete, fleshy mass on the iris should be examined by an ophthalmologist. If malignancy occurs in the choroid, it usually appears as a brown or gray mushroom-shaped lesion. If the lesion is on the iris, an iridectomy is performed. For melanoma of the choroid, enucleation is necessary. Many eye tumors are noninvasive and are not necessarily life-threatening.

DIAGNOSTIC, SYMPTOMATIC, AND RELATED TERMS

Term	Meaning
EYE	
achromatopsia ăh-krō-măh-TŎP-sē-ăh	severe congenital deficiency in color perception; color blindness
conjunctivitis kŏn-jŭnk-tĭ-VĪ-tĭs	inflammation of the conjunctiva with vascular congestion, producing a red or pink eye, and may be secondary to viral, chlamydial, bacterial, or fungal infections or allergy
convergence kŏn-VĚR-jens	medial movement of the two eyeballs so that they are both directed at the object being viewed
ectropion ĕk-TRŌ-pē-ŏn	eversion of the edge of the eyelid
entropion ĕn-TRŌ-pē-ŏn	inversion or turning inward of the edge of the lower eyelid
exophthalmos ĕk-sŏf-THĂL-mŏs	protrusion of one or both eyeballs frequently caused by hyperactive thyroid, trauma or tumors
hordeolum, sty hŏr-dē-ŌL-ŭm	a localized circumscribed inflammatory swelling of one of the several sebaceous glands of the eyelid, generally caused by a bacterial infection
metamorphopsia mĕt-ă-mŏr-FŎP-sē-ăh	distortion of shapes
nyctalopia nĭk-tăh-LŌ-pē-ăh	night-blindness
nystagmus nĭs-TAG-mŭs	involuntary eye movements that appear jerky
papilledema, choked disc păp-ĭl-ĕ-DĒ-măh	edema and hyperemia of the optic disc usually associated with increased ocular pressure resulting from intracranial pressure
trachoma trā-KŌ-măh	chronic contagious form of conjunctivitis found frequently in the southwestern states; often leads to blindness
visual field	area within which objects may be seen when the eye is fixed

DIAGNOSTIC, SYMPTOMATIC, AND RELATED TERMS (Continued)

Term	Meaning
EAR	
anacusis ăn-ăh-KŪ-sĭs	deafness
conduction impairment kŏn-DŬK-shŭn	blocking of sound waves as they are conducted through the external and middle ear (conduction pathway)
labyrinthitis lăb-ĭ-rĭn-THĪ-tĭs	inflammation of the inner ear that usually results from an acute febrile process; may cause progressive vertigo
Ménière's disease měn-ē-ĀRZ	disorder of the labyrinth that leads to progressive loss of hearing, characterized by vertigo, sensorineural hearing loss, and tinnitus
otitis externa ō-TĪ-tĭs eks-TĚR-nă	infection of the external auditory canal
presbyacusia, presbycusis prěz-bē-ă-KŪ-sē-ăh, prěs-bē-KŪ-sĭs	impairment of hearing resulting from old age
tinnitus tĭn-Ī-tŭs	ringing in the ears
vertigo VĚR-tĭ-gō	hallucination of movement; a feeling of spinning or dizziness

Special Procedures

CLINICAL PROCEDURES

Term	Description
EYE	
electronystagmography ē-lěk-trō-nĭs-tăg-MŎG-ră-fē	method of recording nystagmus activity by detecting the electrical activity of the extraocular muscles
ophthalmoscopy ŏf-thăl-MŎS-kō-pē	visual examination of the interior of the eye using an ophthalmoscope; useful in detecting eye disorders as well as disorders of other organs that cause changes in the eye
retinoscopy rět-ĭn-ŎS-kō-pē	visual examination to evaluate refractive errors of the eye

CLINICAL PROCEDURES (Continued)

Term	Description
tonometry tōn-ŎM-ĕ-trē	measurement of tension and pressure, especially of the eye for detection of glaucoma
visual acuity test ă-KŪ-ĭ-tē	part of an eye examination that evaluates the patient's ability to distinguish the form and detail of an object

EAR

Term	Description
audiometry aw-dē-OM-ĕ-trē	measurement of the acuity of hearing for the various frequencies of sound waves
otoscopy o-TOS-kŏ-pē	visual examination of the external auditory canal and the tympanic membrane using an otoscope

SURGICAL PROCEDURES

Term	Description
EYE	
blepharectomy blĕf-ăh-RĔK-tō-mē	excision of a lesion of the eyelid
cyclodialysis sī-klō-dī-ĂL-ĭ-sĭs	formation of an opening between the anterior chamber and the suprachoroidal space for the draining of aqueous humor in glaucoma
enucleation ē-nū-klē-Ā-shŭn	removal of an organ or other mass intact from its supporting tissues; removal of the eyeball from the orbit
evisceration ē-vĭs-ĕr-Ā-shun	removal of the contents of the eye while leaving the sclera and cornea
keratocentesis kĕr-ăh-tō-sĕn-TĒ-sĭs	surgical puncture of the cornea
phacoemulsification făk-ō-ē-MŬL-sĭ-fĭ-kā-shŭn	method of treating cataracts by using ultrasonic waves to disintegrate the cataract, which is then aspirated and removed
sclerostomy sklĕ-RŎS-tō-mē	surgical formation of an opening in the sclera

SURGICAL PROCEDURES (Continued)

Term	Description
EAR	
mastoid antrotomy MĂS-toid ăn-TRŎT-ō-mē	surgical opening of a cavity within the mastoid process
myringoplasty, tympanoplasty mĭ-RĬNG-gō-plăs-tē, tĭm-păh-nō-PLĂS-tē	reconstruction of the eardrum
otoplasty Ō-tō-plăs-tē	corrective surgery for a deformed or excessively large or small pinna

PHARMACOLOGY

Medication	Action
beta-adrenergics	agents that lower intraocular pressure by reducing the production of aqueous humor; used in treatment of glaucoma
cycloplegics	agents that paralyze the ciliary muscles thereby dilating pupils; used to facilitate certain eye examinations
miotics	substances that constrict the pupils; used in treatment of glaucoma
mydriatics	agents that dilate the pupils. In certain eye diseases the pupil must be dilated during treatment to prevent adhesions of the pupils

ABBREVIATIONS

Abbreviation	Term
EYE	
Acc	accommodation
Ast	astigmatism
D	diopter (lens strength)
Em	emmetropia
ENT	ear, nose, and throat
EOM	extraocular movement
IOP	intraocular pressure
mix astig	mixed astigmatism
OD	right eye (oculus dexter)
OS	left eye (oculus sinister)
OU	both eyes (oculi unitas) each eye (oculus uterque)
REM	rapid eye movement
ST	esotropia
VA	visual acuity
VF	visual field
XT	exotropia
EAR	
ABLB	alternate binaural loudness balance
ABR	auditory brain stem response
AC	air conduction
AD	right ear (auris dextra)
AS	left ear (auris sinistra)
PTS	permanent threshold shift
TTS	temporary threshold shift

Case Study

Operative Report

Preoperative Diagnosis. Foreign body, ears

Postoperative Diagnosis. Foreign body, ears

Procedure. Removal of foreign bodies from ears with placement of paper patches

Anesthesia. General

Operative Indications. The patient is a 9-year-old girl who presents with bilateral retained **tympanostomy** tubes. The tubes had been placed for more than 2.5 years.

The risks and alternatives were explained to the mother, and she agreed to the surgery.

Operative Findings. Retained tympanostomy tubes, bilateral

Operative Description. In the **supine** position under satisfactory general anesthesia via mask, the patient was draped in a routine fashion.

The operating microscope was used to inspect the right ear. A previously placed tympanostomy tube was found to be in position and was surrounded with hard **cerumen.** The cerumen and the tube were removed, resulting in a very large **perforation.** The edges of the perforation were freshened sharply with a pick, and a paper patch was applied.

Worksheet 5 provides a dictionary and reading application and an analysis of this case study.

Worksheet 1

Use ophthalm/o (eye) to build a medical word meaning:

1. paralysis of the eye _____

2. instrument to examine the eye _____

3. study of the eye _____

Use pupill/o (pupil) to build a medical word meaning:

4. examination of the pupil _____

5. instrument to measure the pupil _____

Use kerat/o (cornea) to build a medical word meaning:

6. instrument to incise the cornea _____

7. instrument for measuring the cornea _____

Use scler/o (sclera) to build a medical word meaning:

8. inflammation of the sclera _____

9. softening of the sclera _____

Use irid/o (iris) to build a medical word meaning:

10. paralysis of the iris _____

11. herniation of the iris _____

12. softening of the iris _____

Use retin/o (retina) to build a medical word meaning:

13. disease of the retina _____

14. inflammation of the retina _____

Use blephar/o (eyelid) to build a medical word meaning:

15. paralysis of the eyelid _____

16. inflammation of the eyelid and the conjunctiva _____

17. tumor of the gland of the eyelid _____

Use the suffix -opia (vision) to build a medical word meaning:

18. excessive (farsighted) vision _____

19. dim or dull vision _____

Use ot/o (ear) to build a medical word meaning:

20. pain in the ear _____

21. discharge from the ear _____

22. flow of pus from the ear _____

Use audi/o (hearing) to build a medical word meaning:

23. instrument for measuring hearing _____

24. study of hearing _____

Use myring/o (eardrum) to build a medical word meaning:

25. instrument for cutting the eardrum _____

Worksheet 2

Build a surgical term meaning:

1. removal of the stapes _____

2. incision of the labyrinth _____

3. removal of the mastoid process _____

4. surgical repair of the eardrum _____

5. puncture of the eardrum _____

6. incision of the cornea _____

7. surgical repair of an ear (deformity) _____

8. suture of the eyelid _____

Worksheet 3

Match the following words with the definitions in the numbered list.

achromatopsia   metamorphopsia
anacusis   nyctalopia
aphakia   nystagmus
exophthalmos   otitis externa
hordeolum   spina bifida
labyrinthitis   visual field

1. _____ inflammatory swelling of one of the sebaceous glands of the eyelid

2. _____ inflammation of the inner ear; may cause progressive vertigo

3. _____ infection of the external auditory canal

4. _____ area within which objects may be seen when the eye is fixed

5. _____ deficiency in color perception; color blind

6. _____ deafness

7. _____ distortion of shapes

8. _____ night blindness

9. _____ protrusion of one or both eyes

10. _____ involuntary eye movement that appears jerky

Worksheet 4

SPECIAL PROCEDURES, PHARMACOLOGY, AND ABBREVIATIONS

Match the following words with the definitions in the numbered list.

AD
AS
audiometry
cyclodialysis
cycloplegics
electronystagmography
enucleation
evisceration

mastoid antrotomy
miotics
mydriatics
OD
OS
otoplasty
otoscopy
phacoemulsification
retinoscopy

1. _____ medications that dilate pupils

2. _____ formation of an opening in the anterior chamber for draining of aqueous humor

3. _____ surgical opening of a cavity within the mastoid process

4. _____ examination to evaluate refractive errors of the eye by projecting a beam of light into the eye

5. _____ right ear

6. _____ right eye

7. _____ measurement of the acuity of hearing for various sound waves frequencies

8. _____ method of recording nystagmus activity by detecting the electrical activity of the extraocular muscles

9. _____ method of treating cataracts by using ultrasonic waves to disintegrate the cataract, which is then aspirated and removed

10. _____ drugs that constrict the pupils

11. _____ visual examination of the external auditory canal and tympanic membrane

12. _____ removal of the eyeball

13. _____ removal of the contents of the eye while leaving the sclera and cornea intact

14. _____ paralyzes the ciliary muscles thereby dilating the pupils; used to facilitate certain eye examinations

15. _____ corrective surgery for a deformed pinna

Worksheet 5

OPERATIVE REPORT DICTIONARY EXERCISE

Use a medical dictionary or other resource to define the following terms and determine their pronunciation; then practice reading the case study aloud (p. 358).

cerumen _____

perforation _____

supine _____

tympanostomy _____

ANALYSIS OF OPERATIVE REPORT

1. Did the patient's surgery involve one or both ears?

2. What was the nature of the foreign body in the patient's ears?

3. What ear structure was involved?

4. What type of anesthetic was administered?

5. In what position was the face during surgery?

6. What instrument was used to locate the tubes?

7. What was the material in which the tubes were imbedded?

8. What injury was caused by the tubes?

Worksheet 6

Label the following diagram. To check your answers, refer to Figure 16–1.

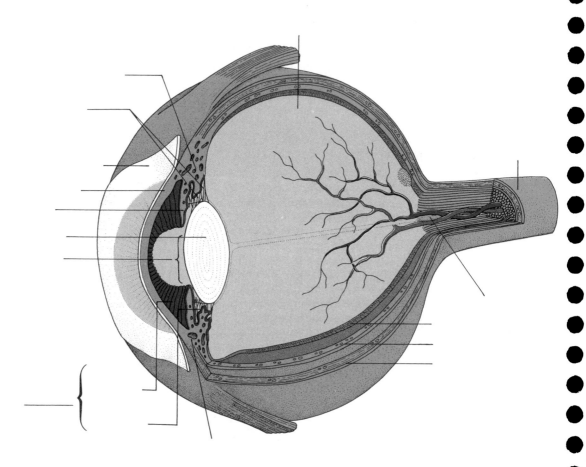

Suspensory ligaments	Pupil	Vitreous humor
Ciliary body (muscles)	Anterior chamber	Optic nerve
Lens		Choroid
	Posterior chamber	Sclera
Cornea		
	Aqueous humor	Optic disc
Conjunctiva		Retina
Iris	Canal of Schlemm	

Worksheet 7

Label the following diagram. To check your answers, refer to Figure 16–2.

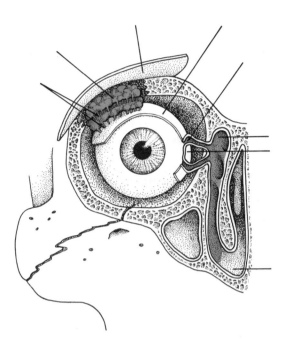

Eyelid

Lacrimal glands

Lacrimal ducts

Conjunctiva

Lacrimal canaliculus

Lacrimal sac

Canthus

Nasolacrimal
duct

Worksheet 8

Label the following diagram. To check your answers, refer to Figure 16–3.

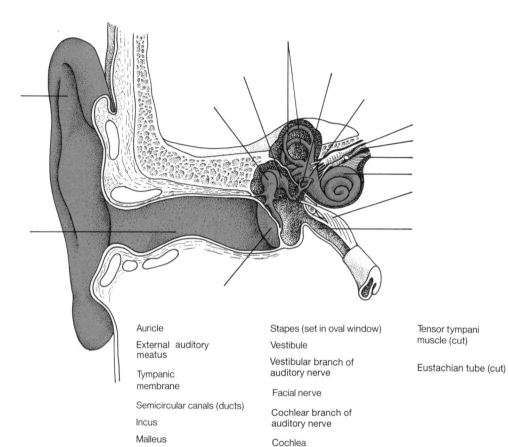

Auricle

External auditory
meatus

Tympanic
membrane

Semicircular canals (ducts)

Incus

Malleus

Stapes (set in oval window)

Vestibule

Vestibular branch of
auditory nerve

Facial nerve

Cochlear branch of
auditory nerve

Cochlea

Tensor tympani
muscle (cut)

Eustachian tube (cut)

Appendix A

Answer Key

WORKSHEET 1

1. root, combining form, suffix, prefix
2. teach
3. False. A combining vowel is usually an "o."
4. True
5. True
6. False. A combining vowel is used before a suffix that begins a consonant.
7. False. To define a medical word, first define the suffix or end of the word. Second, define the prefix or first part of the word. Last, define the middle of the word.

WORKSHEET 2

1. rhin/o
2. splen/o
3. hyster/o
4. enter/o
5. neur/o
6. ot/o
7. dermat/o
8. hydr/o
9. hepat/o
10. toxic/o

WORKSHEET 3

1. nephritis
2. arthrodesis
3. phlebotomy
4. dentist
5. gastrectomy
6. lumpectomy
7. hepatoma
8. cardi/o/logist
9. gastr/ia
10. therm/o/meter

WORKSHEET 4

3. cardi/o
4. oste/o
5. gastr/o
6. nephr/o
9. erythr/o
10. dent/o

WORKSHEET 5

1. mast/o
2. hepat/o
3. arthr/o
4. cyst/o
5. phleb/o
6. thorac/o
7. abdomin/o
8. trache/o
9. leuk/o
10. gastr/o

Chapter 2   *Suffixes: Surgical, Diagnostic, Symptomatic, and Related*

WORKSHEET 1

1. episiotomy
2. colectomy
3. arthrocentesis
4. splenectomy
5. colostomy
6. dermatome
7. tympanotomy
8. tracheostomy
9. mastectomy
10. lithotomy
11. hemorrhoidectomy
12. colostomy
13. colectomy
14. dermatome
15. arthrocentesis
16. lithotomy
17. mastectomy
18. tympanotomy
19. tracheostomy
20. splenectomy

WORKSHEET 2

1. arthrodesis
2. rhinoplasty
3. tenoplasty
4. myorrhaphy
5. mastopexy
6. cystorrhaphy
7. osteoclasis
8. lithotripsy
9. enterolysis
10. neurotripsy
11. rhinoplasty
12. arthrodesis
13. myorrhaphy
14. mastopexy
15. cystorrhaphy
16. tenoplasty
17. osteoclasis
18. lithotripsy
19. enterolysis
20. neurotripsy

WORKSHEET 3

1. bronchiectasis
2. gastrodynia
3. nephrosis

4. cholelith
5. carcinogen
6. psychology
7. osteomalacia
8. hepatomegaly
9. cholelithiasis
10. thermometer
11. hepatocele
12. lipoid
13. neuropathy
14. dermatosis
15. hemiplegia
16. proctoscopy
17. dysphagia
18. aphasia
19. cephalalgia
20. blepharospasm
21. angiorrhexis
22. hemopoiesis
23. hysteroptosis
24. hemiparesis
25. hyperplasia, hypertrophy

WORKSHEET 4

1. lithotripsy
2. arthrocentesis
3. splenectomy
4. colostomy
5. dermatome
6. tracheostomy
7. lithotomy
8. mastectomy
9. hemorrhoidectomy
10. tracheotomy
11. mastopexy
12. colectomy
13. gastrorrhaphy
14. hysteropexy
15. rhinoplasty
16. arthrodesis
17. osteoclasis
18. neurolysis
19. myorrhaphy
20. tympanotomy

WORKSHEET 5

1. bronchiectasis
2. neuralgia, neurodynia
3. gastritis

4. cephalodynia
5. hepatoma
6. carcinogenesis
7. dermatosis
8. lipoid
9. nephromegaly
10. pylorostenosis
11. otorrhea
12. hemopoiesis
13. hysterorrhexis
14. blepharospasm

15. cystocele
16. hemorrhage
17. lithiasis
18. hemiplegia
19. myopathy
20. dysphagia
21. osteomalacia
22. aphasia
23. leukemia
24. erythropenia
25. pelvimetry

Chapter 3 Suffixes: Adjective, Noun, Diminutive, Singular, Plural

WORKSHEET 1

1. thoracic
2. gastric, gastral
3. bacterial
4. aquatic
5. axillary
6. cardiac, cardial
7. spinal, spinous
8. membranous

WORKSHEET 2

1. internist
2. pneumonia
3. sigmoidoscopy
4. alcoholism
5. allergist
6. senilism
7. mania
8. orthopedist

WORKSHEET 3

Plural	Rule
1. diagnoses	Drop is and add es.
2. fornices	Drop ix and add ices.
3. bursae	Retain a and add e.
4. vertebrae	Retain a and add e.
5. keratoses	Drop is and add es.
6. bronchi	Drop us and add i.
7. spermatozoa	Drop on and add a.
8. septa	Drop um and add a.
9. cocci	Drop us and add i.
10. apices	Drop ex and add ices.
11. ganglia	Drop on and add a.
12. prognoses	Drop is and add es.
13. thrombi	Drop us and add i.
14. appendices	Drop ix and add ices.
15. bacteria	Drop um and add a.
16. radii	Drop us and add i.
17. testes	Drop is and add es.
18. nevi	Drop us and add i.

Chapter 4 Prefixes

WORKSHEET 1

Word	Definition of Prefix
1. inter/dental	between
2. hypo/dermic	under, below
3. epi/gastrium	above, upon
4. retro/active	backward, behind
5. sub/nasal	under, below
6. medi/al	middle
7. infra/patellar	under, below
8. post/natal	after, behind

Word	Definition of Prefix
9. quadri/plegia	four
10. hyper/lipidemia	excessive, above normal
11. primi/para	first
12. micro/cephaly	small
13. tri/ceps	three
14. poly/dipsia	many, much
15. im/potent	not
16. an/aerobic	without, not
17. macro/cephaly	large

Word	Definition of Prefix
18. intra/muscular	in, within
19. supra/renal	above, excessive
20. dia/rrhea	through, across
21. circum/renal	around
22. ad/hesion	toward
23. peri/renal	around
24. brady/cardia	slow
25. tachy/pnea	rapid, fast
26. dys/pnea	bad, painful, difficult
27. eu/pnea	good, normal
28. hetero/graft	different
29. mal/function	bad
30. peri/osteum	around

WORKSHEET 2

1. retroperitoneal
2. hypodermic
3. preoperative
4. subnasal
5. postoperative
6. intercostal
7. medial
8. periosteum

9. diarrhea
10. ectoderm
11. suprarenal
12. hemiplegia
13. monocyte
14. quadriplegia
15. macrocephaly
16. microscope
17. polyphobia
18. primigravida

WORKSHEET 3

1. dyspepsia
2. heterosexual
3. pseudomembranous
4. antibacterial
5. bradycardia
6. malnutrition
7. amastia
8. anesthesia
9. eupnea
10. synarthrosis
11. tachycardia
12. contraception
13. homosexual

Chapter 5 **Body Structure**

WORKSHEET 1

1. hist/o
2. -gram
3. ultra-
4. ventr/o
5. home/o
6. -cyte
7. infra-
8. -graphy
9. peri-
10. later/o

WORKSHEET 2

1. lateral
2. medial
3. distal
4. proximal
5. supine
6. prone
7. adduction
8. abduction
9. superior

10. inferior
11. anterior
12. posterior
13. inversion
14. eversion

WORKSHEET 3

1. etiology
2. radiologist
3. pathologist
4. morbid
5. pathogenesis
6. sign
7. symptom
8. prognosis
9. diagnosis
10. homeostasis
11. radiopaque material
12. tomography
13. magnetic resonance imaging
14. ultrasonography
15. x-ray

WORKSHEET 4

1. to determine cervical curvature
2. No, there was no evidence of recent body disease or injury
3. the first cervical vertebra (atlas) and the second cervical vertebra (axis)
4. No, it was intact
5. a muscle spasm

Chapter 6 **Integumentary System**

WORKSHEET 1

1. mastodynia, mastalgia
2. mastitis
3. mastopathy
4. amastia
5. mammogram
6. mammary
7. adipoma, lipoma
8. adipocele, lipocele
9. adipoid, lipoid
10. lipocyte, adipocyte
11. dermatitis
12. dermatologist
13. onychitis
14. onychoma
15. onychopathy
16. onychomycosis
17. onychomalacia
18. onychocryptosis
19. trichopathy
20. trichomycosis

WORKSHEET 2

1. mastectomy, mammectomy
2. mammoplasty, mastoplasty
3. adipectomy, lipectomy
4. onychectomy
5. onychotomy
6. dermatoplasty, dermoplasty

WORKSHEET 3

1. pediculosis
2. vitiligo
3. tinea
4. scabies
5. impetigo
6. urticaria
7. chloasma
8. ecchymosis
9. petechiae
10. alopecia

WORKSHEET 4

1. antipruritics
2. antiseptics, antibacterials
3. astringents
4. dermabrasion
5. parasiticides
6. keratolytics
7. Bx
8. Schick test
9. protectives
10. ung.

WORKSHEET 5

1. stratum germinativum
2. papillary dermis
3. nodular and infiltrating basal cell carcinoma near the elbow
4. Bowen's disease

Chapter 7 **Gastrointestinal System**

WORKSHEET 1

1. esophagodynia, esophagalgia
2. esophagospasm
3. esophagostenosis
4. gastritis
5. gastrodynia, gastralgia
6. gastropathy
7. gastromegaly, megalogastria
8. duodenal
9. ileitis
10. jejunoileal, jejunoiliac
11. enteritis
12. enteropathy
13. colitis

14. coloscopy
15. coloenteritis, enterocolitis
16. coloptosis
17. colopathy
18. proctostenosis, rectostenosis
19. rectocele, proctocele
20. proctoplegia; proctoparalysis
21. cholecystitis
22. cholelithiasis
23. hepatoma
24. hepatomegaly
25. pancreatitis

WORKSHEET 2

1. gingivectomy
2. glossectomy
3. esophagoplasty
4. gastrectomy
5. gastrojejunostomy
6. esophagectomy
7. gastroenterocolostomy
8. enteroplasty
9. enteropexy
10. choledochorrhaphy
11. colostomy
12. hepatopexy
13. proctoplasty, rectoplasty
14. cholecystectomy
15. choledochoplasty

WORKSHEET 3

1. hematemesis
2. dysphagia
3. fecalith
4. halitosis
5. anorexia

6. dyspepsia
7. melena
8. cirrhosis
9. obstipation
10. bulimia

WORKSHEET 4

1. pc, pp
2. occult blood
3. emetics
4. bid
5. choledochoplasty
6. lower GI
7. gastroscopy
8. stomatoplasty
9. cathartics
10. anastomosis
11. oral cholecystography
12. spleen scan
13. antiflatulants
14. antacids
15. FBS
16. intravenous cholangiography
17. qid
18. stat
19. proctosigmoidoscopy
20. upper GI

WORKSHEET 5

1. posteriorly and inferiorly
2. yes
3. appendectomy and cholecystectomy
4. continuous deep right-sided pain, which took a crescendo pattern and then a decrescendo pattern. The initial pain was intermittent and sharp

Chapter 8 **Respiratory System**

WORKSHEET 1

1. rhinopathy
2. rhinitis
3. rhinorrhea
4. laryngitis
5. laryngoscopy
6. laryngospasm
7. laryngostenosis
8. laryngotracheal, tracheolaryngeal
9. laryngopathy
10. bronchoscope

11. bronchitis
12. bronchiectasis
13. bronchiospasm, bronchospasm
14. bronchopathy
15. pneumonitis, pneumonia
16. pneumonography
17. thoracic
18. thoracomyodynia, thoracomyalgia
19. dyspnea
20. orthopena
21. apnea

22. eupnea
23. bradypnea
24. pneumothorax
25. hemothorax

WORKSHEET 2

1. laryngostomy
2. pneumonocentesis, pneumocentesis
3. lobectomy
4. rhinoplasty
5. thoracocentesis, thoracentesis
6. laryngorrhaphy
7. pneumonopexy, pneumopexy
8. bronchoplasty
9. tracheostomy
10. pleurectomy

WORKSHEET 3

1. sputum
2. rales/crackles
3. compliance
4. mucus
5. pulmonary edema
6. Cheyne-Stokes respiration
7. anosmia
8. anoxemia
9. stridor
10. coryza

WORKSHEET 4

1. pulmonary function studies
2. bronchography

3. tomography
4. throat culture
5. AP
6. COPD
7. antitussives
8. antihistamines
9. mucolytics
10. arterial blood gases
11. thoracentesis
12. sweat test
13. sputum culture
14. CXR
15. FEV

WORKSHEET 5

Analysis of Respiratory Evaluation

1. shortness of breath
2. difficult breathing, high blood pressure, chronic obstructive pulmonary disease, and peripheral vascular disease
3. bilateral wheezes and rhonchi heard anteriorly and posteriorly
4. interstitial vascular congestion, superimposed inflammatory change, possibly some pleural reactive change
5. acute exacerbation of chronic obstructive pulmonary disease; congestive heart failure; hypertension; peripheral vascular disease
6. congestive heart failure
7. CHF

Chapter 9   **Cardiovascular System**

WORKSHEET 1

1. atheroma
2. atherosclerosis
3. phlebitis
4. phlebosclerosis
5. phlebothrombosis
6. venosclerosis
7. venospasm
8. venous
9. venostenosis
10. cardiomegaly, megalocardia
11. endocarditis
12. epicarditis
13. cardiopulmonary

14. cardiovascular
15. myocarditis
16. cardiomyopathy, myocardiopathy
17. arteriosclerosis
18. arteriospasm
19. arteriorrhexis
20. arterial

WORKSHEET 2

1. cardiotomy
2. cardiocentesis
3. phlebopexy, venopexy
4. arteriorrhaphy
5. pericardiectomy

6. phlebotomy, venotomy
7. arterioplasty
8. angioplasty
9. embolectomy
10. venorrhaphy, phleborrhaphy

WORKSHEET 3

1. coarctation
2. extravascular
3. hypertension
4. Adams-Stokes syndrome
5. patent
6. thrombus
7. ischemia
8. fibrillations
9. hyperlipidemia
10. aneurysm

WORKSHEET 4

1. echocardiography
2. electrocardiography (ECG, EKG)

3. pericardiocentesis
4. MS
5. antianginals
6. inotropics, cardiotonics
7. cardiac enzyme studies
8. phlebography, venography
9. beta blockers
10. treadmill stress test
11. phonocardiography
12. MI
13. ligation and stripping
14. arterial anastomosis
15. arterial biopsy

WORKSHEET 5

1. approximately 2 hours
2. yes
3. SGOT, CPK, and LDH
4. streptokinase and heparin
5. the front side of the heart
6. no; in the earlier admission, the damage was to the lower part of the heart.

Chapter 10 **Blood and Lymphatic Systems**

WORKSHEET 1

1. erythrocytosis
2. leukocytosis
3. granulocytosis
4. thrombocytosis
5. lymphocytosis
6. reticulocytosis
7. erythrocytopenia, erythropenia
8. leukocytopenia, leukopenia
9. thrombocytopenia, thrombopenia
10. granulocytopenia, granulopenia
11. lymphocytopenia
12. hematopoiesis, hemopoiesis
13. erythropoiesis, erythrocytopoiesis
14. leukopoiesis, leukocytopoiesis
15. lymphopoiesis, lymphocytopoiesis
16. immunologist
17. immunology
18. splenocele
19. splenitis

WORKSHEET 2

1. splenectomy
2. splenotomy
3. thymectomy
4. thymolysis
5. splenolaparotomy, laparosplenotomy
6. splenopexy

WORKSHEET 3

1. serology
2. antigen
3. hemolysis
4. hemostasis
5. anisocytosis
6. antibody
7. lymphosarcoma
8. dyscrasia
9. coagulopathy
10. edema

WORKSHEET 4

1. hemostatics
2. hemoglobin
3. erythrocyte sedimentation rate
4. hematocrit
5. Ig
6. PMN
7. coagulation time
8. Monospot
9. bleeding time
10. complete blood count, CBC
11. fibrinolytics
12. anticoagulants
13. prothrombin time
14. EBV
15. splenography

WORKSHEET 5

1. Cobe Spectra
2. blood pressure, which fell to 90 systolic
3. approximately 12 cups
4. minus 253 mL
5. All were within the reference range, except platelets, which were low.
6. 1 hour and 50 minutes

Chapter 11 **Musculoskeletal System**

WORKSHEET 1

1. osteocytes
2. ostealgia, osteodynia
3. osteoarthropathy
4. osteogenesis
5. cervical
6. cervicobrachial
7. cervicofacial
8. myelocele
9. myelosarcoma
10. myelomalacia
11. myeloblastoma
12. suprasternal
13. sternoid
14. chondroblast
15. arthritis
16. osteoarthritis
17. pelvimeter
18. myoma
19. myosclerosis
20. myorrhexis

WORKSHEET 2

1. phalangectomy
2. thoracotomy
3. vertebrectomy
4. arthrodesis
5. osteoplasty
6. myoplasty
7. laminectomy

WORKSHEET 3

1. subluxation
2. rickets
3. spondylolisthesis
4. claudication
5. muscular dystrophy
6. talipes
7. sequestrum
8. myasthenia gravis
9. prosthesis

WORKSHEET 4

1. myelography
2. open reduction
3. chrysotherapy
4. corticosteroids
5. laminectomy
6. arthrography
7. arthrodesis
8. amputation
9. HNP

WORKSHEET 5

1. AP
2. the fracture caused damage to surrounding tissue
3. to determine if the elbow was fractured
4. the distal shafts of the radius and ulna
5. a single view of the left elbow was obtained in the lateral projection

Chapter 12 **Genitourinary System**

WORKSHEET 1

1. nephrolith
2. nephrologist
3. nephropyosis
4. hydronephrosis, nephrohydrosis
5. pyelectasis, pyelectasia
6. pyelopathy
7. ureterectasis, ureterectasia
8. ureterolith
9. ureteromegaly
10. cystitis
11. cystoscope
12. vesicocele
13. vesicoprostatic
14. urethrostenosis
15. urethrotome
16. urography
17. uropathy
18. hematuria
19. dysuria
20. oliguria
21. orchiopathy
22. orchialgia, orchiodynia, orchidalgia
23. vesiculopathy
24. prostatorrhea
25. balanorrhea

WORKSHEET 2

1. vasectomy
2. urethrorrhaphy
3. ureteropyeloplasty
4. nephroureterectomy, ureteronephrectomy
5. cystolithectomy
6. cystoplasty
7. nephrocystanastomosis
8. prostatectomy
9. prostatolithotomy
10. orchidectomy, orchiectomy

WORKSHEET 3

1. incontinence
2. oliguria
3. epispadias
4. impotence
5. varicocele
6. hypospadias
7. urolithiasis
8. frequency
9. aspermia
10. urgency

WORKSHEET 4

1. intravenous pyelogram (IVP)
2. urinalysis (UA)
3. blood urea nitrogen (BUN)
4. uricosuric agents
5. gonadotropins
6. pH
7. circumcision
8. diuretics
9. spermicidal preparations
10. semen analysis
11. retrograde pyelogram (RP)
12. nephrotomography
13. estrogenic hormones
14. urethroscopy
15. cystography

WORKSHEET 5

1. to examine the bladder
2. number 26 French Van Buren
3. to dilate the urethra
4. longitudinally
5. no, because there was minimal bleeding

Chapter 13 **Female Reproductive System**

WORKSHEET 1

1. gynecopathy
2. gynecology
3. gynecologist
4. cervicovaginitis
5. cervicovesical
6. colposcope
7. colposcopy
8. vaginitis
9. vaginal
10. vaginomycosis

11. vaginolabial
12. hysteromyoma
13. hysteropathy
14. hysterosalpingography
15. metrorrhagia
16. parametritis
17. uterocele
18. uterocervical
19. uterorectal
20. uterovesical
21. oophoritis
22. oophoralgia, oophorodynia
23. oophorosalpingitis
24. salpingocele
25. salpingography

WORKSHEET 2

1. oophoropexy
2. oophorrhaphy
3. colpoplasty, vaginoplasty
4. hystero-oophorectomy
5. colpoperineoplasty, vaginoperineoplasty
6. episiorrhaphy, perineorrhaphy
7. hysterosalpingo-oophorectomy
8. amniocentesis

WORKSHEET 3

1. pyosalpinx
2. primipara
3. gestation
4. LMP

5. hydrocephalus
6. corpus luteum
7. dystocia
8. atresia
9. Down's syndrome
10. pruritus vulvae

WORKSHEET 4

1. Pap smear
2. hysterosalpingography
3. amniocentesis
4. cryosurgery
5. colpocleisis
6. D&C
7. total abdominal hysterectomy (TAH)
8. tubal ligation
9. CPD
10. laparoscopy
11. spermicidals
12. ultrasonography
13. chorionic villus sampling
14. estrogens
15. oxytocin

WORKSHEET 5

1. a brownish discharge
2. severe itching and pain
3. yes
4. the ulcer-like lesion on the right
5. probably from the cold sore when having oral-genital sex

Chapter 14   **Endocrine System**

WORKSHEET 1

1. hyperglycemia
2. hypoglycemia
3. glycogenesis
4. pancreatitis
5. pancreatolysis
6. pancreatopathy
7. thyroiditis
8. thyromegaly

WORKSHEET 2

1. thyroidectomy
2. thyrochondrotomy
3. parathyroidectomy

4. adrenalectomy
5. bilateral adrenalectomy

WORKSHEET 3

1. virile
2. myxedema
3. diuresis
4. hirsutism
5. cretinism
6. insulin
7. Addison's disease
8. exophthalmic goiter
9. hyperkalemia
10. pheochromocytoma

WORKSHEET 4

1. FBS
2. RAIU
3. corticosteroids
4. vasopressin
5. thyroid echogram
6. T_4
7. insulin
8. serum glucose test
9. antihyperlipidemics
10. RAI
11. T_3

WORKSHEET 5

1. The four parathyroid glands are located bilaterally on the thyroid gland
2. four
3. a benign tumor of a gland
4. endocrine, circulatory
5. physician who specializes in treating diseases of the endocrine system
6. excessive amount of calcium in the urine
7. approximately 1.5 packs per day

Chapter 15 **Nervous System**

WORKSHEET 1

1. encephalopathy
2. encephalocele
3. cerebrospinal
4. cerebrosclerosis
5. cerebropathy
6. craniocele
7. craniomalacia
8. craniosclerosis
9. craniometer
10. neuroblast
11. neuralgia, neurodynia
12. neurologist
13. myelography, myelogram
14. myelocele
15. myeloplegia, myeloparalysis
16. meningocele
17. meningomyelocele
18. hemiplegia
19. quadriplegia
20. narcolepsy
21. analgesia
22. dysphasia
23. aphasia
24. hypertrophy
25. atrophy

WORKSHEET 2

1. neurolysis
2. craniotomy
3. cranioplasty
4. neurorrhaphy
5. encephalotomy
6. thalamotomy

WORKSHEET 3

1. concussion
2. coma
3. Huntington's chorea
4. aura
5. paraplegia
6. sciatica
7. transient ischemic attack
8. Reye's syndrome
9. lethargy
10. asthenia

WORKSHEET 4

1. cerebral angiography
2. cryosurgery
3. trephination
4. cisternal puncture
5. electromyogram
6. analgesic
7. tranquilizer
8. laminectomy
9. pneumoencephalograph
10. syncope
11. computed tomography (CT)
12. echoencephalography
13. cordotomy
14. myelography
15. SAH

WORKSHEET 5

1. occipital, the back part of the head
2. CT scan: blood in the cisterna subarachnoidalis and mild acute

hydrocephalus; cerebroangiogram: no aneurysm
3. there is no inflammation in meningismus
4. it confirmed another subarachnoid hemorrhage

5. MRI and angiogram
6. an attempt to exhale forcibly with the glottis, nose, and mouth closed

Chapter 16   **Special Senses**

WORKSHEET 1

1. ophthalmoplegia
2. ophthalmoscope
3. opthalmology
4. pupilloscopy
5. pupillometer
6. keratome, keratatome
7. keratometer
8. scleritis
9. scleromalacia
10. iridoplegia, iridoparalysis
11. iridocele
12. iridomalacia
13. retinopathy
14. retinitis
15. blepharoplegia
16. blepharoconjunctivitis
17. blepharoadenoma
18. hyperopia
19. amblyopia
20. otalgia, otodynia
21. otorrhea
22. otopyorrhea
23. audiometer
24. audiology
25. myringotome

WORKSHEET 2

1. stapedectomy
2. labyrinthotomy
3. mastoidectomy
4. myringoplasty, tympanoplasty
5. tympanocentesis, myringocentesis
6. corneotomy, keratotomy
7. otoplasty
8. blepharorrhaphy

WORKSHEET 3

1. hordeolum
2. labyrinthitis

3. otitis externa
4. visual field
5. achromatopsia
6. anacusis
7. metamorphopsia
8. nyctalopia
9. exophthalmos
10. nystagmus

WORKSHEET 4

1. mydriatic
2. cyclodialysis
3. mastoid antrotomy
4. retinoscopy
5. AD
6. OD
7. audiometry
8. electronystagmography
9. phacoemulsification
10. miotics
11. otoscopy
12. enucleation
13. evisceration
14. cycloplegics
15. otoplasty

WORKSHEET 5

1. both ears
2. tympanostomy tubes inserted 2.5 years ago
3. eardrum
4. general anesthetic
5. the face was upward
6. operating microscope
7. cerumen, earwax
8. perforation of the eardrums

Appendix B

Abbreviations

The use of medical and scientific abbreviations is timesaving and often a standard practice in the health care industry. Note the use of capital and lower case letters.

Abbreviation

AB, ab	abortion
ABC	aspiration biopsy cytology
ABGs	arterial blood gases
ABLB	alternate binaural loudness balance
ABR	auditory brain stem response
ac	before meals (ante cibum)
AC	air conduction; anticoagulant
acc	accommodation
ACG	angiocardiography
ACS	American Cancer Society
ACTH	adrenocorticotropic hormone
AD	right ear (auris dextra)
ad lib	as desired
adeno-CA	adenocarcinoma
ADH	antidiuretic hormone; vasopressin
AE	above the elbow
AFB	acid-fast bacillus (TB organism)
AFP	alpha-fetoprotein
AG	albumin/globulin ratio
AGN	acute glomerulonephritis
AHF	antihemophilic factor VIII
AHG	antihemophilic globulin factor VIII
AI	artificial insemination
AIDS	acquired immunodeficiency syndrome
AK	above the knee
AKA	above-knee amputation
ALL	acute lymphocytic leukemia
AMA	American Medical Association
AMI	acute myocardial infarction
AML	acute myelogenous leukemia
ANS	autonomic nervous system
A&P	auscultation and percussion
AP	anteroposterior
APP	activated partial thromboplastin time

ARDS	adult respiratory distress syndrome
AS	aortic stenosis; left ear (auris sinistra)
ASD	atrial septal defect
ASHD	arteriosclerotic heart disease
AST	aspartate transaminase
Astigm	astigmatism
ATN	acute tubular necrosis
AV	atrioventricular; arteriovenous
AVMs	arteriovenous malformations
AVR	aortic valve replacement
Ba	barium
BaE	barium enema
baso	basophil
BBB	bundle-branch block
BE	below the elbow
bid	twice a day
BIN, bin	twice a night
BK	below the knee
BKA	below-knee amputation
BM	bowel movement
BMR	basal metabolic rate
BNO	bladder neck obstruction
BP	blood pressure
BPH	benign prostatic hypertrophy; benign prostatic hyperplasia
BT	bleeding time
BUN	blood urea nitrogen
Bx	biopsy
$\bar{c}$	with (cum)
C1, C2, etc	first cervical vertebra, second cervical vertebra, etc
CA	cancer
Ca	calcium
CAD	coronary artery disease
CBC	complete blood count
cc	cubic centimeter
CC	cardiac catheterization; chief complaint
CCU	coronary care unit
CDC	Centers for Disease Control
CDH	congenital dislocation of the hip
CEA	carcinoembryonic antigen
CHD	coronary heart disease
CHF	congestive heart failure
CK	creatine kinase
Cl	chlorine
CLL	chronic lymphocytic leukemia
cm	centimeter
CML	chronic myelogenous leukemia
CNS	central nervous system
CO_2	carbon dioxide
COLD	chronic obstructive lung disease
COPD	chronic obstructive pulmonary disease

CP	cerebral palsy
CPD	cephalopelvic disproportion
CPK	creatine phosphokinase
CPR	cardiopulmonary resuscitation
CPT	carpal tunnel syndrome
CS, C-section	cesarean section
CSF	cerebrospinal fluid
CT scan, CAT scan	computed axial tomography
CV	cardiovascular
CVA	cerebrovascular accident
CVD	cardiovascular disease
CVS	chorionic villus sampling
CWP	childbirth without pain
CXR	chest x-ray
cysto	cystoscopy
/d	per day
D	diopter (lens strength)
D&C	dilation and curettage
D&E	dilation and evacuation
dc	discontinue
DC	discharge
DDS	Doctor of Dental Surgery
decub	decubitus
derm	dermatology
DI	diabetes insipidus; diagnostic imaging
diff	differential count (white blood cells)
DJD	degenerative joint disease
DM	diabetes mellitus
DO	doctor of osteopathy
DOA	dead on arrival
DOB	date of birth
DPT	diphtheria, pertussis, tetanus
DRGs	diagnosis-related groups
DUB	dysfunctional uterine bleeding
DVT	deep vein thrombosis
Dx	diagnosis
EBV	Epstein-Barr virus
ECF	extracellular fluid; extended care facility
ECG, EKG	electrocardiogram
EDC	estimated date of confinement
EEG	electroencephalogram
EENT	eye, ear, nose, and throat
EGD	esophagogastroduodenoscopy
Em	emmetropia
EMG	electromyogram
ENT	ear, nose, and throat
EOM	extraocular movement
eos, eosin	eosinophil
ERCP	endoscopic retrograde cholangiopancreatography

ERT	estrogen replacement therapy
ESL	extracorporeal shock-wave lithotripsy
ESR	erythrocyte sedimentation rate
EST	electroshock therapy
ET	esotropia
F	Fahrenheit
FACP	Fellow, American College of Physicians
FACS	Fellow, American College of Surgeons
FBS	fasting blood sugar
FDA	Food and Drug Administration
FEF	forced expiratory flow
FEKG	fetal electrocardiogram
FEV	forced expiratory volume
FH	family history
FHR	fetal heart rate
FHT	fetal heart tone
FS	frozen section
FSH	follicle-stimulating hormone
FTND	full-term normal delivery
FUO	fever of undetermined origin
FVC	forced vital capacity
Fx	fracture
g	gram
GB	gallbladder
GC	gonorrhea
GCSF	granulocyte colony-stimulating factor
GH	growth hormone
GI	gastrointestinal
GOT	glutamic oxaloacetic transaminase (AST)
GPT	glutamic pyruvic transaminase (ALT)
gr	grain
GTT	glucose tolerance test
gtt	drops (guttae)
GU	genitourinary
gyn	gynecology
h	hour
H	hypodermic; hydrogen
HAV	hepatitis A virus
HBV	hepatitis B virus
HCG	human chorionic gonadotropin
HCl	hydrochloric acid
HCO	bicarbonate
HCT, hct	hematocrit
HD	hip disarticulation; hemodialysis; hearing distance
HDL	high-density lipoprotein
HEENT	head, eyes, ears, nose, and throat
Hg	mercury
HGB, Hgb, Hb	hemoglobin
HIV	human immunodeficiency virus

HMD	hyaline membrane disease
HNP	herniated nucleus pulposus (herniated disk)
HP	hemipelvectomy
hs	at bedtime
HSG	hysterosalpingography
HSV	herpes simplex virus
Hx	history
hypo	hypodermically
IAS	interatrial septum
ICF	intracellular fluid
ICSH	interstitial cell-stimulating hormone
ICU	intensive care unit
ID	intradermal
I&D	incision and drainage
IDDM	insulin-dependent diabetes mellitus
Ig	immunoglobulin
IH	infectious hepatitis
IM	intramuscular
inj	injection
IOP	intraocular pressure
IPPB	intermittent positive-pressure breathing
IQ	intelligence quotient
IRDS	infant respiratory distress syndrome
IS	intercostal space
ITP	idiopathic thrombocytopenia purpura
IUD	intrauterine device
IV	intravenous
IVC	inferior vena cava, intravenous cholangiography
IVF	in vitro fertilization
IVP	intravenous pyelogram
IVS	interventricular septum
K	potassium
KD	knee disarticulation
kg	kilogram
KUB	kidney ureter bladder
L, l	liter
L1, L2, etc.	first, second lumbar vertebra, etc.
LA	left atrium
L&A	light and accommodation
LAT, lat	lateral
LB	large bowel
LD	lactic dehydrogenase
LDL	low-density lipoprotein
LE	lupus erythematosus, lower extremity
LH	luteinizing hormone
LLQ	left lower quadrant
LMP	last menstrual period
LP	lumbar puncture
LPN	Licensed Practical Nurse
LRQ	lower right quadrant
lt, L	left

LUQ	left upper quadrant
LV	left ventricle
lymphs	lymphocytes
MCH	mean corpuscular hemoglobin
MCHC	mean corpuscular hemoglobin concentration
MCV	mean corpuscular volume
MD	medical doctor
mets	metastases
mg	milligram (0.001 gram)
MH	marital history
MI	myocardial infarction; mitral insufficiency
mix astig	mixed astigmatism
mL, ml	milliliter (0.001 liter)
mm	millimeter (0.001 meter; 0.039 inch)
mono	monocyte
MRI	magnetic resonance imaging
MS	mitral stenosis; multiple sclerosis; musculoskeletal
MSH	melanocyte-stimulating hormone
MVP	mitral valve prolapse
myop	myopia
Na	sodium
NB	newborn
NIDDM	non–insulin-dependent diabetes mellitus
NPH	neutral protamine Hagedorn (insulin)
npo	nothing by mouth (nulla per os)
NSAID	nonsteroidal anti-inflammatory drug
O_2	oxygen
OA	osteoarthritis
OB	obstetrics
OB-GYN	obstetrics and gynecology
OCPs	oral contraceptive pills
od	once a day
OD	right eye (oculus dexter); overdose
OHS	open heart surgery
OR	operating room
ortho, ORT	orthopedics; orthopaedics
os	mouth; opening; bone
OS	left eye (oculus sinister)
oto	otology
OU	both eyes (oculi unitas); each eye (oculus uterque)
OV	office visit
oz	ounce
P	pulse
PA	posteroanterior
Pap	Papanicolaou
paren	parenterally
PAT	paroxysmal atrial tachycardia
Path	pathology

PBI	protein-bound iodine
pc	after meals
PCP	*Pneumocystis carinii* pneumonia
PCV	packed cell volume (hematocrit)
PD	peritoneal dialysis
PE	physical examination
PET	positron emission tomography
PGH	pituitary growth hormone
pH	hydrogen ion concentration
PH	past history
PID	pelvic inflammatory disease
PKU	phenylketonuria
PMH	past medical history
PMN	polymorphonuclear neutrophil
PMP	previous menstrual period
PMS	premenstrual syndrome
PND	paroxysmal nocturnal dyspnea
PNS	peripheral nervous system
po, PO	orally; by mouth
poly	polymorphonuclear neutrophil; polymorphonuclear leukocyte
pp	postprandial (after meals)
prn	as required
PT	prothrombin time; physical therapy
PTCA	percutaneous transluminal coronary angiography
PTH	parathyroid hormone
PTS	permanent threshold shift
PTT	partial thromboplastin time
PVC	premature ventricular contraction
q	every
qam	every morning
qd	every day (quaque die)
qh	every hour
q2h	every 2 hours
qid	four times a day
qns	quantity not sufficient
qpm	every night
R, rt	right
RA	right atrium, rheumatoid arthritis
rad	radiation absorbed dose
RAI	radioactive iodine
RBC	red blood cell; red blood cell (count)
RD	respiratory disease
REM	rapid eye movement
RLQ	right lower quadrant
RN	registered nurse
RNA	ribonucleic acid
R/O	rule out
ROM	range of motion
RP	retrograde pyelogram
RT	radiation therapy

RUQ	right upper quadrant
RV	right ventricle
Rx	prescription, treatment, therapy
s̄	without
S1, S2, etc	first, second sacral vertebra, etc
SA	sinoatrial (node)
SAH	subarachnoid hemorrhage
sc	subcutaneous
SD	shoulder disarticulation
seg	polymorphonuclear neutrophil
SH	serum hepatitis
SLE	systemic lupus erythematosus
SNS	somatic nervous system
SOB	shortness of breath
sono	sonogram, sonography
sos	if necessary
sp gr	specific gravity
SR	sedimentation rate
ss	half
st	stage (of a disease)
ST	esotropia
staph	staphylococcus
stat	immediately
STD	sexually transmitted diseases
strep	streptococcus
subcu, subq	subcutaneous
SVC	superior vena cava
SVD	spontaneous vaginal delivery
T	temperature
T1, T2, etc	first thoracic vertebra, second thoracic vertebra, etc
T_3	triiodothyronine
T_4	thyroxine
T&A	tonsillectomy and adenoidectomy
TAH	total abdominal hysterectomy
TB	tuberculosis
THA	total hip arthroplasty
THR	total hip replacement
TIA	transient ischemic attack
tid	three times a day
TKA	total knee arthroplasty
TKR	total knee replacement
TNM	tumor, nodes, metastasis
top	topically
TPN	total parenteral nutrition
TPR	temperature, pulse, and respiration
TPUR	transperineal urethral resection
tr, tinct	tincture
TSH	thyroid-stimulating hormone
TSS	toxic shock syndrome
TTH	thyrotrophic hormone
TTS	temporary threshold shift

TUR, TURP	transurethral resection (for prostatectomy)
Tx	tumor cannot be assessed
U	units
UA	urinalysis
UC	uterine contractions
UGI	upper gastrointestinal
U&L, U/L	upper and lower
ULQ	upper left quadrant
ung	ointment
URI	upper respiratory infection
URQ	upper right quadrant
UTI	urinary tract infection
UV	ultraviolet
VA	visual acuity
VC	vital capacity
VCU, VCUG	voiding cystourethrogram
VD	venereal disease
VF	visual field
VHD	ventricular heart disease
VLDL	very-low-density lipoprotein
VSD	ventricular septal defect
WBC	white blood cell; white blood cell (count)
wt	weight
w/v	weight by volume
$\times$	multiplied by
XP	xeroderma pigmentosa
XT	exotropia
XX	female sex chromosomes
XY	male sex chromosomes

Appendix C

Index of Medical Word Elements

Part I: Medical Word Element to English Term

Medical Word Element	Pronunciation	Meaning	Page Numbers
a-	ăh	without, not	36, 185, 326
ab-	ăb	from, away from	36, 53
-ac	ăk	pertaining to	28
acr/o-	ăk-rō	extremity	300
acromi/o	ă-krō-mē-ō	acromion (projection of scapula)	215
ad-	ăd	toward	36, 53
aden/o	ăd-ē-nō	gland	67, 183
adenoid/o	ăd-ē-noid-ō	adenoid	123
adip/o	ăd-ĭ-pō	fat	67
adren/o	ăd-rē-nō	adrenal glands	300
adrenal/o	ă-drĕn-ăl-ō	adrenal glands	300
-al	ăl	pertaining to	28
albin/o	ăl-bĭn-ō	white	68
albumin/o	al-bū-mĭn-ō	albumin (protein)	244
-algesia	ăl-gē-zē-ah	pain	325
-algia	ăl-jē-ah	pain	10, 12, 325
alveol/o	ăl-vē-ōl-ō	alveolus (pl. alveoli)	124
ambly/o	ăm-blē-ō	dull, dim	348
amni/o	ăm-nē-ō	amnion (amniotic sac)	269
an-	ăn	without, not	36, 326
an/o	ā-nō	anus	94
andr/o	ăn-drō	male	244, 300
angi/o	ăn-jē-ō	vessel	151
aniso-	ăn-ī-sō	unequal, dissimilar	185
ankyl/o	ăng-kĭ-lō	stiffness, bent, crooked	215
ante-	ăn-tē	before, in front	34
anter/o	ăn-tĕr-ō	anterior, front	52
anthrac/o	ăn-thrăh-kō	charcoal (coal dust)	68, 124
anti-	ăn-tĭ	against	37
aort/o	ā-ŏr-tō	aorta	151
append/o	ăp-ĕn-dō	appendix	94

391

Medical Word Element	Pronunciation	Meaning	Page Numbers
appendic/o	ăp-ĕn-dĭk-ō	appendix	94
aque/o	ā-kwē-ō	water	348
-ar	ĕr	pertaining to	28
-arche	ăr-kē	beginning	270
arteri/o	ăr-tē-rē-ō	artery	151
arteriol/o	ăr-tĕr-ĭ-ōl-ō	arteriole	151
arthr/o	ăr-thrō	joint	3, 10, 215
-ary	ĕr-ē	pertaining to	28
atel/o	ăt-ē-lō	incomplete, imperfect	125
ather/o	ăth-ĕr-ō	fatty plaque	151
atri/o	ā-trē-ō	atrium	151
audi/o	aw-dē-ō	hearing	349
bacteri/o	băk-tē-rē-ō	bacteria	244
balan/o	bah-lăn-ō	glans penis	244
bi-	bī	two	35
-blast	blăst	embryonic cell	184
blast/o	blăs-tō	embryonic cell	183, 216
blephar/o	blĕf-ah-rō	eyelid	348
brachi/o	brăk-ē-ō	arm	213
brady-	brăd-ē	slow	37, 125, 326
bronch/o	brŏng-kō	bronchus (pl. bronchi)	124
bronchi/o	brŏng-kē-ō	bronchus (pl. bronchi)	124
bucc/o	bŭk-ō	cheek	93
calc/o	kăl-kō	calcium	300
calcane/o	kăl-kā-nē-ō	calcaneum (heel bone)	214
-capnia	kăp-nē-ah	carbon dioxide (CO_2)	125
cardi/o	kăr-dē-ō	heart	2, 151
carp/o	kăr-pō	carpus, wrist bones	213
-cele	sēl	hernia, swelling	12
-centesis	sĕn-tē-sĭs	puncture	3, 10, 11
cephal/o	sĕf-ăl-ō	head	213
cerebr/o	sĕr-ē-brō	cerebrum	325
cervic/o	sĕr-vĭ-kō	neck, cervix uteri (neck of cervix)	213, 269
cheil/o	kī-lō	lip	94
chlor/o	klŏr-ō	green	69
chol/e	kō-lē	bile, gall	95
cholangi/o	kō-lăn-jē-ō	bile vessel	95
cholecyst/o	kō-lē-sĭs-tō	gallbladder	95
choledoch/o	kō-lĕ-dō-kō	bile duct	96
chondr/o	kŏn-drō	cartilage	216
choroid/o	kō-roid-ō	choroid	348
chrom/o	krōm-ō	color	183
circum-	sĕr-kŭm	around	36
cirrh/o	sĭr-rō	yellow	69
-clasis	klăh-sĭs	break, fracture	12, 216
col/o	kō-lō	colon	95
colon/o	kō-lŏn-ō	colon	10, 95

Medical Word Element	Pronunciation	Meaning	Page Numbers
colp/o	kŏl-pō	vagina	269
condyl/o	kŏn-dĭ-lō	condyle	215
coni/o	kō-nē-ō	dust	124
contra-	kŏn-trah	against	37
core/o	kō-rē-ō	pupil	348
corne/o	kŏr-nē-ō	cornea	348
cost/o	kŏs-tō	ribs	213
crani/o	krā-nē-ō	cranium, skull	213, 325
-crine	krĭn/krīn	secrete	301
crypt/o	krĭp-tō	hidden	67, 244
cutane/o	kū-tā-nē-ō	skin	67
cyan/o	sī-ăn-ō	blue	69
cycl/o	sī-klō	ciliary body	348
cyst/o	sĭs-tō	bladder	243
-cyte	sīt	cell	69
cyt/o	sī-tō	cell	52
dacry/o	dăk-rē-ō	tear, lacrimal sac	348
dactyl/o	dăk-tĭ-lō	digit (finger or toe)	213
dent/o	dĕnt-ō	teeth	94
-derma	dĕr-mă	skin	69
derm/o	dĕr-mō	skin	67
dermat/o	dĕr-măh-tō	skin	67
-desis	dē-sĭs	binding, fixation (of a bone or joint)	12, 216
dia-	dī-ăh	through, across	36, 97
diplo-	dĭp-lō	double, twofold	35
-dipsia	dĭp-sē-ăh	thirst	301
duoden/o	dū-ŏd-ē-nō	duodenum	95
-dynia	dĭn-ē-ăh	pain	12
dys-	dĭs	bad, painful, difficult	37, 97
-eal	ē-ăl	pertaining to	28
ec-	ĕk	out, out from	36
-ectasis	ĕk-tăh-sĭs	dilation, expansion	12
ecto-	ĕk-tō	outside	36
-ectomy	ĕk-tŏ-mē	excision, removal	10, 11
-emesis	ĕm-ĕ-sĭs	vomiting	12, 96
-emia	ē-mē-ăh	blood	13, 184
encephal/o	ĕn-sĕf-ah-lō	brain	11, 325
endo-	ĕn-dō	in, within	36, 152
enter/o	ĕn-tĕr-ō	intestine (usually small intestine)	95
eosin/o	ē-ō-sĭn-ō	dawn (rose colored)	183
epi-	ĕp-ĭ	above, upon	34, 70, 217
epididym/o	ĕp-ĭ-dĭd-ĭ-mō	epididymis	244
episi/o	ē-pĭz-ē-ō	vulva	269
erythem/o	ĕr-ĭ-thē-mō	red	69
erythr/o	ē-rĭth-rō	red	2, 69, 183
eso-	ĕ-sō	inward	350

Medical Word Element	Pronunciation	Meaning	Page Numbers
esophag/o	ē-sŏf-ah-gō	esophagus	94
-esthesia	ĕs-thē-zē-ah	feeling, sensation	325
eu-	ū	good, normal	37, 125
ex-	ĕks	out, out from	36
exo-	ĕks-ō	outside	36, 350
extra-	ĕks-trah	outside	36, 152
femor/o	fĕm-ō-rō	femur (thigh bone)	214
fibul/o	fĭb-ū-lō	fibula (smaller, outer bone of lower leg)	214
galact/o	gă-lăk-tō	milk	269
gastr/o	găs-trō	stomach	2, 3, 11, 94
-gen	jĕn	forming, producing, origin	13, 53
-genesis	jĕn-ĕ-sĭs	forming, producing, origin	13, 53, 245
gingiv/o	jĭn-jĭ-vō	gum(s)	94
gli/o	glī-ō	glue, neuroglia	325
-globin	glō-bĭn	protein	184
glomerul/o	glō-mĕr-ū-lō	glomerulus	243
gloss/o	glŏs-ō	tongue	93
gluc/o	gloo-kō	sugar, sweetness	300
glyc/o	glī-kō	sugar, sweetness	300
-gnosis	nō-sĭs	knowing	53
gonad/o	gō-năd-ō	sex glands	300
-gram	grăm	a writing, record	13, 53, 69, 152
granul/o	grăn-ū-lō	granule	183
-graph	grăf	instrument for recording	13, 53, 69, 152
-graphy	gră-fē	process of recording	13, 53, 69
-gravida	grăv-ĭ-dah	pregnancy	270
gynec/o	jĭn-ē-kō/gĭ-nē-kō	woman, female	269
hem/o	hĕm-o	blood	183
hemangi/o	hē-măn-jē-ō	blood vessel	151
hemat/o	hĕm-ăh-tō	blood	183
hemi-	hĕm-ē	one half	35
hepat/o	hĕp-ăh-tō	liver	96
hetero-	hĕt-ĕr-ō	different	37, 185
hidr/o	hī-drō	sweat	67
hist/o	hĭs-tō	tissue	52
home/o	hō-mē-ō	same	52, 300
homo-	hō-mō	same	37, 185
humer/o	hū-mĕr-ō	humerus	213
hyper-	hī-pĕr	excessive, above normal	3, 35, 70, 97
hypo-	hī-pō	under, below	34, 70
hyster/o	hĭs-tĕr-ō	uterus, womb	270
-ia	ē-ah	condition	3, 28
-iasis	ī-ă-sĭs	abnormal condition (produced by something specified)	13, 96, 245

Medical Word Element	Pronunciation	Meaning	Page Numbers
iatry	ī-ă-trē	treatment, medicine	28
-ic	ĭk	pertaining to	28
-ical	ĭk-ăl	pertaining to	28
ichthy/o	ĭk-thē-ō	dry, scaly	67
-icle	ĭk-ăl	small, minute	29
idi/o	ĭd-ē-ō	unknown, peculiar	52
ile/o	ĭl-ē-ō	ileum	95
ili/o	ĭl-ē-ō	ilium (lateral, flaring portion of hip bone)	214
im-	ĭm	not	36
immun/o	ĭm-ū-nō	safe	183
in-	ĭn	in, not	36
infra-	ĭn-frah	under, below	34, 53
inter-	ĭn-těr	between	34
intra-	ĭn-trah	in, within	36
irid/o	ĭr-ĭ-dō	iris	348
is/o	ī-sō	same	185
ischi/o	ĭs-kē-ō	ischium (lower portion of hip bone)	214
-ism	ĭzm	condition	28
-ist	ĭst	specialist	28
-itis	ī-tĭs	inflammation	10, 11, 13
jaund/o	jawn-dō	yellow	69
jejun/o	jě-joo-nō	jejunum	95
kary/o	kăr-ē-ō	nucleus	183
kerat/o	kěr-ăh-tō	horny tissue, hard, cornea	67, 348
kinesi/o	kĭ-nē-sē-ō	movement	325
labi/o	lā-bē-ō	lip	94, 270
labyrinth/o	lăb-ĭ-rĭn-thō	labyrinth, inner ear	349
lact/o	lăk-tō	milk	68, 269
lamin/o	lăm-ĭ-nō	lamina	215
lapar/o	lăp-ăr-ō	abdomen	270
laryng/o	lăh-rĭng-ō	larynx (voice box)	123
later/o	lăt-ěr-ō	side, to one side	52
leiomy/o	lī-ō-mī-ō	smooth muscle (visceral)	216
-lepsy	lěp-sē	seizure	326
leuc/o	loo-kō	white	68
leuk/o	loo-kō	white	68, 183
lingu/o	lĭng-gwō	tongue	93
lip/o	lĭ-pō	fat	67
-lith	lĭth	stone, calculus	13, 96
lob/o	lō-bō	lobe	124
-logist	lō-jĭst	specialist in the study of	13, 69
-logy	lō-jē	study of	13, 69
lumb/o	lŭm-bō	loins	214
lymph/o	lĭm-fō	lymph	183
-lysis	lī-sĭs	separation, destruction, loosening	12

Medical Word Element	Pronunciation	Meaning	Page Numbers
macro-	măk-rō	large	3, 35, 185
mal-	măl	bad	37
-malacia	măh-lā-shē-ăh	softening	13, 216
mamm/o	mă-mō	breast	68, 270
mast/o	măs-tō	breast	68, 270
medi-	mē-dē	middle	34
medi/o	mē-dē-ō	middle	52
-megaly	mĕg-ăh-lē	enlargement	3, 13, 96
melan/o	mĕl-ăh-nō	black	69
mening/o	mĕ-nĭng-gō	meninges	325
men/o	mĕn-ō	menses, menstruation	270
mes/o	mĕs-ō	middle	34
metacarp/o	mĕt-ăh-kăr-pō	metacarpus (bones of the hand)	213
-meter	mē-tĕr	instrument for measuring	13, 152
metr/o	mĕ-trō	uterus, womb	270
-metry	mĕt-rē	act of measuring	13
micro-	mī-krō	small	3, 35, 185
mono-	mŏn-ō	one	35, 185
morph/o	mŏr-fō	shape	183
multi-	mŭl-tē	many, much	35
my/o	mī-ō	muscle	216
myc/o	mī-kō	fungus	68
myel/o	mī-ē-lō	bone marrow, spinal cord	183, 215
myring/o	mĭ-rĭng-gō	tympanic membrane, eardrum	349
narc/o	năr-kō	stupor, numbing	325
nas/o	nā-zō	nose	123
nat/a	nā-tă	birth	270
nephr/o	nĕf-rō	kidney	2, 243
neur/o	nū-rō	nerve, nervous system	325
noct/o	nŏk-tō	night	244
nucle/o	nū-klē-ō	nucleus	52, 183, 244
ocul/o	ŏk-ū-lō	eye	348
odont/o	ō-dŏn-tō	teeth	94
-oid	oid	resembling	13
-ole	ŏl	small, minute	29
olig/o	ō-lĭ-gō	scanty	244
-oma	ō-măh	tumor	13
onych/o	ŏn-ĭ-kō	nail	68
oophor/o	ō-ŏf-ō-rō	ovary	270
ophthalm/o	ŏf-thăl-mō	eye	348
-opia	ō-pē-ah	vision	349
opt/o	ŏp-tō	eye, vision	348
orch/i	ŏr-kē	testes	244
orchi/o	ŏr-kē-ō	testes	244
orchid/o	ŏr-kĭ-dō	testes	244
or/o	ŏr-ō	mouth	93

Medical Word Element	**Pronunciation**	**Meaning**	**Page Numbers**
orth/o	ŏr-thō	straight	125, 216
-ory	ŏr-ē	pertaining to	28
-osis	ō-sĭs	abnormal condition, increase (used primarily with blood cells)	14, 184
-osmia	ŏz-mē-ah	smell	125
oste/o	ŏs-tē-ō	bone	2, 11, 216
ot/o	ō-tō	ear	349
-ous	ŭs	pertaining to	28
ovari/o	ō-vǎr-ē-ō	ovary	270
ox/o	ŏks-ō	oxygen (O_2)	124
pan-	pǎn	all	37
pancreat/o	pǎn-krē-ǎ-tō	pancreas	96, 300
para-	pǎr-ah	near, along the side of	37
-para	pǎr-ah	to bear (offspring)	14, 270
parathyroid/o	pǎr-ah-thī-roi-dō	parathyroid glands	300
-paresis	pah-rē-sĭs	partial paralysis	14
patell/o	pah-tĕl-ō	patella (kneecap)	215
path/o	pǎth-ō	disease	52
-pathy	pǎh-thē	disease	14, 53
pector/o	pĕk-tō-rō	chest	124
ped/i	pĕd-ē	foot	215
-penia	pē-nē-ǎh	decrease, deficiency	14, 184
-pepsia	pĕp-sē-ǎh	digestion	96
peri-	pĕr-ē	around	36, 53, 97, 152
perine/o	pĕr-ĭ-nē-ō	perineum	270
-pexy	pĕk-sē	fixation (of an organ)	12
phac/o	fā-kō	lens	348
phag/o	fǎg-ō	swallowing, eating	184
-phagia	fā-jē-ah	eating, swallowing	14, 96, 301
phalang/o	fǎl-ǎn-jō	phalanges (bones of fingers and toes)	214
pharyng/o	fǎh-rĭng-gō	pharynx, throat	94, 123
-phasia	fā-zē-ǎh	speech	326
-phil	fĭl	attraction to	184
-philia	fĭl-ē-ǎh	attraction	14
phleb/o	flĕb-ō	vein	10, 151
-phobia	fō-bē-ǎh	fear	14
-phonia	fō-nē-ah	voice	125
-phoresis	fō-rē-sĭs	borne, carried	184
-physis	fī-sĭs	growth	217, 301
pil/o	pī-lō	hair	68
-plasia	plā-zē-ǎh	formation, growth	14
-plasty	plǎs-tē	surgical repair	12, 96, 217
-plegia	plē-jē-ah	paralysis	14
pleur/o	ploo-rō	pleura	124
-pnea	nē-ah	breathing	125
pneum/o	nū-mō	air, gas	124
pneumat/o	nū-mah-tō	air, gas	124

Medical Word Element	Pronunciation	Meaning	Page Numbers
salpinx	săl-pĭnks	fallopian tubes, oviducts, uterine tubes	271
-schisis	skĭ-sĭs	a splitting	217
scler/o	sklĕ-rō	hardening, sclera	68, 349
-scope	skōp	instrument to view or examine	15
-scopy	skō-pē	visual examination	10, 15, 217
semi-	sĕm-ē	one half	35
sial/o	sī-ăh-lō	saliva, salivary gland	96
sider/o	sĭd-ĕr-ō	iron	184
sigmoid/o	sĭg-moi-dō	sigmoid colon	95
somat/o	sō-măt-ō	body	301
-spasm	spăzm	involuntary contraction, twitching	15
spermat/o	spĕr-măh-tō	sperm	244
sphygm/o	sfĭg-mō	pulse	152
spir/o	spī-rō	breathe	124
splen/o	splē-nō	spleen	184
spondyl/o	spŏn-dĭ-lō	vertebrae (backbone)	214
squam/o	skwā-mō	scale	68
staped/o	stā-pē-dō	stapes	349
-stasis	stā-sĭs	standing still	15, 185
steat/o	stē-ă-tō	fat	67
-stenosis	stĕ-nō-sĭs	narrowing, stricture	16
stern/o	stĕr-nō	sternum (breastbone)	214
steth/o	stĕth-ō	chest	124
stomat/o	stō-măh-tō	mouth	93
-stomy	stō-mē	forming an opening (mouth)	11
sub-	sŭb	under, below	34, 70, 97, 217
super-	soo-pĕr	above, excessive	37
supra-	soo-prah	above, excessive	37
sym-	sĭm	union, together, joined	37
syn-	sĭn	union, together, joined	37
tachy-	tăk-ē	rapid	37, 125
ten/o	tĕn-ō	tendon	216
tend/o	tĕnd-ō	tendon	216
tendin/o	tĕn-dĭn-ō	tendon	216
thalam/o	thăl-ăh-mō	thalamus, chamber	325
thel/o	thē-lō	nipple	68
-therapy	thĕr-ăh-pē	treatment	69
therm/o	thĕr-mō	heat	3, 4
thorac/o	thō-rah-kō	chest	3, 10, 124, 214
-thorax	thō-răks	chest	125
thromb/o	thrŏm-bō	blood clot	152, 184
thym/o	thī-mō	thymus	184, 301
thyr/o	thī-rō	thyroid	301
thyroid/o	thī-roi-dō	thyroid	301

Part II: English Term to Medical Word Element

English Term	Medical Word Element	Pronunciation	Page Numbers
abdomen	lapar/o	lăp-ăr-ō	270
abnormal condition	-iasis	ī-ă-sĭs	13, 96, 245
	-osis	ō-sĭs	14, 184
above	epi-	ĕp-ĭ	34, 70, 217
	super-	soo-pĕr	37
	supra-	soo-prăh	37
above normal	hyper-	hī-pĕr	3, 35, 70, 97
acromion	acromi/o	ă-krō-mē-ō	215
across	-dia	dī-ăh	36, 97
	trans-	trănz	36, 53, 152
art of measuring	-metry	mĕt-rē	13
adenoid	adenoid/o	ăd-ē-noid-ō	123
adrenal glands	adren/o	ăd-rē-nō	300
	adrenal/o	ă-drĕn-ăl-ō	300
after	post-	pōst	35
against	anti-	ăn-tĭ	37
	contra-	kŏn-trăh	37
air	pneum/o	nū-mō	124
	pneumat/o	nū-măh-tō	124
albumin (protein)	albumin/o	ăl-bū-mĭn-ō	244
all	pan-	păn	37
alveolus (pl. alveoli)	alveol/o	ăl-vē-ōl-ō	124
amnion (amniotic sac)	amni/o	am-nē-ō	269
anterior	anter/o	ăn-tĕr-ō	52
anus	an/o	ā-nō	94
	proct/o	prŏk-tō	95
appendix	append/o	ăp-ĕn-dō	94
	appendic/o	ăp-ĕn-dĭk-ō	94
aorta	aort/o	ā-ŏr-tō	151
arm	brachi/o	brăk-ē-ō	213
around	circum-	sĕr-kŭm	36
	peri-	pĕr-ē	36, 53, 97, 152
arteriole	arteriol/o	ar-tēr-ĭ-ōl-ō	151
artery	arteri/o	ăr-tē-rē-ō	151
atrium	atri/o	ā-trē-ō	151
attraction to	-phil	fĭl	184
	-philia	fĭl-ē-ăh	14
away from	ab-	ăb	36, 53
back	poster/o	pŏs-tĕr-ō	56
backbone	spondyl/o	spŏn-dĭl-ō	214
	vertebr/o	vĕr-tĕ-brō	214
backward	retro-	rĕt-rō	35
bacteria	bacteri/o	băk-tē-rē-ō	244
bad	dys-	dĭs	37, 97
	mal-	măl	37
bear (offspring), to	-para	păr-ăh	14

English Term	Medical Word Element	Pronunciation	Page Numbers
carpus	carp/o	kăr-pō	213
carried	-phoresis	fō-rē-sĭs	184
cartilage	chondr/o	kŏn-drō	216
cell	-cyte	sīt	69
	cyt/o	sī-tō	52
cerebrum	cerebr/o	sĕr-ē-brō	325
cervix uteri (neck of cervix)	cervic/o	sĕr-vĭ-kō	213, 269
chamber	thalam/o	thăl-ăh-mō	325
charcoal (coal dust)	anthrac/o	ăn-thrăh-kō	68, 124
cheek	bucc/o	bŭk-ō	93
chest	pector/o	pĕk-tō-rō	124
	steth/o	stĕth-ō	124
	thorac/o	thŏr-ăh-kō	3, 10, 124, 214
	-thorax	thō-răks	125
childbirth	-tocia	tō-sē-ăh	271
choroid	choroid/o	kō-roid-ō	348
clot (blood)	thromb/o	thrŏm-bō	152, 184
ciliary body	cycl/o	sī-klō	348
colon	col/o	kō-lō	95
	colon/o	kō-lŏn-ō	10, 95
color	chrom/o	krōm-ō	183
condition	-ia	ē-ah	3, 28
	-iasis	ī-ă-sĭs	13, 96, 245
	-ism	ĭzm	28
	-y	ē	28
condyle	condyl/o	kŏn-dĭ-lō	215
contraction, involuntary	-spasm	spăzm	15
control	-stasis	stā-sĭs	15, 185
cornea	corne/o	kŏr-nē-nō	348
	kerat/o	kĕr-ah-tō	67, 348
cranium	crani/o	krā-nē-ō	213, 325
crooked	ankyl/o	ăng-kĭ-lō	215
crushing	-tripsy	trĭp-sē	12
cut into	-tomy	tō-mē	13
dawn (rose colored)	eosin/o	ē-ō-sĭn-ō	183
decrease	-penia	pē-nē-ăh	14, 184
deficiency	-penia	pē-nē-ăh	14, 184
destruction	-lysis	lī-sĭs	12
development	-trophy	trō-fē	15, 301
different	hetero-	hĕt-ĕr-ō	41, 185
difficult	dys-	dĭs	37, 97
digestion	-pepsia	pĕp-sē-ăh	96
digit (finger or toe)	dactyl/o	dăk-tĭ-lō	213
dilation	-ectasis	ĕk-tăh-sĭs	12
dim	ambly/o	ăm-blē-ō	348
discharge	-rrhea	rē-ăh	15

English Term	Medical Word Element	Pronunciation	Page Numbers
heel bone	calcane/o	kăl-kā-nē-ō	214
hernia	-cele	sēl	12
hidden	crypt/o	krĭp-tō	67, 244
horny tissue	kerat/o	kĕr-ăh-tō	67, 348
humerus	humer/o	hū-mĕr-ō	213
ileum	ile/o	ĭl-ē-ō	95
ilium	ili/o	ĭl-ē-ō	214
imperfect	atel/o	ăt-ē-lō	125
in	endo-	ĕn-dō	36, 152
	in-	ĭn	36
	intra-	ĭn-trah	36
in front	ante-	ăn-tē	34
	pre-	prē	34
	pro-	prō	34
incision	-tomy	tō-mē	3, 10, 11
incomplete	atel/o	ăt-ē-lō	125
increase, abnormal	-osis	ō-sĭs	14, 184
inflammation	-itis	ī-tĭs	10, 11, 13
inner ear	labyrinth/o	lăb-ĭ-rĭn-thō	349
instrument to cut	-tome	tōm	11
instrument for measuring	-meter	mē-tĕr	13, 152
instrument for recording	-graph	grăf	13, 53, 69, 152
instrument to view or examine	-scope	skōp	15
intestine (usually small intestine)	enter/o	ĕn-tĕr-ō	95
involuntary contraction	-spasm	spăzm	15
inward	eso-	ĕ-sō	350
iris	irid/o	ĭr-ĭ-dō	348
iron	sider/o	sĭd-ĕr-ō	184
irregular	poikil/o	poi-kĭ-lō	184
ischium	ischi/o	ĭs-kē-ō	214
jejunum	jejun/o	jĕ-joo-nō	95
joined	sym-	sĭm	37
	syn-	sĭn	37
joint	arthr/o	ăr-thrō	3, 10, 215
kidney	nephr/o	nĕf-rō	2, 243
	ren/o	rē-nō	243
kneecap	patell/o	păh-tĕl-ō	215
knowing	-gnosis	nō-sĭs	53
labor	-tocia	tō-sē-ăh	271
labyrinth	labyrinth/o	lăb-ĭ-rĭn-thō	349
lacrimal sac	dacry	dăk-rē-ō	348

English Term	Medical Word Element	Pronunciation	Page Numbers
paralysis	-plegia	plē-jē-ăh	14
parathyroid glands	parathyroid/o	păr-ah-thī-roi-dō	300
partial paralysis	-paresis	pah-rē-sĭs	14
patella	patell/o	pah-tĕl-ō	215
peculiar	idi/o	ĭd-ē-ō	52
pelvic bone (anterior)	pub/o	pū-bō	215
perineum	perine/o	pĕr-ĭ-nē-ō	270
pertaining to	-ac	ăk	28
	-al	ăl	28
	-ar	ĕr	28
	-ary	ĕr-ē	28
	-eal	ē-ăl	28
	-ic	ĭk	28
	-ical	ĭk-ăl	28
	-ory	ŏr-ē	28
	-ous	ŭs	28
	-tic	tĭk	28
phalanges (bones of fingers and toes)	phalang/o	făl-ăn-jō	214
pharynx	pharyng/o	făh-rīng-gō	94, 123
pleura	pleur/o	ploo-rō	124
poison	-toxic	tŏks-ĭk	15, 301
porous	-porosis	pō-rō-sĭs	217
posterior	poster/o	pŏs-tĕr-ō	52
pregnancy	-gravida	grăv-ĭ-dah	270
pressure	ton/o	tŏn-ō	325
process	-ia	ē-ăh	28
	-y	ē	28
producing	-gen	jĕn	13, 53
	-genesis	jĕn-ĕ-sĭs	13, 53
production	-poiesis	poy-ē-sĭs	14, 185
prolapse	-ptosis	tō-sĭs	14
prostate	prostat/o	prŏs-tăh-tō	244
protein	-globin	glō-bĭn	184
pulse	sphygm/o	sfĭg-mō	152
puncture	-centesis	sĕn-tē-sĭs	3, 10, 11
pupil	core/o	kō-rē-ō	348
	pupill/o	pū-pĭ-lō	348
pus	py/o	pī-ō	244
pylorus	pylor/o	pī-lō-rō	94
radiation	radi/o	rā-dē-ō	52
rapid	tachy-	tăk-ē	37, 125
record	-gram	grăm	13, 53, 69, 152
recording (instrument used for)	-graph	grăf	14, 70
recording (process of)	-graphy	gră-fē	14, 70
rectum	proct/o	prŏk-tō	95
	rect/o	rĕk-tō	95

English Term	Medical Word Element	Pronunciation	Page Numbers
red	erythem/o	ĕr-ĭ-thē-mō	69
	erythr/o	ē-rĭth-rō	2, 69, 183
	rube/o	roo-bē-ō	69
refracture	-clasis	klăh-sĭs	216
relating to	-ac	ăk	28
	-al	ăl	28
	-ar	ĕr	28
	-ary	ĕr-ē	28
	-eal	ē-ăl	28
	-ic	ĭk	28
	-ical	ĭk-āl	28
	-ory	ŏr-ē	28
	-ous	ŭs	28
	-tic	tĭk	28
removal	-ectomy	ĕk-tō-mē	10, 11
resembling	-oid	oid	13
retina	retin/o	rĕt-ĭ-nō	349
ribs	cost/o	kŏs-tō	213
rod-shaped (striated)	rhabd/o	răb-dō	216
rod-shaped muscle (striated)	rhabdomy/o	răb-dō-mī-ō	216
rose colored	eosin/o	ē-ō-sĭn-ō	183
rupture	-rrhexis	rĕk-sĭs	15
safe	immun/o	īm-ū-nō	183
saliva	sial/o	sī-ăh-lō	96
salivary gland	sial/o	sī-ăh-lō	96
same	home/o	hō-mē-ō	52, 300
	hom/o	hō-mō	37, 185
	is/o	ī-sō	185
scale	squam/o	skwă-mō	68
scaly	ichthy/o	ĭk-thē-ō	67
scanty	olig/o	ō-lĭg-ō	244
sclera	scler/o	sklĕ-rō	68, 349
secrete	-crine	krĭn/krīn	301
seizure	-lepsy	lĕp-sē	326
seminal vesicle	vesicul/o	vē-sĭk-ū-lō	244
sensation	-esthesia	ĕs-thē-zē-ah	325
separation	-lysis	lī-sĭs	12
sex glands	gonad/o	gō-năd-ō	300
shape	morph/o	mŏr-fō	183
side	later/o	lăt-ĕr-ō	52
sigmoid colon	sigmoid/o	sĭg-moi-dō	95
skin	cutane/o	kū-tā-nē-ō	67
	-derma	dĕr-măh	69
	derm/o	dĕr-mō	67
	dermat/o	dĕr-măh-tō	67
skull	crani/o	krā-nē-ō	213, 325
slow	brady-	brăd-ē	37, 126, 326

English Term	Medical Word Element	Pronunciation	Page Numbers
small	-icle	ĭk-ăl	29
	-ole	ōl	29
	micro-	mī-krō	3, 35, 185
	-ula	ū-lā	29
	-ule	yool	29
smell	-osmia	ŏz-mē-ah	125
smooth muscle	leiomy/o	lī-ō-mī-ō	216
softening	-malacia	măh-lā-shē-ăh	13, 216
specialist in the study of	-logist	lō-jĭst	13, 69
speech	-phasia	fā-zē-ăh	326
sperm	spermat/o	spĕr-măh-tō	244
spinal cord	myel/o	mī-ē-lō	183, 215
spine	rachi/o	răk-ē-ō	214
spitting	-ptysis	tĭ-sĭs	125
spleen	splen/o	splē-nō	184
splitting	-schisis	skĭ-sĭs	217
stabilization	-desis	dē-sĭs	13, 216
standing still	-stasis	stā-sĭs	15, 185
stapes	staped/o	stā-pē-dō	249
sternum (breastbone)	stern/o	stĕr-nō	214
stiffness	ankyl/o	ăng-kĭ-lō	215
stimulate	-tropin	trō-pĭn	301
stomach	gastr/o	găs-trō	2, 3, 11, 94
stone	-lith	lĭth	13, 96
straight	orth/o	ŏr-thō	125, 216
striated (rod-shaped) muscle	rhabdomy/o	răb-dō-mī-ō	216
stricture	-stenosis	stĕ-nō-sĭs	16
stroke	-plegia	plē-jē-ăh	15
study of	-logy	lō-jē	13, 69
stupor	narc/o	năr-kō	325
sugar	gluc/o	gloo-kō	300
	glyc/o	glī-kō	300
surgical repair	-plasty	plăs-tē	12, 96, 217
suspension	-pexy	pĕk-sē	13
suture	-rrhaphy	răf-ē	12
swallowing	phag/o	făg-ō	184
	-phagia	fā-jē-ăh	14, 96, 301
sweat	hidr/o	hī-drō	67
sweetness	gluc/o	gloo-kō	300
	glyc/o	glī-kō	300
swelling	-cele	sēl	12
tear	dacry/o	dăk-rē-ō	348
teeth	dent/o	dĕn-tō	94
	odont/o	ŏ-dŏn-tō	94
tendon	ten/o	tĕn-ō	216
	tend/o	tĕnd-ō	216
	tendin/o	tĕn-dĭn-ō	216

English Term	Medical Word Element	Pronunciation	Page Numbers
urine	ur/o	ū-rō	243
	-uria	ū-rē-ah	245, 301
uterine tubes	salping/o	săl-pĭng-gō/săl-pĭn-	270, 349
	-salpinx	jō	271
		săl-pĭnks	
uterus	hyster/o	hĭs-tĕr-ō	270
	metr/o	mĕ-trō	270
	uter/o	ū-tĕr-ō	270
vagina	colp/o	kŏl-pō	269
	vagin/o	vă-jĭn-ō	269
varied	poikil/o	poi-kĭ-lō	184
vas deferens	vas/o	văs-ō	244
vein	phleb/o	flĕb-ō	10, 151
	ven/o	vē-nō	151
ventricles	ventricul/o	vĕn-trĭk-ū-lō	325
venule	venul/o	vĕn-ū-lō	153
vertebrae	spondyl/o	spŏn-dĭ-lō	214
	vertebr/o	vĕr-tē-brō	214
vesicle, seminal	vesicul/o	vĕ-sĭk-ū-lō	244
vessel	angi/o	ăn-jē-ō	151
	vas/o	văs-ō	151, 244
vision	-opia	ō-pē-ah	349
	opt/o	ŏp-tō	348
visual examination	-scopy	skō-pē	10, 15, 217
voice	-phonia	fō-nē-ah	125
vomiting	-emesis	ĕm-ĕ-sĭs	12, 96
vulva	episi/o	ē-pĭz-ē-ō	269
	vulv/o	vŭl-vō	269
water	aque/o	ā-kwē-ō	348
white	albin/o	ăl-bĭn-ō	68
	leuc/o	loo-kō	68
	leuk/o	loo-kō	68, 183
within	endo-	ĕn-dō	36, 152
	intra-	ĭn-trah	36
without	a-	ăh	36, 185, 326
	an-	ăn	36, 326
woman	gynec/o	gĭ-nĕ-kō/jĭn-ē-kō	269
womb	hyster/o	hĭs-ter-ō	270
	metr/o	mĕ-trō	270
	uter/o	ū-tĕr-ō	270
wrist bones	carp/o	kăr-pō	213
a writing, record	-gram	grăm	13, 53, 69, 152
yellow	cirrh/o	sĭr-rō	69
	jaund/o	jawn-dō	69
	xanth/o	zăn-thō	69

Index of Genetic Disorders

Appendix E

Index of Diagnostic Imaging Procedures

Appendix F

Index of Pharmacology

Appendix G

Index of Oncological Terms

Index

Page numbers followed by "f" indicate figures; those followed by "t" indicate tables.

HOW TO USE THE FLASH CARDS

The following pages include flash cards for word elements introduced in Chapters 2, 3, 5 and 6. Remove the pages from the book before you cut the cards.

The flash cards are labeled according to the chapter that the element was first presented and can be arranged in various ways for study purposes. For example, the surgical, diagnostic and symptomatic, and grammatical suffixes can be organized in three separate packets. The flash cards can also be separated according to basic elements (combining forms, suffixes, prefixes) or body systems.

WHEN TO USE THE FLASH CARDS

Use the cards to learn the elements after they are presented in the chapter. Also, use the cards to reinforce retention of word elements before and after you complete the worksheets or take a test. This procedure will help you master the medical terminology covered in the chapters.

PREPARE ADDITIONAL FLASHCARDS

Additional flash cards can be produced on 3 × 5 index cards. You can also use the flash cards for study purposes either in group activities or as a self-tutorial activity.

-centesis

-ectomy

-stomy

-tome

-tomy

-desis

-pexy

-rrhaphy

-plasty

-clasis

-lysis

-tripsy

-algia, -dynia

-cele

suture

puncture

surgical repair

excision, removal

break,
fracture

forming an opening
(mouth)

separation,
destruction,
loosening

instrument to cut

crushing

incision, cut into

pain

binding, fixation
(of a bone or joint)

hernia, swelling

fixation
(of an organ)

-ectasis

-emesis

Chapter 2

-emia

Chapter 2

-gen, -genesis

Chapter 2

-gram

Chapter 2

-graph

Chapter 2

-graphy

Chapter 2

-iasis

Chapter 2

-itis

Chapter 2

-lith

Chapter 2

-logist

Chapter 2

-logy

Chapter 2

-malacia

Chapter 2

-megaly

Chapter 2

abnormal condition (produced by something specified)	dilation, expansion
inflammation	vomiting
stone, calculus	blood
specialist in the study of	forming, producing, origin
study of	record, a writing
softening	instrument for recording
enlargement	process of recording

-meter

-metry

-oid

-oma

-osis

-para

-paresis

-pathy

-penia

-phagia

-phasia

-philia

-phobia

-plasia

disease	instrument for measuring
decrease, deficiency	act of measuring
eating, swallowing	resembling
speech	tumor
attraction for	abnormal condition, increase (used primarily with blood cells)
fear	to bear (offspring)
formation, growth	partial paralysis

-plegia

Chapter 2

-poiesis

Chapter 2

-ptosis

Chapter 2

-rrhage, -rrhagia

Chapter 2

-rrhea

Chapter 2

-rrhexis

Chapter 2

-scope

Chapter 2

-scopy

Chapter 2

-spasm

Chapter 2

-stasis

Chapter 2

-stenosis

Chapter 2

-trophy

Chapter 2

-toxic

Chapter 2

-ac, -al, -ar, -ary, -eal

Chapter 3

visual examination

paralysis

involuntary
contraction,
twitching

formation,
production

standing still

prolapse,
downward
displacement

narrowing,
stricture

bursting forth

development,
nourishment

discharge, flow

poison

rupture

adjective suffixes
meaning pertaining
or relating to

instrument to view
or examine

-ic, -ical, -ory, -ous, -tic

Chapter 3

hist/o

Chapter 5

-ia, -ism, -y

Chapter 3

home/o

Chapter 5

-ist

Chapter 3

idi/o

Chapter 5

-iatry

Chapter 3

later/o

Chapter 5

-ole, icle, -ula, -ule

Chapter 3

medi/o

Chapter 5

anter/o

Chapter 5

nucle/o

Chapter 5

cyt/o

Chapter 5

path/o

Chapter 5

tissue

adjective suffixes
meaning pertaining
or relating to

same

noun endings
meaning
condition of

unknown, peculiar

noun ending

to one side, side

noun ending
meaning treatment,
medicine

middle, median

diminutive suffixes
meaning small,
minute

nucleus

anterior, front

disease

cell

poster/o

proxim/o

radi/o

ventr/o

viscer/o

-gnosis

ab-

ad-

infra-

peri-

trans-

ultra-

aden/o

adip/o, lip/o, steat/o

toward	back (of body), behind, posterior
below, under	near, nearest
around	radiation, x-ray
across, through	belly, belly-side
excess, beyond	internal organs
gland	knowing
fat	away from

crypt/o

cutane/o, dermat/o, derm/o

hidr/o

ichthy/o

kerat/o

lact/o

mamm/o, mast/o

myc/o

onych/o, ungu/o

pil/o, trich/o

scler/o

thel/o

xer/o

albin/o, leuk/o, leuc/o

cell	charcoal (coal dust)
skin	green
treatment	yellow
above, upon	blue
excessive	red
under, below	black
	scaly